MODERN
METHODS IN
PHARMACOLOGY
Volume 4

METHODS FOR STUDYING PLATELETS AND MEGAKARYOCYTES

MODERN METHODS IN PHARMACOLOGY

SERIES EDITORS

Sydney Spector
Roche Institute of Molecular Biology
Nutley, New Jersey

Nathan Back
State University of New York
Buffalo, New York

TITLES IN THE SERIES

Modern Methods in Pharmacology, Volume 1
Sydney Spector and Nathan Back, *Editors*

Modern Methods in Pharmacology, Volume 2
Sydney Spector and Nathan Back, *Editors*

Modern Methods in Pharmacology, Volume 3
Electrophysiological Techniques in Pharmacology
Herbert M. Geller, *Editor*

Modern Methods in Pharmacology, Volume 4
Methods for Studying Platelets and Megakaryocytes
Robert W. Colman and J. Bryan Smith, *Editors*

MODERN
METHODS IN
PHARMACOLOGY
Volume 4

METHODS FOR STUDYING PLATELETS AND MEGAKARYOCYTES

Editors

Robert W. Colman

Thrombosis Research Center
Temple University School of Medicine
Philadelphia, Pennsylvania

J. Bryan Smith

Department of Pharmacology
Temple University School of Medicine
Philadelphia, Pennsylvania

Alan R. Liss, Inc., New York

Address all Inquiries to the Publisher
Alan R. Liss, Inc., 41 East 11th Street, New York, NY 10003

Printed in the United States of America

Library of Congress Cataloging-in-Publication Data

Methods for studying platelets and megakaryocytes.
(Modern methods in pharmacology ; v. 4)
Includes bibliographies and index.
1. Blood platelets—Research—Methodology.
2. Megakaryocytes—Research—Methodology. I. Colman, Robert W. II. Series. [DNLM: 1. Blood Platelets—physiology. 2. Megakaryocytes—physiology.
W1 MO166M v.4 / WH 300 M592]
RM301.M63 vol. 4 615'.1'072 s 87-3208
[QP97] [612'.117'072]
ISBN 0-8451-2503-6

Contents

Contributors

Barrie Ashby, Thrombosis Research Center, Temple University School of Medicine, Philadelphia, PA 19140 **[157]**

Joel S. Bennett, Hematology/ Oncology Section, Hospital of the University of Pennsylvania, Philadelphia, PA 19140 **[89]**

Robert W. Colman, Hematology/ Oncology Section, Department of Medicine and Thrombosis Research Center, Temple University School of Medicine, Philadelphia, PA 19140 **[ix,33]**

James L. Daniel, Department of Pharmacology and Thrombosis Research Center, Temple University School of Medicine, Philadelphia, PA 19140 **[185]**

Alan M. Gewirtz, Hematology/ Oncology Section, Department of Medicine and Thrombosis Research Center, Temple University School of Medicine, Philadelphia, PA 19140 **[1]**

Paul Grant, Thrombosis Research Center, Temple University School of Medicine, Philadelphia, PA 19140 **[157]**

Holm Holmsen, Department of Biochemistry, University of Bergen, N-5000 Bergen, Norway **[133]**

Edward P. Kirby, Department of Biochemistry and Thrombosis Research Center, Temple University School of Medicine, Philadelphia, PA 19140 **[65]**

Karen Knudsen, Department of Cell Biology, Lankenau Medical Research Center, Philadelphia, PA 19151 **[267]**

David C.B. Mills, Department of Pharmacology and Thrombosis Research Center, Temple University School of Medicine, Philadelphia, PA 19140 **[65]**

A. David Purdon, Department of Pharmacology and Thrombosis Research Center, Temple University School of Medicine, Philadelphia, PA 19140 **[185,229]**

Leon Salganicoff, Department of Pharmacology and Thrombosis Research Center, Temple University School of Medicine, Philadelphia, PA 19140 **[185,287]**

Barbara Schick, Department of Biochemistry and Thrombosis Research Center, Temple University School of Medicine, Philadelphia, PA 19140 **[19]**

Paul K . Schick, Hematology/Oncology Section, Department of Medicine and Thrombosis Research Center, Temple University School of Medicine, Philadelphia, PA 19140 **[19]**

The numbers in brackets are the opening page numbers of the contributors' articles.

Alvin H. Schmaier, Hematology/Oncology Section, Department of Medicine and Thrombosis Research Center, Temple University School of Medicine, Philadelphia, PA 19140 **[109]**

Mary A. Selak, Department of Pharmacology, Temple University School of Medicine, Philadelphia, PA 19140 **[185]**

J. Bryan Smith, Department of Pharmacology and Thrombosis Research Center, Temple University School of Medicine, Philadelphia, PA 19140 **[ix,217]**

Hanna I. Switalska, Department of Platelet Hematology, Lankenau Medical Research Center, Philadelphia, PA 19151; present address: Institute of Hypertension and Angiology, Academy of Medicine, Warsaw, Poland **[267]**

George P. Tuszynski, Department of Platelet Hematology, Lankenau Medical Research Center, Philadelphia, PA 19151 **[267]**

Adrie J.M. Verhoeven, Department of Biochemistry, University of Bergen, N-5000 Bergen, Norway; present address: Department of Biochemistry, Dutch Cancer Institute, 1066 CX Amsterdam, The Netherlands **[133]**

Peter N. Walsh, Departments of Medicine and Biochemistry and Thrombosis Research Center, Temple University School of Medicine, Philadelphia, PA 19140 **[41]**

Preface

Pharmacologists are becoming increasingly interested in platelets. Thromboxane A_2 synthesized and released by platelets probably contributes to the pathophysiology of unstable angina by causing platelet aggregation and vessel constriction. Platelet aggregates may occlude coronary and cerebral vessels. Platelet-derived growth factor is a potent mitogen released from platelets which stimulates smooth muscle cell proliferation, a central pathologic lesion in atherosclerosis. Pharmacologists are involved in developing new agents and studying existing compounds as candidates for effective antiplatelet therapy.

The platelet is also an easily isolated cell fragment which allows detailed study of fundamental cell biology including receptors, stimulus-response coupling, intracellular messengers, and contractile proteins. Megakaryocytes, the progenitors of platelets, expand the area of research to allow consideration of the control of biosynthesis, development of organelles, and proliferative responses.

Thus, it is timely to collect into a single volume useful techniques adapted to the platelet for the study of such critical intracellular regulators as products of phospholipid and arachidonate metabolism, intracellular calcium, and cAMP. Methods of studying important platelet proteins, such as receptors, cytoskeletal elements, contractile components, and coagulant proteins are detailed. Approaches to elucidating megakaryocyte function, development, and biochemistry are outlined. The powerful technology of modern research is illustrated by the panoply of techniques discussed, including the application of high pressure liquid chromatography, monoclonal antibodies, affinity labeling ELISA, and radioimmunoassays, as well as more classical biochemical and pharmacological approaches. We hope this volume will be of use to the pharmacologist involved in research in hemostasis and thrombosis as well as those interested in basic problems of cell biology.

Robert W. Colman
J. Bryan Smith

Modern Methods in Pharmacology, Volume 4
Methods for Studying Platelets and Megakaryocytes, pages 1–17

Recent Methodologic Advances in the Study of Human Megakaryocyte Development and Function

ALAN M. GEWIRTZ

INTRODUCTION

Megakaryocytes are unusual bone marrow cells whose major function is the production of platelets. It is less well appreciated that megakaryocytes synthesize coagulant proteins such as fibrinogen [1,2], FVIIIR:Ag [3], platelet factor 4 [4], and factor V [5,6]. Tracy et al. [7] suggest that the production of factor V by these cells may be of clinical importance since deficiency of platelet associated factor V is associated with a clinically significant bleeding diathesis. Accordingly, these cells play a critical role in the maintenance of normal hemostatic mechanisms.

In comparison to other hematopoietic cells in the marrow, megakaryocytes are unique by virtue of the large size and polyploid complement of DNA they typically acquire upon complete maturation. Unfixed cells in suspension have a mean diameter of ~35 μm [8] and a mean ploidy level of 8 N [9]. Megakaryocytes, in spite of their importance, are infrequent in human bone marrow, comprising only 0.05% of all nucleated cells found in the marrow [10].

The rarity of these cells in the marrow, combined with their apparent fragility, has posed a considerable obstacle to the study of human megakaryocyte biology and function. Indeed, until recently the study of these cells was restricted to observations made on morphologically recognizable cells present in bone marrow aspirates and biopsies [11,12]. New techniques allowing for the isolation and enrichment of relatively pure populations of mature human megakaryocytes, as well as for the cloning of megakaryocyte progenitor cells in tissue culture, have dramatically altered this situation. In the 7 years that these methods have been

From the Department of Internal Medicine and the Thrombosis Research Center, Temple University School of Medicine, Philadelphia, Pennsylvania 19140.

available, progress in understanding human megakaryocyte ontogeny and function has been rapid. Nevertheless, relatively few laboratories in the country appear to be utilizing these techniques. It is clear that many of the functional properties of platelets are determined by the megakaryocyte. Platelets are known to play important roles not only in blood clotting, but in atherogenesis [13] and perhaps metastasis of tumor cells [14]. Thus the importance of learning more about the biology of this cell cannot be overstated. The goal of this chapter is to describe methods of isolation and progenitor cell cloning in sufficient detail so that the interested investigator will be able to establish them in his or her laboratory without undue difficulty, allowing the rapid progress being made in this field to continue unabated.

HUMAN MEGAKARYOCYTE ISOLATION AND ENRICHMENT

To study megakaryocyte function at the biochemical and molecular level, large numbers of highly purified cells are required. In rodent species, several techniques are available for isolating and enriching megakaryocytes [15–18]. Relying on the physical differences between megakaryocytes and other marrow cells, these techniques are quite reproducible and are relatively easy to perform. Obtaining such populations of megakaryocytes from human bone marrow has proven to be difficult. Nonetheless, techniques based on the same physical principles which govern other cell separations are available and have been used with some success [8–10,19–21]. Flow cytometry has also been applied for megakaryocyte separations [17,22,23] but, to my knowledge, has not been used for separation of viable human cells.

Rabellino and coworkers described the first separation technique for human megakaryocytes [19]. This method involves an initial density sedimentation through discontinuous polyvinyl-pyrrolidine coated silica particle gradients (Percoll, Pharmacia), followed by a velocity sedimentation through a continuous gradient of the same material. The density sedimentation has been reported to yield up to 240,000 megakaryocytes representing ~85% of the total number of megakaryocytes in the starting material. However, the purity of megakaryocytes after this initial density separation is ~2%. After a velocity sedimentation, 180,000 megakaryocytes remained in a suspension ~70% pure. Levine has reported obtaining similar results using a technique employing bovine serum albumin gradients [9]. Rabellino has pointed out, however, that it is possible for albumin to enter megakaryocytes through their demarcation membrane system [19]. This alteration might render the cells less sensitive to the separation forces of centrifugation alone and therefore give poorer separation. Percoll does not enter cells and therefore does not have this problem. A variation of both techniques, which relies on the use of a specially constructed gradient maker to give good separations, was reported by Sitar [10].

A different technique has recently been described by Berkow and coworkers [8], which employs the process of counterflow centrifugal elutriation (CCE). The theoretical basis and initial instrumentation for this procedure was first described by Lindahl [24]. CCE also takes advantage of physical differences between cells in order to separate them one from another. In the case of CCE, however, and in contrast to the methods just described, cell separation is based primarily on size and, to a much lesser degree, on cell density. The cell separations take place in a centrifuge rotor specially designed to hold a hollow chamber with both fluid inlet and outlet channels (Fig. 1). The channels allow fluid to be pumped through the separation chamber as it spins in the centrifuge rotor. Cells suspended in the separation chamber line up by size, from smaller to larger, away from the rotational axis, with their location being fixed by the opposing forces of gravity and an oppositely directed fluid flow. By slowing the rotor speed or increasing the fluid flow, cells will begin to flow out of the chamber (and rotor) from smallest to largest allowing them to be effectively separated.

CCE was first used successfully for the isolation of murine megakaryocytes [17]. When applied to human cells, Berkow et al. [8] reported that approximately 63% of the megakaryocytes available in bone marrow aspirates could be recovered by this technique in a cell suspension of ~20% purity. An average yield of 2.4×10^5 megakaryocytes (>95% viable) was obtained. Since most human megakaryocytes have a density $\leqslant$1.050 g/ml (in Percoll) whereas most other nucleated marrow cells have a density greater than this, a combination of CCE and density centrifugation through Percoll might be expected to yield the greatest number of purified megakaryocytes with the least number of manipulations in the shortest period of time. The separation procedure we employ [6] is a modification and combination of those described by Berkow et al. [8] and Rabellino et al. [20]. It is detailed below.

Human megakaryocytes may be enriched from marrow obtained from a number of sources including the resected ribs of patients undergoing thoracotomy, femoral marrow removed at the time of total hip replacement, and from iliac crest aspirates. In terms of yield, fewer cells are derived from aspirates (50–75% less in the author's experience) than whole marrow, but they may be adequate for certain purposes.

Marrow removed from bone should be placed immediately in a specifically formulated collection medium designed to inhibit blood clotting as well as megakaryocyte aggregation and release. A number of formulations have been published and most are modifications of the "CATCH" medium originally described by Levine and Fedorko [15]. In our laboratory a modified version of

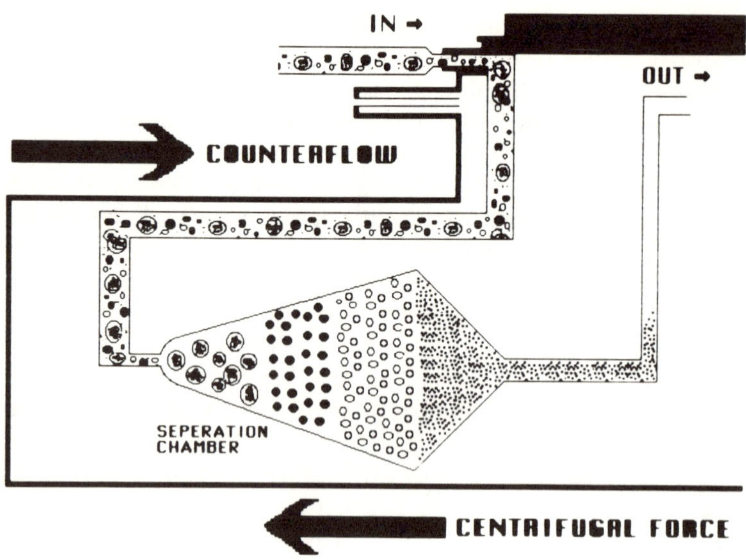

ROTOR

Fig. 1. Schematic representation of cell separation by the process of counterflow centrifugal elutriation. A heterogeneous cell suspension is pumped into a separation chamber, which is housed in a specially designed centrifuge rotor. As the rotor spins, cells sediment in the chamber according to their size so that the largest cells are farthest, and smallest cells closest, to the rotational axis. The position of any size cohort of cells in the separation chamber is a function of the net force exerted on the population by the process of centrifugation and the pumping of fluid into the chamber (counterflow). As the relative counterflow force is increased over centrifugal force, cells begin to move out of the separation chamber allowing for the collection of highly enriched cell fractions.

the medium of Berkow et al. [8] is used. DNAase I, added to prevent cell clumping, is left out of the formulation, since it adds to the expense and, in our hands at least, does not seem to significantly improve yield or purity. We also add lidocaine (Sigma Chemical Corp., St. Louis, MO) at a final concentration of 5×10^{-5}M, and $PGE_{1\alpha}$ (Sigma Chemical Corp., St. Louis, MO) at a final concentration of 2×10^{-7}M in order to inhibit neutrophil and platelet release reactions, respectively. We have also used a formulation, described by Thompson et al., for the elutriation of platelets [25] to which is added adenosine (1 mmol/1) and theophyline (2 mmol/1). Both appear equally efficacious so that the choice of megakaryocyte collection medium (MKCM) ultimately depends on the results obtained by the individual investigator and the purpose for which the cells are being collected.

Marrow tissue scraped from bone should be minced in MKCM and then filtered through a 100 μm pore sized nylon filter (Nytex, Tetko, Inc., Elmsford, NY) to remove bone particle and cell clumps. At this point we have routinely removed erythrocytes by either ammonium chloride lysis or by dextran sedimentation [6,26]. More recently, however, we have found that this step is unnecessary and that the cells may be loaded directly into the elutriation apparatus (J2-21M centrifuge; JE-6B rotor; standard or Sanderson separation chamber, Beckman Instruments, Spinco Division, Palo Alto, CA) after being filtered.

After priming the system with buffer, and making sure *all* air bubbles are purged from the system, cells may be loaded into the centrifuge in a number of ways [8,27]. We have designed a gravity feed system which enables us to load a large number of cells at relatively low concentrations, and with a minimum of mechanical manipulation. A schematic representation of this system is shown in Figure 2.

The conditions of each run will vary with the particular centrifuge and separation chamber employed (it should be noted that many investigators prefer a Sanderson separation chamber to the standard chamber). In contrast to our earlier report [6] we are now keeping centrifuge speed at 1,500 rpm to reduce nonspecific megakaryocyte loss during the loading procedure.

Buffer counterflow rate is controlled with a roller pump (Masterflex, Cole Palmer, Chicago, IL). During loading we use a pump speed designed to give a flow rate of 7 ml/min. After loading is completed, and distinct cell boundaries have formed in the chamber, the flow rate is then increased to 12, 15, and then 16 ml/min. After each increase in flow rate ~200 ml of buffer is collected. Prior to incrementing flow rate the afferent fluid line is also pinched a few times in order to help break up the cell clump that invariably forms in the distal end of the separation chamber. Finally, the flow rate is increased to 20 ml/min and flow is allowed to continue until the separation chamber effluent is free of cells and debris. The pump is then turned off, the centrifuge stopped, and the rotor unshipped. The megakaryocyte rich cell suspension is then removed from the chamber by gentle aspiration. We routinely load from 2 to 5 $\times$ 10^8 nucleated marrow cells into the chamber. Purity of specimens obtained from the elutriator varies between 5% and 15%. Bone marrow aspirates usually yield 20,000–50,000 megakaryocytes. Marrow obtained from femurs yields between 80,000 and 200,000 megakaryocytes. Cell viability as assessed by trypan blue exclusion is >90%, though Rabellino cautions that this method of judging viability may be inaccurate [20]. Total preparation time is on the order of 1.5 to 2 hours if erythrocytes are not removed from the specimen prior to elutriation. A photomicrograph of a very pure preparation is shown in Figure 3.

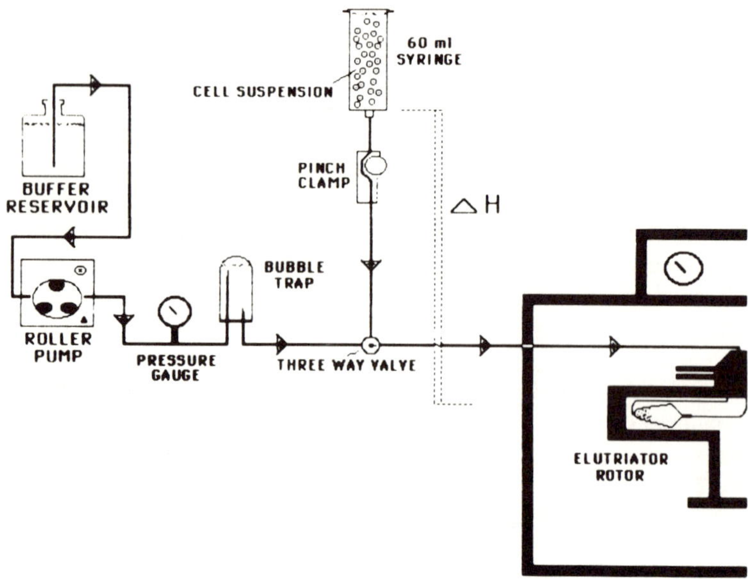

Fig. 2. Flow schematic for construction of gravity feed cell loading system. Roller pump moves fluid from buffer reservoir into (and out of) separation chamber housed in the elutriator rotor. The cells are allowed to enter this circuit via a three-way valve, which is spliced into the tubing distal to the roller pump and bubble trap and proximal to the rotor. Allowing cells to enter the circuit at this location prevents mechanical damage to the cells by the roller pump and loss of cells in the shoulders of the bubble trap. By changing the height of the syringe relative to the plane of the rotor (ΔH) the rate of all loading can be adjusted.

Megakaryocytes enriched by elutriation may be further purified by density gradient centrifugation with Percoll. The megakaryocyte rich preparation is layered over a stock Percoll solution adjusted to a density of 1.050 g/cm^3 [19] by dilution with MKCM. The cells are then centrifuged at 750 × g for 25 min. This maneuver increases megakaryocyte purity to >85% but, at least in our hands, at the expense of considerable cell loss.

One significant disadvantage of the CCE method is the expense of the equipment utilized. Therefore, less expensive alternatives would be highly desirable. Successful use of monoclonal antibodies with a panning procedure has recently been described [28], and if successful in other laboratories, could prove to be such an alternative. In the meantime, CCE and the previously described isolation procedures are currently being used to further understand the synthetic functions of the megakaryocyte and expression of various cell surface markers in normal disease states [1,6,21].

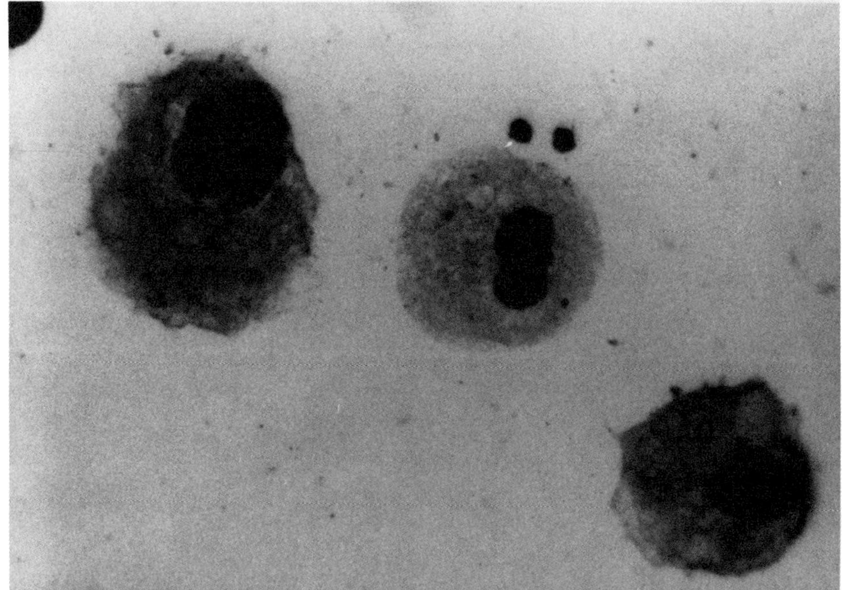

Fig. 3. Example of highly enriched preparation of human megakaryocytes enriched by a combination of counterflow centrifugal elutriation and Percoll density gradient sedimentation.

MEGAKARYOCYTE PROGENITOR CELL CLONING TECHNIQUES

It has been known since 1961 [29] that primitive hematopoietic cells are contained within the bone marrow. The function of these cells is to regenerate the mature, formed elements of the blood that have no ability to reproduce themselves. These blood-forming cells exist in a developmental continuum [30]. The most primitive, or stem cells [31], have great ability to renew themselves and are essentially undifferentiated. They therefore have the potential to develop along any of the hematopoietic differentiation pathways. As stem cells mature, they give rise to more differentiated cells characterized by decreased self-renewal capacity, increased proliferative activity, and increasing commitment to development along one of these specific pathways. As maturation proceeds, cells with decreasing proliferative and no self-renewal capacity are generated. Finally, progeny that are morphologically identifiable as belonging to a given lineage are produced. Such cells are capable of only one or two divisions as they complete their maturation process.

Methodologies for studying the growth and development of primitive hematopoietic cells in vitro were established in the mid-1960s [32–34] with the notable exception of those cells that gave rise to megakaryocytes. Indeed, it was not until 1975 that the first animal culture system for megakaryocytes was described [35,36]. Four years after this event, the first human megakaryocyte progenitor cell assay was established by Vainchenker and his collaborators, in 1979 [37]. This assay represented an important technological advance for the study of human megakaryocytopoiesis in vitro. Nonetheless, it was hampered by the fact that megakaryocyte identification was accomplished by morphologic means. Accordingly, the ability to directly view and study immature, morphologically unrecognizable megakaryocytes was greatly restricted. At the same time, Rabellino and coworkers demonstrated that mature megakaryocytes and a population of putative megakaryocyte precursor cells expressed platelet glycoproteins on their surface [19]. Mazur and his collaborators, using an immunochemical probe capable of recognizing these glycoproteins, subsequently identified both mature and immature megakaryocytes in colonies formed from primitive megakaryocyte cells in vitro [38]. An example of such a colony is shown in Figure 4. The merging of the techniques for cloning megakaryocytes from progenitor cells in vitro and for immunochemically identifying the progeny of these cells has provided a very powerful tool for the study of human megakaryocyte development in vitro.

Different culture techniques are now available for studying human megakaryocytopoiesis in vitro [37–39]. They are similar in that they involve suspending light density mononuclear cells (LDMNC) derived from either bone marrow or peripheral blood in a semisolid matrix bathed in nutrient medium. They differ primarily in the nature of the supporting matrix and nutrient medium employed.

The method originally described by Vainchenker et al. [37,40] and Mazur et al. [38] are modifications of a technique for cloning murine megakaryocytes described by McLeod et al. [41]. Progenitor cells-enriched LDMNC are suspended in a fibrin matrix derived from clotted plasma; hence, giving this technique its name, the plasma clot culture method. This is the method we employ in our laboratory [42,43], and it is described in some detail below. It should be clear that strict sterile culture technique is required. Virtually the entire procedure is carried out in a tissue culture hood.

PREPARATION OF TISSUE CULTURE MEDIA

Three primary media formulations are utilized. Each is modified for a specific purpose. For cell harvesting and preparation Minimal Essential Medium is used. For cell culture, alpha modification of Eagles medium is employed in a specifically formulated megakaryocyte culture medium.

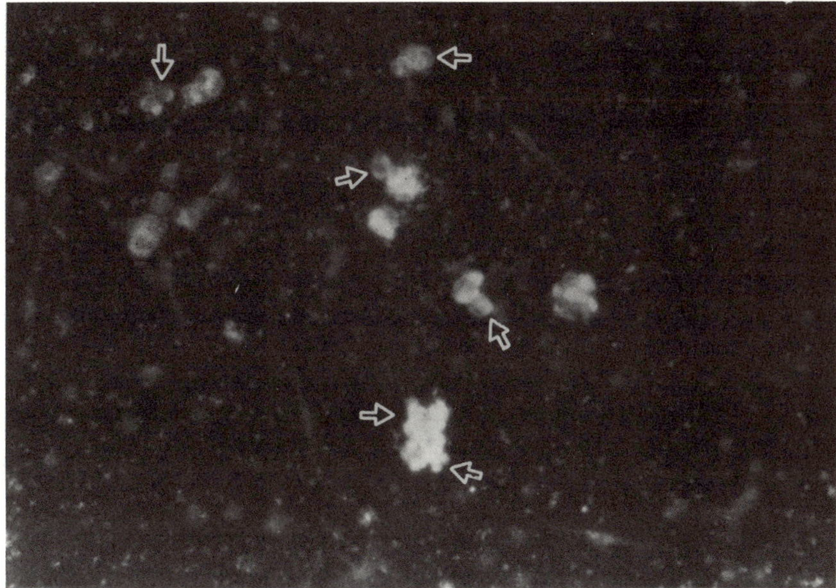

Fig. 4. Human megakaryocyte colony labeled in situ by indirect immunofluorescence technique employing a rabbit antihuman antiplatelet glycoprotein antiserum. Note that cells of different maturational stages are present in the colony, which consists of several scattered cells (arrows).

1. Collection medium I: Minimal Essential Medium with Earles salts (Flow Laboratories, Mclean, VA). To every 100 ml add:
   a. L-glutamine (200 mmol solution)—1 ml*
   b. Sodium pyruvate (100×)—1 ml*
   c. Nonessential aminoacids (100×)—1 ml*
   d. Sodium bicarbonate (7.5%)—0.8 ml*
   e. Penicillin-Streptomycin solution—0.7 ml*
   f. Preservative-free heparin (10,000 U/ml)—0.2/ml**
   g. Fetal calf serum—2 ml**
      *Hazelton Dutchland, Denver, PA
      **Gibco, Grand Island, NY
2. Collection medium II: Same as CM I above but without heparin.
3. Alpha medium: Alpha modification of Eagles medium (with Earles salts and glutamine; without ribosides, deoxyribosides, or sodium bicarbonate. To every 100 ml add:
   a. Pen-Strep solution—0.75 ml
   b. L-glutamine—1 ml

c. Sodium bicarbonate (7.5%)−0.8 ml

4. Supplemented Alpha medium: Alpha medium is prepared as described in #3. In addition, to every 100 ml add:

a. Sodium pyruvate (100%)—1 ml

b. Nonessential aminoacids (100%)−1 ml

5. Megakaryocyte culture medium base: This is composed of five ingredients, each used in equal proportion (20% v/v). When prepared, slightly more than needed should be made to allow for pipetting error and/or loss. We calculate the amount of each constituent required by multiplying the number of culture tubes desired by 0.2, and then adding 0.1 to the number obtained. Therefore to prepare q.s. for five tubes, ([5 × 0.2] + 0.1) or 1.1 ml of each ingredient listed below is needed.

a. Alpha medium

b. Supplemented alpha medium

c. Bovine serum albumin (BSA): Fraction V, Grade B (Calbiochem-Behring, San Diego, CA). To prepare the BSA, the following steps should be carried out:

Day 1

Slowly add 50 g to powder to 91 ml of sterile distilled water in a 500 ml flask. Allow to dissolve overnight at 4°C with slow constant stirring.

Day 2

Add ~5–6 g of deionizing resin [AG 501−× 8(D), Bio-Rad, Rockville Center, NY]. DO NOT STIR. Resin will change from blue to tan in color as reaction proceeds overnight at 4°C.

Day 3

Cover top of a sterile graduated cylinder with a 4 × 4 piece of sterile gauze. Pour BSA through to filter resin. Measure volume of BSA recovered and make isotonic by adding 1.1 ml of 10X phosphate buffered saline (PBS) for each 15 ml of BSA. Use 1× PBS to adjust final concentration to 10% from the 37% concentration that exists at this step. Sterilize by ultrafiltration through a 0.45 μm filter. Aliquot into 5 ml tubes and freeze at −80°C until needed. Upon thawing, 0.1 ml of 7.5% sodium bicarbonate should be added to each 5 ml aliquot.

d. Alpha thioglycerol (3 mercapto-1,2 propanediol) (Aldrich Chemical Co., Milwaukee, WI): A stock solution is prepared by taking 0.1 ml of liquid and diluting in 10 ml of Alpha medium to give a 10^{-1}M solution. Sterilize by ultrafiltration. This may be stored at 4°C for 1 month. For culture use, 0.1 ml of stock is diluted in 9.9 ml of Alpha medium.

e. L-asparagine with $CaCl_2$ (Monohydrate A grade, Calbiochem-Behring, San Diego, CA): To prepare a stock solution dissolve L-asparagine powder in Alpha medium to give a concentration of 2 mg/ml. Sterilize by ultrafiltration and aliquot in 0.5 ml volumes. Store at −80°C. Dilute stock with 4.5 ml of Alpha medium containing $CaCl_2$ at a final concentration of 370 μg/ml. This is most easily prepared by dissolving 370 mg of $CaCl_2$ in 10 ml of deionized water. This is millipore filtered and stored frozen. One milliliter of this solution can be added to 100 ml of Alpha medium.

PREPARATION OF CELLS FOR CLONING

Peripheral blood (PB) of bone marrow (BM) cells may be used for this purpose. The freshly obtained specimen is immediately diluted 1:1 in Collection medium I, pipetted up and down ~5 times and then carefully layered over an equal volume of Ficoll-Hypaque. The cells are then centrifuged at 18°C for 30 min at 500 g. The progenitor cell-rich LDMNC are found at the Ficoll-Medium interface. These interface cells are washed (500 g for 7 min) three times in Collection medium II; and after the third wash are resuspended to a concentration of 1×10^7 or 5×10^6 cells/ml (for PB or BM, respectively) in supplemented Alpha medium containing 2% heat-inactivated (56°C × 30 min) normal human AB serum. 0.2 ml of cells prepared in this manner are then added to sterile tubes (12 × 5 mm) containing 1 ml of megakaryocyte culture medium based, 0.2 ml of Alpha medium, and a total of 0.6 ml of human serum. The human serum employed is usually derived from two sources. Ninety to ninety-five percent of the serum used per culture tube (0.4 or 0.5 ml) is obtained from normal AB blood donors. In addition, serum from patients with markedly decreased or absent bone marrow megakaryocytes is also used at a final concentration of 5% to 10% of the final plated culture volume (0.2 or 0.1 ml). Such serum is a recognized source of Megakaryocyte Colony Stimulating Factor (Meg-CSF), which is needed to maximize progenitor cell cloning efficiency [44,45]. Finally, 0.2 ml of bovine plasma (Hazelton Dutchland, Denver, PA) is added, the mixture is pipetted several times with a 2 ml borosilicate glass pipette, and then dispensed in 1 ml aliquots into two 35 mm plastic culture dishes. The two dishes are covered and placed inside a 100 mm culture dish along with a third uncovered 35 mm dish that is filled with water. The 100 mm dish is covered and the mixture in the 35 mm dishes is allowed to gel (clot). The dish is then ready to be incubated. The dishes are placed in a 5% CO_2 incubator, at >95% humidity for 12 days [46]. The cultures are then ready for harvesting.

PRESERVATION OF CULTURES AND MEGAKARYOCYTE COLONY ENUMERATION

Culture dishes are removed from the incubator and any liquid that has accumulated in the culture is gently aspirated off. Care should be taken not to disturb the clot itself. The dish is then flooded with a mixture of methanol:acetone (1:3) for 10 min. Great care should also be taken not to allow the fixative to contact the underside of the culture dish since it will dissolve the plastic and render it totally unsuitable for any evaluation. After 10 min the fixative is aspirated from the dishes and a second 10 min exposure is started. The methanol:acetone is aspirated again and the dish is washed for 5 min with PBS and the distilled water. The clot is finally dried into a thin, translucent film at the bottom of the dish, after which it may be stored for long periods of time at −20°C.

In my laboratory, megakaryocyte colonies are identified in the cultures using an indirect immunofluorescence assay, but an immunoperoxidase technique has also been described [47]. The probe antibody in our system is a polyvalent rabbit serum which recognized the three major human platelet glycoproteins [38]. Monoclonal antibodies against the major platelet glycoproteins have also been used as probes [21], as have antibodies against von Willebrand factor [39]. The antibody or antiserum employed should be diluted in PBS and then layered over in dried clot in a humidified environment. The antibody titer and time of incubation are functions of the particular antibody employed. One hour at room temperature is a reasonable starting point. After incubation with the probe antibody, the dish is washed × 3 with PBS. A fluorescein-tagged antibody (preferably affinity purified) directed against the probe antibody is then added and incubation repeated for another hour. Again, the dilution of the conjugated antibody should be low enough so that a clear signal is visualized but not so low that background fluorescence is unacceptable. The conjugate is rinsed away, and the plate washed consecutively with PBS followed by two washings with distilled water. The clot is then dried again. After drying, 0.125% Evans blue dye in distilled water is added to the dish for ~ 1 min. This is done to reduce nonspecific fluorescence, especially in heavily granulated cells like eosinophils. The Evans blue dye is rinsed from the dishes with two distilled water washes of 5 min each. Three drops of isotonic glycerol barbital buffer, pH8.6, is added to the dish, which is then covered with a round glass coverslip specifically cut to fit the 35 mm dish (Belco Glass, Vineland, NJ).

Megakaryocyte colonies are enumerated with an epifluorescent microscope by placing the inverted dish on the microscope stage and then completely scanning the base area at a total magnification of 100×. Megakaryocytes are readily identified by their bright yellow-green fluorescence. A cluster of at least three cells is the minimal definition of a colony. They tend to grow in a disperse manner and are usually composed of cells at different stages of maturation. We have found UVfluorite lenses to be particularly useful for this task, since they are much more sensitive to fluorescent light and dramatically improve signal acquisition.

Dual labeling techniques have been described [48] and are useful for detecting more than one antigen or marker on a given cell simultaneously. This system is also ideally suited for testing the effects of various drugs on megakaryocyte progenitor cell maturation and cloning efficiency. The advantages of this system are that 1) it is technically easy to work with; 2) a "permanent" record of the experiment exists in that plates can be stored, refrigerated, or frozen, for long periods of time, and 3) cells fixed in the plasma clot can be analyzed by a variety of immunohistochemical means in situ.

Another culture system, described by Messner et al., involves suspending LDMC in medium made viscous by the addition of methylcellulose [39]. Megakaryocyte colonies grown in methylcellulose have a different morphology from those grown in plasma clot in that they consist of tight, dense clusters of cells. The cells of colonies cloned in plasma clot tend to be more scattered [39]. In addition, colonies cloned in methylcellulose tend to consist of many more cells and to exist in culture longer [39]. Accordingly, it is conceivable that each culture system could promote the growth of a different megakaryocyte progenitor. Regardless, the major advantage of this system is that colonies of viable megakaryocyte may be aspirated from the medium for biochemical, genetic, or other analysis [49,50]. This is usually not possible with cells grown in plasma clot. Disadvantages of this system are that only morphologic identification of colonies in situ is possible and thus some colonies, especially those containing immature cells will be missed. In addition methylcellulose cultures cannot be stored.

In the methylcellulose system, human plasma seems to afford better growth of cells than human serum and is therefore used as a source of essential nutrients not found in the culture medium. The reason for this phenomenon is unclear, but could be explained by the findings of Nissen and her collaborators [51–53]. These investigators have suggested that normal human serum contains an inhibitor that decreases the production of some colony-stimulating activities. This observation may explain the apparent serum inhibition of megakaryocyte colony formation seen in plasma clot cultures when cells are cloned at low concentrations [39]. At the higher cell concentrations usually employed in the plasma clot system, ancillary marrow cells presumably elaborate higher local concentrations of growth factors, which may offset the effect of putative serum inhibitors. It has also been suggested that platelets contain an inhibitor which is released when blood clots [54]. Therefore use of platelet-poor plasma or serum derived from same is recommended.

CONCLUSIONS

The techniques described above have already been exploited in the study of megakaryocyte developmental biology and possess the potential to further elucidate the functional properties of individual mature and immature cells. The prospect of being able to manipulate megakaryocytes pharmacologically, to augment desirable properties such as coagulation factor synthesis, or to diminish the atherogenic and prometastatic properties of their platelet progeny, is exciting. The methods detailed here should help to realize this promise. It should be recognized that the methods discussed in this chapter are in fact the sum of the efforts of numerous investigators. The vital information which should be accrued with their use will be a fitting testimony to all who have participated in the investigation of the properties of megakaryocytes.

ACKNOWLEDGMENTS

Supported in part by grants from the DDHS, National Cancer Institute (R23 CA 36896), a Biomedical Research Support Grant S07 RR05417 from the Division of Research Resources, National Institutes of Health, and a grant-in-aid from the Northwest Central Affiliate, Pennsylvania Chapter of the American Heart Association. Dr. Gewirtz is recipient of a New Investigator Research Award, and is a Special Fellow (101SF) of the Leukemia Society of America.

REFERENCES

1. Belloc F, Hourdille P, Fialon P, Boisseau MR, Sorria J (1985). Fibrinogen synthesis by megakaryocyte rich human marrow cell concentrations. Thromb Res 38:341–351.
2. Leven RM, Schick PK, Budzynski AZ (1985). Fibrinogen biosynthesis in isolated guinea pig megakaryocytes. Blood 65:501–504.
3. Nachman RL, Levine R, Jaffe EA (1977). Synthesis of factor VIII antigen by cultured guinea pig megakaryocytes. J Clin Invest 60:914–921.
4. Ryo R, Nakeff A, Huang SS, Ginsberg M, Deuel TF (1983). New synthesis of platelet specific protein. Platelet factor 4 synthesis in a megakaryocyte enriched rabbit bone marrow culture system. J Cell Biol 96:515–520.
5. Chiu HC, Schick PK, Colman RW (1985). Biosynthesis of factor V in isolated guinea pig megakaryocytes. J Clin Invest 75:339–346.
6. Gewirtz A, Keefer M, Doshi K, Annamali A, Chiu JC, Colman RW (1986). Biology of human megakaryocyte factor V. Blood 67:1639–1648.
7. Tracy PB, Giles AR, Mann KG, Eide LL, Hoogerdoorn H, Rivard GE (1984). Factor V (Quebec): A bleeding diathesis associated with a qualitative platelet FV deficiency. J Clin Invest 74:1221–1228.
8. Berkow RL, Straneva J, Bruno E, Beyer GS, Burgess JS, Hoffman R (1984). Isolation of human megakaryocytes by density centrifugation and counterflow centrifugal elutriation. J Lab Clin Med 103:811–818.
9. Levine RF (1980). Isolation and characterization of normal human megakaryocytes. Br J Haematol 45:487–497.
10. Sitar G (1984). Isolation of normal human megakaryocytes. Br J Haematol 59:465–472.

11. Branehog I, Kutti J, Ridell B, Swolin B, Weinfeld N (1975). The relation of thrombokinetics to bone marrow megakaryocytes in idiopathic thrombocytopenia purpura (ITP). Blood 45:551–561.
12. Queisser V, Queisser W, Spiertz B (1971). Polypoidization of megakaryocytes in normal humans, in patients with idiopathic thrombocytopenia and with pernicious anemia. Br J Haematol 20:489–501.
13. Ross R, Glomset JA (1976). The pathogenesis of atherosclerosis. N Engl J Med 295:369–377;420–425.
14. Karpatkin S, Pearlstein E (1981). Role of platelets in tumor cell metastasis. Ann Int Med 95:636–641.
15. Levine RF, Fedorko ME (1976). Isolation of intact megakaryocytes from guinea pig femoral marrow. J Cell Biol 69:159–172.
16. Nakeff A, Mant B (1974). Separation of megakaryocytes from mouse bone marrow by velocity sedimentation. Blood 213:591–595.
17. Nakeff A, Valeriote F, Gray JW, Grabska R (1979). Application of flow cytometry and cell sorting to megakaryocytopoiesis. Blood 35:732–745.
18. Pretlow TG, Stinson AJ (1976). Separation of megakaryocytes from rat bone marrow cells using velocity sedimentation in a isokinetic gradient of Ficoll in tissue culture medium. J Cell Physiol 88:317–322.
19. Rabellino EM, Nachman RL, Williams N, Winchester RJ, Ross G (1979). Human megakaryocytes: I. Characterization of the membrane and cytoplasmic components of isolated marrow megakaryocytes. J Exp Med 149:1273–1287.
20. Rabellino EM, Levene RB, Leung LLK, Nachman RL (1981). Human megakaryocytes. II. Expression of platelet proteins in early marrow megakaryocytes. J Exp Med 154:88–100.
21. Rabellino EM, Levene RB, Nachman RL, Leung LLK (1984). Human megakaryocytes III: Characterization in myeloproliferative disorders. Blood 63:615–622.
22. Bunn PA, Levine RF, Schlam M, Hazzard KC (1981). Analysis of megakaryocyte DNA content: Comparison of Feulgen microdensitometry and flow cytometry. In Evatt BL, Levine RF, Williams NT (eds): "Megakaryocyte Biology and Precursors: In Vitro Cloning and Cellular Properties." New York: Elsevier North Holland, pp 217–232.
23. Jackson CW, Brown KL, Somerville BC, Lyles SA, Look AT (1984). Two-color flow cytometric measurement of DNA distributions of rat megakaryocytes in unfixed, unfractionated marrow cell suspensions. Blood 63:768–778.
24. Lindahl PE (1956). On counterstreaming centrifugation in the separation of cells and cell fragments. Biochem Biophys Acta 21:411–415.
25. Thompson CB, Eaton KA, Princiotta SM, Rushin CA, Valeri CR (1982). Size dependent platelet subpopulations: Relationship of platelet volume to ultrastructure, enzymatic activity and function. Br J Haematol 50:509–519.
26. Skoog WA, Beck WS (1956). Studies on the fibrinogen, dextran and phytohemagglutinin methods of isolating leucocytes. Blood 11:436–454.
27. Worthington RE, Nakeff A (1981). Thromboxane synthesis in megakaryocytes isolated by centrifugal elutriation. Blood 58:175–178.
28. Damiani G, Zocchi E, Fabbi M, Bargellesi A, Patrone F (1983). A monoclonal antibody to platelet glycoproteins IIb and IIIa complex: Its use in purifying human megakaryocytes from sternal bone marrow aspirates for immunofluorescence studies of Ia-like antigens. Exp Haematol 11:169–177.
29. Till JE, McCulloch EA (1961). A direct measurement of the radiation sensitivity of normal mouse bone marrow cells. Radiat Res 14:213–222.

30. Hellman S, Reincke U, Botnick L, Mauch P (1983). Functional organization of the hematopoietic stem cell compartment: Implication for cancer and its therapy. J Clin Oncol 1:277–284.
31. Ogawa M, Porter PN, Nakahata T (1983). Renewal and commitment to differentiation of hematopoietic stem cells (An interpretive review). Blood 61:823–829.
32. Bradley TR, Metcalf D (1966). The growth of mouse bone marrow cells in vitro. Austr J Exp Biol Med 44:287–300.
33. Pluzik DH, Sachs L (1965). The cloning of normal "mast" cells in tissue culture. J Cell Physiol 66:319–324.
34. Stephenson JR, Axelrod AA, McLeod DL, Shreeve MM (1971). Induction of colonies of hemoglobin-synthesizing cells by erythropoietin in vitro. Proc Natl Acad Sci USA 68:1542–1546.
35. Metcalf D, MacDonald HR, Odartchenko N, Sordat B (1975). Growth of mouse megakaryocyte colonies in vitro. Proc Natl Acad Sci USA 72:1744–1748.
36. Nakeff A, Daniels-McQueen S (1976). In vitro colony assay for a new class of megakaryocyte precursor: Colony forming unit megakaryocyte (CFU-M). Proc Soc Exp Biol Med 151:587–590.
37. Vainchenker W, Bouget J, Guichard J, Breton-Gorius J (1979). Megakaryocyte colony formation from human bone marrow precursors. Blood 54:940–945.
38. Mazur EM, Hoffman R, Bruno E, Marchesi S, Chasis JE (1981). Immunofluorescent identification of human megakaryocyte colonies using an antiplatelet glycoprotein antiserum. Blood 57:277–286.
39. Messner HA, Jamal N, Izaguirre C (1982). The growth of large megakaryocyte colonies from human bone marrow. J Cell Physiol Suppl 1:45–51.
40. Vainchenker W, Guichard J, Breton-Gorius J (1979). Growth of human megakaryocyte colonies in cultures from fetal, neonatal and adult peripheral blood cells. Ultrastructural analysis. Blood Cells 5:23–39.
41. McLeod DL, Shreeve MM, Axelrod AA (1976). Induction of megakaryocyte colonies with platelet formation in vitro. Nature 261:492–494.
42. Gewirtz AM, Bruno E, Elwell J, Hoffman R (1983). In vitro studies of megakaryocytopoiesis in thrombocytotic disorders of man. Blood 61:384–389.
43. Gewirtz AM, Hoffman R (1986). Transitory hypomegakaryocytic thrombocytopenic purpura: Etiologic association with ethanol abuse and implications regarding regulation of human megakaryocytopoiesis. Br J Haematol (In Press).
44. Hoffman R, Mazur E, Bruno E, Floyd V (1984). Assay of an activity in the serum of patients with disorders of thrombopoiesis that stimulates formation of megakaryocytic colonies. N Engl J Med 305:533–538.
45. Hoffman R, Yang HH, Bruno E, Straneva J (1985). Purification and partial characterization of a megakaryocyte colony-stimulating factor from human plasma. J Clin Invest 75:1174–1182.
46. Mazur EM, Hoffman R, Bruno E (1981). Regulation of human megakaryocytopoiesis. An in vitro analysis. J Clin Invest 68:733–741.
47. Clark DA, Dessypris EN (1985). Quantitation of human megakaryocyte progenitors (CFU-M) in plasma clot culture by an indirect immunoperoxidase method. Exp Hematol 13:736–740.
48. Vinci G. Tabilio A, Deschamps JF, VanHaeke D, Henri A, Guichard J, Tetteroo P, Lansdorp PM, Herceno T, Vainchenker W, Breton-Gorius J (1984). Immunological study of in vitro maturation of human megakaryocytes. Br J Haematol 56:589–605.

49. Jenkins RB, Gonchoroff NJ, Oles KJ, Nichols WL, Solberg LA (1984). Analysis of DNA synthesis in human megakaryocytic colonies using a monoclonal antibody reactive with bromodeoxyuridine. Blood 64 (Suppl 1):122a.
50. Jenkins RB, Nichols W, Mann KG, Solberg LA (1986). CFU-M derived human megakaryocytes synthesize glycoproteins IIb/IIIa. Blood 67:682–688.
51. Nissen C, Moser B, Speck B, Burgin M, Bendy H (1983). Dexamethasone enhances "CSA" release and depresses "DPA" release. Br J Haematol 53:301–310.
52. Nissen C, Moser Y, Speck B (1982). Effects of human serum in the release of haemopoietic growth factors. Br J Haematol 51:385–390.
53. Nissen C, Moser Y, Speck B, Brendy J (1983). Haemopoietic stimulations and inhibitors of aplastic anemia serum. Br J Haematol 54:519–530.
54. Kimura H, Burstein SA, Thorning D, Powell JS, Harker L, Fialkow PJ, Adamson JW (1984). Human megakaryocyte progenitors (CFU-M) assayed in methycellulose: Physical characteristics and requirements for growth. J Cell Physiol 118:87–96.

Modern Methods in Pharmacology, Volume 4
Methods for Studying Platelets and Megakaryocytes, pages 19–31

Methods for Studying the Biochemistry of Recognizable Megakaryocytes

PAUL K. SCHICK and BARBARA SCHICK

Megakaryocytes are large multinucleated cells found in bone marrow and give rise to circulating blood platelets. Megakaryocytes are unique in comparison to other blood cell precursors in several respects. Megakaryocytes undergo endomitosis, which results in an increase in DNA content and cell size. Megakaryocytes are heterogeneous in respect to ploidy, size, and cytoplasmic and nuclear morphology. Each megakaryocyte is thought to have the capacity to produce from 1,000 to 4,000 platelets.

Megakaryocytes determine the protein and most likely the lipid composition of platelets. It is important to assess the effects of agents and drugs on megakaryocytes to fully understand the action of antiplatelet drugs on the development and function of circulating platelets.

Until recently it had not been possible to carry out biochemical and pharmacological studies in megakaryocytes since it had been difficult to isolate megakaryocytes in sufficient purity. A method for the isolation of guinea pig megakaryocytes to high yield and purity has provided the means to determine the biochemistry of these bone marrow cells and is described in this chapter. A multiparameter cytological approach for the investigation of subgroups of megakaryocytes that can be applied to the investigation of the biochemistry of individual megakaryocytes is also outlined in this chapter.

It should be emphasized that both of these methods provide a means for the investigation of recognizable megakaryocytes which are critical for the assembly and synthesis of circulating platelets. The techniques used to study the early phase of megakaryopoiesis and the regulation of CFU-M and megakaryocyte progenitors are discussed in the preceding chapter.

METHODS FOR THE PURIFICATION OF MEGAKARYOCYTES

Megakaryocytes have been purified from the marrow of humans [1,2], guinea pigs [3], rabbits [4], rodents [5], and calves and monkeys [6]. Several methods

From the Thrombosis Research Center and the Department of Medicine, Temple University School of Medicine, Philadelphia, Pennsylvania 19140.

have used elutriation to separate megakaryocytes from other bone marrow hemopoietic cells on the basis of size [2,4] and the application of this approach to human cells is described in the preceding chapter. The purification of guinea pig megakaryocytes results in the isolation of large yields of cells up to 85% purity. The yield and purity of megakaryocyte isolated from guinea pigs is considerably greater than that from humans, rabbits, and rodents and thus well suited for biochemical and pharmacological studies. One reason for the high yield is that there are tenfold more megakaryocytes per other bone marrow cells in guinea pig marrow than in other species.

The method for purifying guinea pig megakaryocytes has been developed by Levine and Fedorko [3]. The essential details of the procedure follow.

Animals and Materials

Fort Detrick Dunkin Hartley guinea pigs (300–400 g)
Bovine serum albumin (Cohn Fraction V powder)
Adenosine
Theophylline
Hank's Balanced Salt Solution, Ca^{++}- and Mg^{++}-Free

Collection of Bone Marrow

The animals are sacrificed and marrow is scraped from femora, humeri, and tibiae and placed in a siliconized petri dish containing calcium-free and magnesium-free Hank's Balanced Salt Solution (CMFH), at pH 7.4, which contains 3.8% NaCitrate (10/1 v:v), adenosine (1 mM), and theophylline (2 mM). Bone marrow cells are disaggregated by gently resuspending with a siliconized pasteur pipette whose tip has been cut to enlarge the orifice. The marrow cells are then filtered through nylon mesh (100 microns) into a nalgene beaker to remove stromal cells and bone particles.

Washing Bone Marrow Cells

The bone marrow cells that had been filtered are centrifuged at about 300 × g for 8 min. The supernatant, which contains fat cells, is aspirated and the pellet is suspended in CMFH, which contains albumin (23%) 7/1 (v:v), adenosine (1 mM), and theophylline (2 mM). The resuspended bone marrow cells are centrifuged again at 300 × g for 8 min.

Albumin Density Gradient Centrifugation

The pellet is resuspended in CMFH, which contains 1/7 volume albumin (23%), adenosine (1 mM), and theophylline (2 mM), and layered on an albumin density gradient.[1] The resuspended cells are centrifuged at 10,000 × g for 30 min at 4°C. A separate gradient should be used for each guinea pig. Four distinct bands of megakaryocytes are separated by this step. The majority of megakaryocytes are found in the four bands, which are formed at density layers from 1.035 g/ml to 1.050 g/ml. Some leukocyte and erythrocyte precursors are also found in these four bands. The pellet contains primarily leukocytes and erythrocytes, especially more mature cells, and a few megakaryocytes.

Preparation of Cells for and Use of Albumin Velocity Gradients

All cells in the supernatant of the albumin density gradient to about 1/2 cm above pellet are removed with a siliconized pasteur pipette whose orifice had been enlarged and diluted with CMFH at pH 7.4 with adenosine (1 mM) and theophylline (2 mM) and washed twice by centrifugation at 300 × g for 8 min. The cells are then layered on an albumin velocity gradient,[2] and megakaryocytes were separated from contaminating bone marrow cells by sedimentation at 1 × g for 30 min. Since megakaryocytes are larger than most bone marrow cells, megakaryocytes sediment more rapidly than other bone marrow cells. The larger cells, which are primarily megakaryocytes, are present in the lower half of the velocity gradient after about 30 min and are collected and passed through a second albumin velocity gradient at 1 × g for 30 min. Again cells in the lower half of the albumin velocity are harvested.

Cell counts are performed in duplicate in several aliquots of cell suspension after the second velocity gradient. Viability is assessed by morphological appearance, trypan blue exclusion, and the ability to take up serotonin. Megakaryocyte viability can also be determined by using acridine orange inclusion and ethidium bromide exclusion [7]. About 95% of megakaryocytes are viable following the isolation procedure, which represents excellent viability. Ninety percent viability would be satisfactory for most experiments.

[1]Albumin density gradient: A discontinuous gradient in which the densities of the albumin are 1.030, 1.035, 1.040, 1.045, and 1.050 g/ml (refractive indices of 1.3598, 1.3630, 1.3662, 1.3694, respectively) is used as described by Levine and Fedorko [3] in their original article on megakaryocyte isolation and in the description of subsequent modifications of the methodology [14]. We have found that the addition of adenosine (1mM) and theophylline (2 mM) to the gradients improved megakaryocyte viability and recovery.

[2]Albumin velocity gradient: Discontinuous gradient of three albumin densities is used. One with a refractive index of 1.3430 was prepared and was diluted 1:2 and 2:1 with CMFH to prepare the other two components of the gradient. Adenosine (1 mM) and theophylline (2 mM) are present in the gradients.

There are about 2.5 million megakaryocytes in the bone marrow of two guinea pigs and the method recovers from 1/3 to 1/2 of these cells. Our yield has been greater than reported by Levine and Fedorko [3]. The purity of megakaryocytes following the albumin density is about 4%, following the first velocity gradient is about 30%, and after the second velocity gradient, ranges from 60% to 90% with an acceptable average of about 85% of the total cells.

The purification procedure takes about 5 hours, and the megakaryocytes remain viable for at least 24 hours. Thus, there is sufficient time to carry out metabolic studies as well as the biochemical analyses of these cells. The cells are resuspended in culture medium with gentamycin and incubated at 37°C. We have harvested from 8×10^5 to 1.2×10^6 megakaryocytes from two guinea pigs. There is about 1 mg of protein per million megakaryocytes, which is an ample amount for biochemical analysis using currently available methodology. There is a loss of younger megakaryocytes during the purification procedure, but megakaryocytes at all stages of development are present in the final preparation of purified megakaryocytes [8]. Guinea pig megakaryocytes have recently been prepared by elutriation, and this approach may increase the recovery of younger megakaryocytes [9].

THE INVESTIGATION OF MEGAKARYOCYTES AT VARIOUS STAGES OF MATURATION

It would be very valuable to study younger versus more mature megakaryocytes in respect to composition and metabolic activities. Several obstacles have retarded progress toward this goal. Megakaryocytes comprise a diverse group of cells in respect to morphological appearance, ploidy (DNA content), and size. The relationship of these parameters to maturity is not clear at this time. Therefore, it is difficult to study the biochemistry of megakaryocytes at various stages of maturation when the criteria for maturity have not been definitively established. We have begun to relate serotonin uptake, lectin binding, and other biochemical parameters to the morphological stage, ploidy, and size of megakaryocytes.

A description of a cytological approach for the investigation of individual megakaryocytes follows.

Equipment and Materials

Microscope equipped with fluorescence and phase-contrast microscopy and a photodensitometer
Computer-assisted program to analyze the data
Chromomycin A3

Guinea pig megakaryocytes are isolated by the method described in the previous section.

Centrifugation and Fixation

About 8,000 megakaryocytes are cytocentrifuged at 460 g × 4 min on a glass microscope slide, the slide is adequately air-dried, fixed with 60% acetone, and stored at 4°C.

Exposure to Chromomycin A3

Cytocentrifuged megakaryocytes are immersed in Chromomycin A3 (5×10^{-5} M) at 37°C for 30 min. Chromomycin A3 in PBS, pH 8.0, containing $MgCl_2$ (1.5×10^{-3} M), is made up fresh monthly and stored at 4°C. In order to avoid rapid quenching, megakaryocytes exposed to Chromomycin A3 are illuminated with a 150 watt tungsten lamp at a distance of 50 cm for 3 hours prior to the determination of ploidy (Chatalain and Burstein [10]).

Determination of Ploidy

Chromomycin A3 reacts almost exclusively with cellular DNA to produce a fluorescent DNA-Chromomycin A3 complex. This characteristic of the antibiotic permits the accurate assessment of megakaryocyte ploidy. Relative intensity of fluorescence in megakaryocytes is quantitated by using the transmittance mode of a photodensitometer with filters for FITC fluorescence. The readings are determined in the transmission mode with a 4N cell having a relative fluorescence intensity of 5%. The readings were linear for the assessment of 2N neutrophils, which served as 2N standards, and 8N, 16N, 32N, and 64N megakaryocytes. The data are analyzed by a computer-assisted program and used to produce a histogram of the frequency distribution of megakaryocytes according to relative fluorescent intensity (relative DNA content). Figure 1 demonstrates a representative histogram of the analysis of 200 megakaryocytes. Examination of the histogram demonstrates three distinct groups of megakaryocytes and the mean relative fluorescence intensities of the three groups correlate with ploidy of 8N, 16N, and 32N, respectively. A small percentage of megakaryocytes appears to fall outside of these ploidy groups and represents 4N and 64N cells. If necessary, the number of cells in the three major ploidy classes can be defined by a Gaussian curve fitting program to determine the midpoint of the curve for each ploidy class and then determining the limits for each ploidy class. The histogram, therefore, provides the means to determine upper and lower limits for relative fluorescent intensity for each major ploidy group. This information is needed for the multiparameter computer-assisted analysis described below.

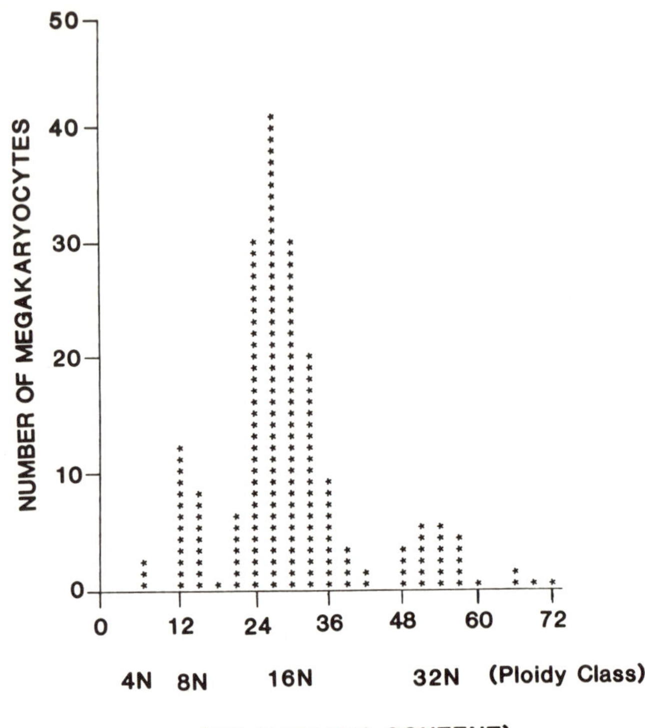

Fig. 1. DNA histogram. A frequency histogram of the relative DNA content of 200 megakaryocytes is shown. Megakaryocytes had been purified from guinea pig marrow and cytocentrifuged onto glass slides and subjected to Chromomycin A3. The relative fluorescent intensity of the Chromomycin-DNA complex in individual megakaryocytes was measured by a Zeiss photodensitometer. The histogram was generated by a computer-assisted program. Neutrophils were also assessed and served as a 2N standard reference (not shown). The three major peaks appeared to represent the three major ploidy classes, 8N, 16N, and 32N. Three 4N megakaryocytes were detected and were distinguished from other megakaryocytes by their morphological appearance and content of fibrinogen and factor VIII:R by immunological methods. Purified megakaryocytes usually contain less than 2% 4N or 64N megakaryocytes.

Assessment of Morphological Stage

The morphological stage of megakaryocytes is determined by examining the nuclear configuration and nuclear/cytoplasmic ratio of megakaryocytes, which had been exposed to Chromomycin A3, under fluorescence microscopy. Since Chromomycin A3 does not react with cytoplasmic components, there is no cytoplasmic fluorescence. In order to accurately evaluate the cytoplasmic/nuclear morphology, the megakaryocytes are examined by both phase-contrast and fluorescence microscopy. Four morphological stages are determined by these criteria with stage I and II representing cells with a large nuclear/cytoplasmic ratio and nuclear configuration. For example, a stage I or II megakaryocyte has a large nuclear/cytoplasmic ratio with an immature nucleus, while more advanced stages have a nuclear/cytoplasmic ratio of less than one. A stage III cell has multilobulated nucleus and a stage IV megakaryocyte has a small involuted nucleus [8]. The four morphological stages of megakaryocytes are shown in Figure 2, in which the nuclei in these cells were visualized by Chromomycin A3. This approach for evaluating megakaryocyte nuclei appears to be superior to that under Wright's stains, since the nuclear patterns are more easily visualized.

Megakaryocyte Size

The diameter of megakaryocytes is determined by using an optical micrometer. In the case of elliptical megakaryocytes, the mean of the longest and shortest diameter is used.

Multiparameter Analysis of Ploidy, Morphological Stage, and Megakaryocyte Size

These parameters were determined in each of 200 megakaryocytes. In order to avoid sample error megakaryocytes were assessed in a random manner on at

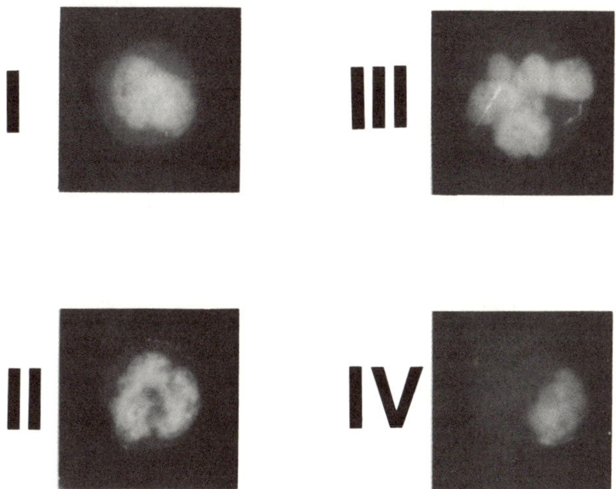

Fig. 2. Morphological stages of megakaryocytes. Cytocentrifuged megakaryocytes had been reacted with Chromomycin A3, which reacts primarily with DNA. The fluorescence of the DNA-Chromomycin A3 complex permitted the characterization of the nucloear configuration and nuclear-cytoplasmic ratio, which served as criteria for the determination of morphological stage. Stage I megakaryocytes are the most immature recognizable megakaryocytes, whereas Stage III and IV are the most mature [8]. The DNA fluorescence was used to determine the ploidy of these megakaryocytes as described in Figure 1.

least three slides. The ploidy was established first, followed by morphological staging and estimation of size to avoid quenching of fluorescence during assessment of morphology. The data were analyzed by a computer assisted program.

RESULTS FROM THE INVESTIGATION OF ISOLATED MEGAKARYOCYTES

The investigation of isolated megakaryocytes have clearly shown that they can synthesize alpha granule proteins, factor V [11], fibrinogen [12,13], factor VIIIag [14]. These experiments were performed by incubating purified megakaryocytes with radiolabeled precursors, e.g., [^{35}S]methionine, and then separating the immunoprecipitated or immunity affinity purified newly synthesized platelet coagulant or platelet specific proteins by SDS gel electrophoresis. It is evident that platelets are endowed with alpha granules which had been packaged in megakaryocytes.

Guinea pig megakaryocytes have extensive capacity to take up serotonin, which is comparable to that in platelets but cannot synthesize the amine [15,16]. The physiological role of serotonin in megakaryocytes is as yet not defined. Megakaryocytes contain both storage and cytoplasmic pool adenine nucleotides, but unlike platelet, megakaryocytes possess a salvage pathway for the synthesis of adenine nucleotides from hypoxanthine [17,18]. These data suggest that storage compartments or granules, which are equivalent to platelet dense bodies, are present in megakaryocytes.

The lipid composition of megakaryocytes with minor exceptions is similar to that in platelets [19]. However, there are certain distinct differences, since only megakaryocytes have the capacity for cholesterol synthesis [20]. Platelets cannot take up significant amounts of cholesterol and thus the synthesis of cholesterol in megakaryocytes may be the principal source for the cholesterol content of platelets [21]. Diet-induced hypercholesterolemia leads to the formation of large megakaryocytes and platelets with abnormal cholesterol content [22]. Megakaryocytes, however, rather than platelets appear to be the target of the modified cholesterol diet, which results in the production of abnormal platelets.

The metabolism of arachidonic acid has been investigated in isolated guinea pig megakaryocytes [23]. Megakaryocytes, unlike platelets, can synthesize arachidonic acid by the desaturation of eicosatrienoic acid by a delta 5 desaturase. The distribution of arachidonic acid synthesized or taken up by megakaryocytes appears to reflect the endogenous distribution of arachidonic acid in megakaryocyte phospholipids. These data indicate that megakaryocytes incorporate arachidonate into all pools of phospholipid arachidonic acid. In contrast, platelets do not readily incorporate exogenous arachidonate into all lipid pools, since only small amounts of the radiolabeled unsaturated fatty acid are incorporated into phosphatidylethanolamine, which contains over 63% of endogenous platelet arachidonic acid. This information suggests that megakaryocytes can establish the content of certain pools of platelets lipids.

Several other aspects of megakaryocyte physiology and biochemistry are currently being investigated, which will provide new insights into the role of megakaryocytes. There is evidence that megakaryocytes have platelet derived growth factor activity [24,25]. Contractile proteins in resting and stimulated megakaryocytes have been investigated. Megakaryocytes can be stimulated to spread and the metabolic basis for this event has been explored [26]. Advances in understanding the biochemistry of megakaryocytes have been recently reviewed [27,28].

RESULTS AND APPLICATION OF THE MULTIPARAMETER APPROACH TO DETERMINING THE BIOCHEMISTRY OF INDIVIDUAL MEGAKARYOCYTES

The results of these analyses are shown in Tables I and II. The data demonstrate that 14% of megakaryocytes are morphological stage I cells, 20% are stage

TABLE I. Percent of Megakaryocytes in Subgroups

Stage	8N	16N	32N	All
I	2.0	8.8	3.4	14.2
II	2.3	14.2	3.5	20.0
III	4.0	32.3	12.3	48.6
IV	3.4	12.2	1.6	17.2
All	11.7	67.5	20.8	100.0

The multiparameter analyses of 200 megakaryocytes in four separate experiments (total of 800 cells) are shown. The ploidy of each cell was determined as described in Figure 1, the morphologic stage as shown in Figure 2, and the size was determined by an optical micrometer. The data were analyzed by a computer-assisted program.

TABLE II. Diameters of Megakaryocyte Subgroups

		Microns		
Stage	8N	16N	32N	All
I	27	36	40	35
II	33	36	43	37
III	33	40	46	40
IV	35	43	40	41
All	32	39	44	39

II, 48% are stage III, and 16% are stage IV cells. Eleven percent are 8N, 67% are 16N, and 21% are 32N megakaryocytes. Only minor differences in the distribution of ploidy classes in each of the four morphological stages were observed, but 8N megakaryocytes were more likely to be stage I cells, while 16N cells were more likely to be stage III and IV megakaryocytes. The size of megakaryocytes was directly related to ploidy with 8N cells being smaller than 32N cells. Stage I and II megakaryocytes are smaller than stage III and IV megakaryocytes.

This information is consistent with the concept that the ploidy of megakaryocytes is established early in their development and that cytoplasmic and nuclear differentiation, which determines morphological stage, occurs at a later phase in megakaryocyte maturation. Most likely, morphological stage is the best parameter for megakaryocyte maturation.

In order to obtain information about the biochemical and metabolic characteristics of megakaryocytes at different stages of maturation, the multiparameter method described above was expanded. For example, wheat-germ agglutinin (WGA) binding was studied in individual megakaryocytes and related to morphological stage, ploidy, and size.

Rhodamine-WGA was incubated with megakaryocytes and was found to bind to only about 50% of megakaryocytes [29]. Since Chromomycin A3 fluorescence can be visualized by using filters for FITC fluorescence, both Rhodamine-WGA and Chromomycin A3 fluorescence could be measured in the same cell using a fluorescence microscope with filters that can discriminate between rhodamine and FITC fluorescence. Thus, WGA binding could be related to ploidy, morphological stage, and size by the multiparameter approach. In these experiments, ploidy was examined first, followed by estimation of morphological stage and size, but to avoid bias Rhodamine-WGA binding was determined last. The results of this study are shown in Table III. WGA binding, which most likely represents the exposure of sialoglycoproteins on the megakaryocyte surface, was primarily detected in stage III and IV megakaryocytes. 8N megakaryocytes were less likely to be labeled by WGA than higher ploidy cells. There was no correlation of lectin binding to megakaryocyte size. Therefore, the primary determinant of WGA binding to megakaryocytes was morphological stage. The study indicated that sialoglycoproteins are primarily expressed on the surface of mature megakaryocytes [29].

In addition to showing that earlier stage and more advanced stage megakaryocytes possessed different biochemical capacities, the studies suggested that the exposure of sialoglycoproteins was virtually exclusively related to the megakaryocyte morphological stage and not to ploidy or size. Thus, biochemical differentiation best correlates with megakaryocyte stage and appears to represent a new parameter for megakaryocyte maturation.

TABLE III. Labeling of Megakaryocytes by WGA in Relation to Morphological Stage and Ploidy

Percentage of megakaryocytes labeled in each morphological stage	
I	35.1 ± 11.1
II	28.7 ± 6.2
III	71.9 ± 8.6
IV	76.7 ± 8.6
Percentage of megakaryocytes labeled in each ploidy class	
8N	44.1 ±8.4
16N	60.4 ± 7.0
32N	58.5 ± 9.7

Isolated megakaryocytes were incubated with rhodamine-WGA (1 μmol/L) at 23°C for 5 min, cytocentrifuged, and incubated with Chromomycin A3. Each megakaryocyte was assessed by the multiparameter analysis described in Tables I and II and the labeling of megakaryocytes by WGA was correlated with the cell's morphologic stage and ploidy. The data were analyzed by a computer-assisted program. The means and S.D. of 4 separate experiments in which 200 cells were counted in each experiment (total 800 cells) are shown.

CONCLUSION

Two methodological advances have permitted the biochemical assessment of megakaryocytes. The ability to isolate highly purified megakaryocytes and to study characteristics of individual megakaryocytes has provided new and important information about the biochemical aspects of megakaryocyte maturation. The expression of sialoglycoproteins on the megakaryocytes occurs primarily in more mature megakaryocytes. Serotonin uptake occurs in megakaryocytes at all stages of maturation and indicates that the storage capacity for serotonin is established early in the course of megakaryocyte development. These methodological approaches can be used to determine the effects of antiplatelet drugs on the megakaryocyte. Therefore, we are in a better position to develop a new generation of antiplatelet drugs and to obtain a more complete understanding of the effects of certain drugs on platelet function.

ACKNOWLEDGMENTS

The studies were supported by NIH Grants HL25455, HL22633, and HL29282, Grant-in-Aid from the American Heart Association, and BRSG support from Temple University.

REFERENCES

1. Rabellino EM, Nachman RL, Williams N, Winchester RJ, Ross GD (1979). Human megakaryocytes I. Characterization of the membrane and cytoplasmic components of isolated marrow megakaryocytes. J Exp Med 149:1273–1287.
2. Berkow RL, Straneva J, Bruno E, Beyer GS, Burgess JS, Hoffman R (1984). Isolation of human megakaryocytes by density centrifugation and counterflow centrifugal elutriation. J Lab Clin Med 103:811–818.
3. Levine RF, Fedorko ME (1976). Isolation of intact megakaryocytes from guinea pig femoral marrow. J Cell Biol 69:159–172.
4. Ryo R, Nakeff A, Huang SS, Ginsburg M, Deuel TF (1983). New synthesis of a platelet-specific protein: Platelet factor 4 synthesis in a megakaryocyte-enriched rabbit bone marrow culture system. J Cell Biol 96:515–520.
5. Wesemann W, Raha S, McDonald TP (1985). Isolation of mouse megakaryocytes II. Functional and metabolic aspects of two different maturation stages. Eur J Cell Biol 37:117–121.
6. Levine RF, Bunn PA, Hazzard KC, Schlamm ML (1980). Flow cytometric analysis of megakaryocyte ploidy. Comparison with Feulgen microdensitometry and discovery that 8N is the predominant ploidy class in guinea pig and monkey marrow. Blood 56:210–217.
7. Ishibashi T, Burstein SA (1985). Separation of murine megakaryocytes and their progenitors on continuous gradients of Percoll. J Cell Physiol 125:559–566.
8. Levine RF, Hazzard KC, Lamberg JD (1982). The significance of megakaryocyte size. Blood 60:1122–1131.
9. Levine RF (1986). Old and new aspects of megakaryocyte development. In Levine RF, Williams N, Levin J, Evatt BL (eds): Megakarocyte Development and Function. Prog Clin Biological Res 215:1–20.
10. Chatalain C, Burstein SA (1984). Fluorescence cytophotometric analysis of megakaryocyte ploidy in culture: Study of normal and thrombocytopenic mice. Blood 61:1193.
11. Chiu HC, Schick PK, Colman RW (1985). Biosynthesis of Factor V in isolated guinea pig megakaryocytes. J Clin Invest 75:339–346.
12. Leven RM, Schick PK, Budzynski AZ (1985). Fibrinogen biosynthesis in isolated guinea pig megakaryocytes. Blood: 65:501–504.
13. Belloc F, Hourdouille P, Fialon MR, Boisseau MR, Soria J (1985). Fibrinogen synthesis by megakaryocyte-rich human marrow cell concentrates. Thromb Res 38:341–351.
14. Nachman RL, Levine RF, Jaffe EA (1977). Synthesis of factor VIII antigen by cultured guinea pig megakaryocytes. J Clin Invest 60:914–921.
15. Schick PK, Weinstein M (1981). A marker for megakaryocytes: Serotonin accumulation in guinea pig megakaryocytes. J Lab Clin Med 98:607–615.
16. Fedorko ME (1977). The functional capacity of guinea pig megakaryocytes. I. Uptake of [3H]-serotonin by megakaryocytes and their physiologic and morphological responses to stimuli for the platelet release reaction. Lab Invest 36:310–320.
17. Levine RF, Webster HK (1981). Purine metabolism in megakaryocytes and platelets. Throm Haemost 6:22.
18. Miller JL (1983). Characterization of the megakaryocyte secretory response: Studies of continuously monitored release of endogenous ATP. Blood 61:967–972.
19. Schick BP, Schick PK, Chase PR (1984). Lipid composition of guinea pig megakaryocytes: The megakaryocyte as a probable source of platelet lipids. Biochim Biophys Acta 663:239–248.

20. Schick BP, Schick PK (1981). Cholesterol and phospholipid biosynthesis in guinea pig megakaryocytes. Biochim Biophys Acta 663:249–254.
21. Schick BP, Schick PK (1984). Cholesterol exchange in platelets, erythrocytes and megakaryocytes. Biochim Biophys Acta 833:281–290.
22. Schick BP, Schick PK (1984). The effect of hypercholestrolemia on guinea pig platelets, erythrocytes and megakaryocytes. Biochim Biophys Acta 833:291–302.
23. Schick PK, Schick BP, Foster KA, Block AB (1984). Arachidonate synthesis and uptake in isolated guinea pig megakaryocytes and platelets. Biochim Biophys Acta 795:341–347.
24. Castro-Malaspina H, Rabellino ER, Yen A, Nachman RL, Moore MA (1981). Human megakaryocyte stimulation of proliferation of bone marrow fibroblasts. Blood 57:781–787.
25. Chernoff A, Levine RF, Goodman DS (1980). Origin of platelet-derived growth factor in megakaryocytes in guinea pigs. J Clin Invest 65:926–930.
26. Leven RM, Millikin WH, Nachmias VT (1983). Role of sodium in ADP- and thrombin-induced megakaryocyte spreading. J Cell Biol 96:1234–1240.
27. Schick PK, Schick PB (1986). Megakaryocyte Biochemistry. In Megakaryocyte Development and Function. RF Levine, N Williams, J Levin, and BL Evatt (eds): Prog Clin Biological Res 215:265–279.
28. Schick BP, Schick PK (1986). Megakaryocyte Biochemistry. Sem Hematol 23:68–87.
29. Schick PK, Filmyer WG, Jr. (1985). Sialic acid in mature megakaryocytes: Detection by wheat germ agglutinin. Blood 65:1120–1126.

Modern Methods in Pharmacology, Volume 4
Methods for Studying Platelets and Megakaryocytes, pages 33–40

Methods for Studying Platelet Shape Change, Aggregation, and Fibrinogen Binding

ROBERT W. COLMAN

OVERVIEW

Platelets initially respond to various soluble agonists such as ADP, thrombin, collagen, and prostaglandin endoperoxides by a morphological change from disks to spheres, decoraled with pseudopic cytoplasmic projections [Born, 1962]. This process may occur on subendothelium exposed by endothelial injury to which platelets adhere. The combination of release of platelet intracellular contents such as ADP, serotonin, and fibrinogen and rheologic condition resulting in collision of inactivated platelets with those which have undergone shape change allows interplatelet contact and the formation of platelet aggregates. Fibrinogen is required for platelet aggregation [Cross, 1964; McLean et al., 1964]. Fibrinogen is believed to bind to a calcium requiring complex of platelet membrane glycoproteins IIb and IIIa [Nachman and Leung, 1982]. The dimeric structure and twofold symmetry renders fibrinogen uniquely well suited to serve as a molecular bridge from platelet to platelet. Since fibrinogen does not bind to unactivated platelets, chemical substances that activate platelets are responsible for exposing these latent receptors. Evidence is accumulating that this process depends on the binding of ADP to a cell surface receptor [Bennett et al., 1978] and/or proteolytic cleavage of that same protein [Figures et al., 1981], which in its intact state may be responsible for the latency of the fibrinogen receptor complex. Research into the importance of ADP in the mechanism of platelet aggregation requires methods for measuring platelet shape change, platelet aggregation, fibrinogen binding, and a probe to identify the ADP receptor responsible for platelet aggregation. These approaches are detailed in this chapter. Study of platelet release reaction, intracellular calcium changes, prostaglandin metabolism, and agonist binding are dealt with in other chapters in this book.

From the Thrombosis Research Center, Temple University School of Medicine, Philadelphia, Pennsylvania 19140.

METHODS

Isolation of Platelets From Blood

Platelet-rich plasma (PRP) is prepared from whole human blood anticoagulated with ACD (sodium citrate 0.085 M, citric acid 0.079 M, dextrose 0.180 M) by differential centrifugation (120 × g, 15 min, 37°C). The top layer containing platelet-rich plasma is separated from the red cell layer and used as a source of platelets.

Removal of Plasma From Platelets

Method 1. Potato apyrase is prepared by extraction of potatoes using the method of Molnar and Lorand [1961]. These preparations contain both ADPase and ATPase activities as well as a platelet aggregation lectin. The lectin was separated from the apyrase using fetuin-agarose affinity chromatography [Winham et al, 1976]. Washed platelets were prepared from platelet-rich plasma by the method of Mustard et al. [1972]. Platelets are sedimented from platelet-rich plasma (1,100 × g, 20 min) and resuspended in Tyrode-albumin buffer (NaH_2PO_4 0.02 mM, NaCl 136 mM, KCl 2.68 mM, $NaHCO_3$ 11.9 mM, dextrose 5.4 mM, bovine serum albumin [Cohn fraction V] 0.35%, pH 7.35) containing heparin (25 U/ml), apyrase (50 U/ml), calcium chloride (2.0 mM), and magnesium chloride (1.0 mM). The use of apyrase prevents the action of ADP on platelets during preparation and the use of heparin minimizes exposure of thrombin. After 20 min incubation at 37°C, the cells are sedimented (1,100 × g, 20 min) and resuspended without the addition of heparin. After incubation (20 min, 37°C), the cells are resedimented and suspended in the same buffer in the absence of apyrase and heparin.

Method 2. Plasma can be removed efficiently by gel-filtration using Sepharose 2B. The plastic column is equilibrated with Tyrode-albumin buffer (as above but without apyrase, heparin, or calcium) and buffered with Hepes [Timmons and Harviger, 1978], to a volume of PRP, not greater than one-sixth of the volume of the column. Typically, 4 ml PRP is applied to a 24 ml column in a 30 ml plastic syringe barrel and the platelets appear in the void volume-free of plasma fibrinogen.

Platelet Shape Change and Aggregation

For measurement of shape change, platelet suspensions (0.5 ml, 2 × 10^8 cells/ml) are diluted immediately prior to use with 5 mM EDTA in 0.15 M NaCl, incubated at 37°C in siliconized glass cuvettes in a dual channel Chronolog Lumi-Aggregometer (Chronolog Corp., Havertown, PA). The reference channel contains platelets that had been incubated with 10 μM ADP. Platelet suspensions for shape change measurements are incubated with an agonist or carrier solvent alone and the maximum change in optical density in millivolts measured 20 sec after addition of agonist [Mills et al., 1985]. For platelet aggregations the EDTA is omitted and the reference channel does not contain ADP.

The greatest decrease in light transmittance is defined as 100% of maximum shape change. All other measurements on similar platelet suspensions are given in relation to this value. In addition to the extent, the rate of the decrease in light transmittance is measured with the slope of the tracings. The greatest rate of change is defined as 100% of maximum rate of shape change, and all other rates for a specific compound and platelet suspension are expressed in terms of the maximum. Platelet aggregation is measured in the same instrument as an increase in light transmittance of the platelet suspension. Either the maximum rate of aggregation or the extent of aggregation can be recorded. Platelet shape change can also be assessed by scanning electron microscopy, by adding 2.5% glutaraldehyde to Tyrode's buffer. The samples were fixed for 30 min at 25°C and kept overnight at 4°C. After 18 hours, the platelets are deposited with suction (10 mm Hg) on a 1 μm pore nucleopore membrane. The cells on the membrane are then postfixed in 1% osmium tetroxide, dehydrated through graded alcohol, dried at the critical point, and coated with gold. Photomicrographs are made at 5,000X magnification and coded samples are classified as discoid, spiny spheres, or intermediate forms.

Preparation of ^{125}I-Fibrinogen and Binding of ^{125}I-Fibrinogen to Platelets

Fibrinogen (Kabi, Stockholm, Sweden) is purified by ammonium sulfate precipitation as described by Niewiarowski et al. [1981]. Prior to purification, solutions of fibrinogen (10 mg/ml) are treated with diisopropylfluorophosphate (10 mM, 1 h) to inhibit any protease activity associated with the fibrinogen. The clottability of fibrinogen prepared by this method is >93%. The purified fibrinogen is labeled with ^{125}I by the Iodine monochloride technique. Excess ^{125}I is removed by gel-filtration of the sample on Bio-Gel P2. The clottability of the labeled fibrinogen is usually >90% and the specific activity ranges from 3.1–50 μCi/nmol fibrinogen.

The measurement of fibrinogen binding to platelet receptors is carried out using a silicone oil centrifugation technique in which the binding of ^{125}I-fibrinogen to these sites is measured. Platelets (3×10^8 cells/ml) are incubated with ADP (10 μM) and fibrinogen at concentrations ranging from 0–50 μg/ml. The cells are incubated for 20 min, at which time an aliquot of reaction mixture is layered on top of silicone oil in an Eppendorf centrifuge tube with a constricted tip. The silicone oil consists of a mixture of DC550 (8 parts) and DC250 (2 parts) (William F. Nye Inc., New Bedford, MA). The tubes are then centrifuged for 2 min in an Eppendorf centrifuge. The pellets are then counted for ^{125}I in a LKB gamma counter. In order to determine specific binding of ^{125}I-fibrinogen, identical samples containing an excess of unlabeled fibrinogen (1%) are evaluated in the same system. Specific binding is then calculated as the total binding - nonspecific binding.

Identification of an ADP Receptor Responsible for Platelet Activation

Properties of FSBA. The nucleotide affinity analog, 5′-p-fluorosulfonyl benzoyl adenosine (FSBA), has been demonstrated to covalently modify active and allosteric regulatory sites in many enzymes [Colman et al., 1977] requiring nucleotides as well as the ATP binding sites of actin and myosin on the internal surface of the platelet membrane [Bennett et al., 1981]. Bennett et al. [1978] have presented evidence that FSBA can covalently incorporate into a single polypeptide (M_r 100,000) on the external surface of the platelet membrane. The labeling of this protein demonstrates considerable specificity, as it is protected by ADP and its competitive inhibitor, ATP, but not by adenosine, AMP, or epinephrine, in experiments carried out with platelet membranes. In the same study, FSBA was shown to induce a rapid inhibition of ADP-induced shape change, which was progressive with time of incubation with FSBA. Figures et al. [1981] have demonstrated that incubation of intact washed platelets with FSBA resulted in the inhibition of ADP mediated aggregation as well as exposure by ADP of latent fibrinogen binding sites. A single site of covalent incorporation was observed concomitantly in the washed platelet preparation. Mills et al. [1985] demonstrated that FSBA in the presence of adenosine deaminase and under conditions where covalent incorporation was achieved did not block inhibition of cAMP accumulation by ADP and had no effect in binding of 2-methyl thio ADP, which binds to adenylate cyclase. The inhibition of ADP-induced platelet activation coupled with the modification of an externally oriented membrane protein makes this protein an attractive candidate for an adenine nucleotide receptor site, which mediates shape change and aggregation as well as exposure of fibrinogen receptors in human platelets.

Preparation of FSBA. FSBA is synthesized by the method of Wyatt and Colman [1977]. The synthesis involves the condensation of adenosine with fluorosulfonylbenzoyl chloride. For the synthesis of radiolabeled FSBA, [^3H]-adenosine (New England Nuclear) was utilized. Typical radiolabeled preparations have specific radioactivities of 20 Ci/mol. Once isolated, the compound is stored in solid form at $-70°C$ in a desiccated environment. When needed, the stored sample is thawed and a small amount (~ 1 mg) dissolved in dimethylformamide (DMF). The concentration of FSBA is then determined by absorbance measurement of an aliquot of DMF solution diluted in ethanol (1:3,000). The absorbance (259 nm) is read versus a blank sample containing the same volume of pure DMF diluted in ethanol. The molar extinction coefficient for FSBA is $1.35 \times 10^4\ M^{-1}\ cm^{-1}$ at 259 nm.

Labeling of platelets with FSBA. A stock solution of FSBA dissolved in DMF is added to suspensions of washed platelets to give a desired final concentration of FSBA. All control samples are treated with DMF alone. The DMF concentration should never exceed 1.0% of the volume of platelet suspensions 5×10^8 cells/ml. In order to completely block ADP-induced activation of platelets, 100 μM FSBA is incubated with the platelets for 20 min at 37°C. At the conclusion of the incubation period, the cells are sedimented (1,200 × g, 20 min) to separate them from the excess FSBA and then resuspended in fresh Tyrode buffer. Since FSBA inhibits ADP aggregation of platelets, even gel-filtered platelets can be sedimented in this fashion without clumping of the cells caused by centrifugation-induced ADP leakage. All incubations are carried out in the presence of adenosine deaminase (2 U/ml) to prevent the effects of any contaminating adenosine in the preparation [Mills et al., 1985].

Incorporation of the affinity label into platelet membrane protein. Method 1 involves the labeling of cells with FSBA as described above, followed by the isolation of platelet membranes, solubilization of membrane proteins, and separation of proteins by SDS polyacrylamide gel electrophoresis [Bennett et al., 1978; Figures et al., 1981]. The glycerol lysis method of Barber and Jamieson [1970] is used for the lysis of cells and isolation of platelet membranes. The membrane proteins are then solubilized in SDS (10%), urea (8 M), DTT(0.2 M), and DFP (10 mM). The solubilized platelet membrane proteins are then separated by SDS-PAGE using the method of Weber and Osborn [1975]. The system is used because of the neutral pH of the running gel, thus stabilizing the ester bond at the 5′ position of the ribose ring in FSBA, which is quite susceptible to hydrolysis at pH levels <6.0 and >8.0. The gels are then sliced, the slices counted, extracted in a mixture of toluene-water-Protosol (New England Nuclear) (9:1:10), and then counted in a liquid scintillation cocktail (Econofluor-New England) to localize the radiolabeled protein. FSBA has been shown to label a single membrane polypeptide in platelet membranes with M_r 100,000. This method renders reproducible results but requires large number of platelets.

An alternate method is used to measure the effect of FSBA concentration on covalent incorporation of FSBA into the cell surface receptor. In these assays, cells were incubated at 37°C for 40 min. In order to stop the reaction, cells were then added to dithiothreitol (200 mM final conc). The DTT causes rapid hydrolysis of the sulfonyl fluoride, thus rendering any residual FSBA incapable of further reaction with platelets. In order to measure the extent of incorporation in the receptor, cells are removed by centrifugation (8,000 × g, 20 min) in an

Eppendorf microfuge and supernatants are carefully aspirated. The pellets are then dissolved in phosphate buffer (0.1 M, pH 7.2) containing SDS (10%), urea (8 M), and EDTA (10 mM). The dissolution of cells is allowed to proceed overnight (18 hours, 23°C). The solutions of solubilized platelet proteins are then dialyzed in a multiple chamber continuous flow dialysis chamber (Bethesda Research Laboratories, MD #1200) for 3 days. The dialysis buffer consisted of phosphate (0.05 M, pH 7.2) containing SDS (0.1%) and EDTA (10 mM). The dialysis step is necessary to remove any radiolabeled material that had not covalently bound to membrane protein. In order to assure complete removal of unbound radiolabel, a number of samples at the highest concentration is included and tested on a daily basis. As mentioned above, it is important to maintain proteins labeled with SBA-protein in a pH range between 7.0 and 8.0, since the ester bond at the 5′ position is quite susceptible to hydrolysis at pH outside these ranges. Dialysis is considered complete when the amount of radiolabel in a sample remained constant for 24 hours. Samples are then removed from the dialysis chamber and counted in a liquid scintillation cocktail (ACSII-Amersham). The amount of radiolabel in the sample is evaluated and the specific activity is calculated in terms of molecules incorporated per platelet. Nonspecific binding to nonnucleotide binding sites is determined by use of an ADP (10 mM) chase. Specific binding can then be calculated by the difference between total binding and nonspecific binding.

RESULTS AND DISCUSSION

The result of using FSBA to label nucleotide binding sites on the external surface of the platelet membrane is consistent with the results expected if the reagent covalently incorporated into an ADP receptor mediating shape change and aggregation. Cells treated with FSBA for 20–40 min fail to respond to ADP such that both shape change and aggregation responses produced by this nucleotide in control cells is inhibited [Bennett et al., 1978; Figures et al., 1981]. Thus, this procedure can be used to render platelets permanently incapable of responding to ADP by activation. In addition, the inhibition of ADP-mediated fibrinogen binding to fibrinogen receptors is also inhibited by pretreatment of platelets with nucleotide analog. The specificity of this inhibition is demonstrated by the lack of inhibition of shape change induced by prostracyclin endoperoxide analog azo-PGH_2 [Morinelli et al., 1983]. In contrast, FSBA inhibits azo-PGH_2 induced aggregation, suggesting an ADP requirement for platelet aggregation induced by prostaglandin endoperoxides and thromboxane A_2. It is interesting to note that in all systems tested, FSBA acts in a functionally identical manner to ADP metabolizing enzymes, apyrase, and CP/CPK, in their effect on platelets. In addition, we have recently demonstrated that guanosine derivative FSBG has no such effect [Mills et al., 1985]. The use of FSBA has indicated the initial site of action of ADP to be a cell surface protein with M_r 100,000. This protein may represent the platelet ADP receptor mediating shape change, aggregation, and fibrinogen binding.

One of the major functions of the receptor is to prevent access of fibrinogen to its receptor GPIIb/IIIa. When ADP binds to the receptor a conformational change in the 100K Dalton membrane protein may expose the latent fibrinogen receptor. Thus, the action of epinephrine to aggregate platelets and expose fibrinogen binding sites is completely inhibited by FSBA [Figures et al., 1986]. Epinephrine indirectly potentiates platelet activation by increasing the affinity for ADP. Collagen-induced shape change, aggregation, and fibrinogen binding are also inhibited by FSBA, indicating a requirement for ADP [Colman et al., 1986]. Further evidence in favor of this concept is the ability of chymotrypsin [Figures et al., 1981] not only to induce platelet aggregation even after FSBA is incorporated covalently but to cleave the SBA-labeled protein. Thus proteolysis of ADP receptor can take the place of the alteration induced by ADP binding. This finding suggests other proteolytic enzymes such as thrombin may work in a similar way.

A recent study by Mills et al. [1985] has demonstrated this site is distinct from ADP binding site on the platelet surface that controls cyclic AMP (cAMP) levels in platelets. In this study, pretreatment of platelets with FSBA under conditions known to inhibit ADP-mediated shape change and aggregation failed to impair the ability of ADP to lower cAMP levels. This observation strongly suggests that there are two types of binding sites on the cell surface for ADP: one site controlling aggregation and shape change and the other controlling cAMP levels in the cell. Apparently FSBA interacts with the former site only.

ACKNOWLEDGMENTS

Supported in part by grants from NIH HL36359, HL14217 and HL36579.

REFERENCES

Barber AJ, Jamieson GA (1970). Isolation and characterization of plasma membranes from human blood platelets. J Biol Chem 245:6357–6365.

Bennett JS, Colman RF, Colman RW (1978). Identification of adenine nucleotide binding proteins in human platelet membranes by affinity labeling with 5′-p-fluorosulfonylbenzoyl adenosine. J Biol Chem 253:7346–7354.

Bennett JS, Vilaire G, Colman RF, Colman RW (1981). Localization of human platelet membrane-associated actomyosin using the affinity label 5′-p-fluorosulfonylbenzoyl adenosine. J Biol Chem 256:1185–1190.

Born GVR (1962). Aggregation of blood platelets by adenosine diphosphate and its reversal. Nature 194:927–929.

Colman RW, Figures WR, Scearce LM, Strumpler AM, Zhou F, Rao AK (1986). Inhibition of collagen-induced platelet activation by 5′-p- fluorosulfonylbenzoyl adenosine: Evidence for an ADP requirement and the synergistic influence of prostaglandin endoperoxidases. Blood (In Press).

Colman RF, Pal PK, Wyatt J (1977). Adenosine derivatives for dehydrogenases and kinases. Meth Enzymol 46:240.

Cross MJ (1964) Effect of fibrinogen on the aggregation of platelets by adenosine diphosphate. Thromb Diath Haemorrh 12:524–527.

Figures WR, Niewiarowski S, Morinelli TA, Colman RF, Colman RW (1981). Affinity labeling of a human platelet membrane protein with 5′-p-fluorosulfonylbenzoyl adenosine. J Biol Chem 256:7789–7795.

Figures WR, Scearce LM, Wachtfogel Y, Chen J, Colman RF, Colman RW (1986). Platelet ADP receptor and α_2- adrenoreceptor interaction: Evidence for an ADP requirement for epinephrine induced platelet activation and an influence of epinephrine or ADP binding. J Biol Chem (In Press).

Mclean JR, Maxwell RE, Hartler D (1964). Fibrinogen and adenosine diphosphate-induced aggregation of platelets. Nature 202:605–606.

Mills DCB, Figures WR, Scearce LM, Colman RF, Colman RW (1985). Two mechanisms for inhibition of ADP-induced platelet shape change by 5′-p-fluorosulfonylbenzoyl adenosine: Conversion to adenosine and covalent modification at an ADP binding site distinct from that which inhibits adenylate cyclase. J Biol Chem 260:8078–8083.

Molnar J, Lorand L (1961). Studies on apyrases. Arch Biochem Biophys 93:353–363.

Morinelli TA, Niewiarowski S, Kornecki E, Figures W, Wachtfogel T, Colman RW (1983). Platelet aggregation and exposure of fibrinogen receptors by prostaglandin endoperoxide analogues. Blood 61:41–49.

Mustard JF, Perry DW, Ardlie NG, Packham MA (1972). Preparations of suspensions of washed platelets from humans. Br J Haematol 22:193–204.

Nachman RL, Leung LLK (1982). Complex formation of platelet membrane glycoproteins IIb and IIIa with fibrinogen. J Clin Invest 69:263–269.

Niewiarowski S, Budzynski AZ, Morinelli TA, Brudzynski TM, Stewart GJ (1981). Exposure of fibrinogen receptor on human platelets by proteolytic enzymes. J Biol Chem 256:917–925.

Timmons S, Hawiger J (1978). Separation of human platelets from plasma proteins including factor VIII combined albumin density gradient-gel filtration method using HEPES buffer. Thromb Res 12:297–306.

Weber K, Osborn M (1975). Proteins and sodium dodecyl sulfate molecular weight determination on polyacrylamide gels and related procedures. Neurath H, Hill R (eds): "The Proteins" New York: Academic Press, 3rd ed., Vol. 1., pp. 179–223.

Winham KAE, Drummond AH, Edgar W, Prentice CRM (1976). A method for the removal of platelet aggregating activity of commercial apyrase. Thromb Haem 36:652–653.

Wyatt JL, Colman RF (1977). Affinity labeling of a lysine residue in the coenzyme binding site of a pig heart mitrochondrial dehydrogenose. Biochemistry 16:1333–1342.

Modern Methods in Pharmacology, Volume 4
Methods for Studying Platelets and Megakaryocytes, pages 41–63

Methods for Studying Interactions of Platelets With Coagulation Proteins

PETER N. WALSH

INTRODUCTION

During the last several decades, studies of the events comprising normal hemostasis have focused on coagulation proteins, platelets, and other blood and vascular cells. Purification, characterization, and elucidation of interactions between coagulation proteins have yielded a large body of information concerning the cascade of events leading to the formation of fibrin at sites of vascular injury. On the other hand, the separate study of platelet physiology, biochemistry, and pharmacology, generally viewed as comprising primary hemostasis, have provided a great deal of information concerning mechanisms of cell activation, membrane structure and function, prostanoid metabolism, energy metabolism, cytoskeletal protein biochemistry, and mechanisms of platelet adhesion, shape change, aggregation, and secretion. An alternative approach to studying hemostatic mechanisms arises from the view, which has received increasing emphasis during the past decade, that platelet plug formation and blood coagulation are inseparable processes, the elucidation of which requires an investigation of interactions between coagulation proteins and platelets as well as other cells. The study of platelet-coagulation protein interactions has resulted in the view that platelets have plasma membrane receptors for coagulation proteins that result in specific effects upon the platelets themselves or upon other coagulation substrates.

It has become apparent that the platelet surface membrane and those of other cells provide a locus for the assembly of coagulation protein complexes with resultant acceleration of enzymatic reactions leading to the proteolytic activation of coagulation proteins at all stages of coagulation [Walsh, 1974; Majerus and Miletich, 1978; Walsh 1982]. Thus, studies of interactions of thrombin with platelets initially suggested that some of the effects of thrombin on platelets were catalytic, whereas others indicated a stoichiometric interaction between thrombin

From the Thrombosis Research Center and the Departments of Medicine and Biochemistry, Temple University School of Medicine, Philadelphia, Pennsylvania 19140.

and platelets [Tollefsen et al., 1975]. Other models [Detwiler and Feinman, 1973] have combined these two lines of evidence and have given rise to the concept that platelets have specific, high-affinity receptors to which coagulation enzymes can bind reversibly with defined physiological and biochemical consequences. This approach was subsequently extended to the study of prothrombin activation [Miletich et al., 1978]. Human factor Xa has been shown to bind specifically and reversibly in the presence of calcium ions to high-affinity receptors on platelets, and factor Xa binding has been closely correlated with prothrombin activation. The functional consequence of the assembly of the prothrombinase complex on platelets is a 300,000-fold acceleration of the rate of prothrombin activation by factor Xa. Furthermore, it has been demonstrated that this reversible, saturable, high-affinity binding of factor Xa to platelets depends on the presence of factor Va [Kane et al., 1980]. Coordinate binding studies of factor Xa and factor Va to platelets indicate that a stoichiometric complex is bound [Tracy et al., 1981]. It has further been demonstrated that fibrinogen is a cofactor for aggregation of platelets by ADP, which can induce specific, saturable binding sites for fibrinogen on platelets [Marguerie et al., 1979; Bennett and Vilaire, 1979]. Thus, the platelet membrane appears to possess specific receptors for various coagulation proteins that have regulatory functions in zymogen activations and platelet physiology.

Additional evidence supports the view that platelets participate in the events of the early stages of intrinsic coagulation leading to the activation of factor IX and factor X. Platelets, activated by ADP, collagen, or thrombin can promote the proteolytic activation of purified factor XII by kallikrein in the presence of high molecular weight kininogen [Walsh, 1972a; Walsh, 1972b; Walsh and Griffin, 1981]. Thereafter, activated platelets can specifically and tightly bind factor XI in the presence of high molecular weight kininogen and zinc ions [Greengard et al., 1986] and can promote the proteolytic activation of factor XI in the presence of either factor XIIa or kallikrein in the absence of factor XII [Walsh and Griffin, 1981]. A molecule has been identified in platelet membranes with functional and immunological similarity to plasma factor XI from which it differs in molecular weight, charge, and subunit structure [Lipscomb and Walsh, 1979; Tuszynski et al., 1982]. This molecule has also been found in platelets from hemostatically normal individuals without detectable plasma factor XI. Recent studies indicate that factor XIa in the presence of high molecular weight kininogen also binds tightly and specifically to a site on the activated platelet surface distinct from the binding site for factor XI [Sinha et al., 1984b]. These interactions can therefore be viewed as localizing the activation of factor XI and the activity of factor XIa to the hemostatic plug where coagulation enzymes including factor XIa and factor Xa have been reported to be protected from inactivation by plasma protease inhibitors [Walsh, 1972b; Walsh and Biggs, 1972d; Marciniak, 1973; Miletich et al., 1977]. Kinetic analysis of the factor XIa-catalyzed activation of factor IX suggests that this is a kinetically favorable reaction [Walsh et al., 1984], the rates of which are similar when factor XIa is bound to the platelet surface and when it is free in solution [Sinha et al., 1984a; Walsh et al., 1986]. This and subsequent reactions may occur preferentially on the platelet surface since factor XIa as well as factor Xa can be protected from inactivation by plasma protease inhibitors [Walsh, 1972b; Walsh and Biggs, 1972d; Marciniak, 1973; Miletich et al., 1977]. Thereafter, factor IX and factor IXa appear to be bound specifically to the platelet membrane [Heeb et al., 1985; Ahmad et al., 1985] where the factor-IXa catalyzed activation of factor X is greatly accelerated [Walsh and Biggs, 1972d; Walsh, 1978; Lundblad and Davie, 1965; Schiffman et al., 1966; Hultin, 1982; Rosing et al., 1985] as is the factor Xa catalyzed activation of prothrombin [Miletich et al., 1978; Kane et al., 1980; Tracy et al., 1981; Miletich et al., 1977]. Thus, the platelet membrane contains highly specific receptor sites for the assembly of coagulation proteins and for the acceleration of enzymatic reactions at all stages of intrinsic coagulation leading eventually to the conversion of fibringen to fibrin and the formation of the hemostatic plug [Walsh, 1974; Majerus and Miletich, 1978; Walsh, 1982].

Some of the methods utilized in the study of the assembly of these coagulation protein complexes on the platelet surface and in the study of conversions of coagulation zymogens to enzymes are reviewed in this chapter.

GENERAL METHODS

Preparation and Characterization of Washed Platelet Suspensions

The study of the interaction between platelets and coagulation proteins requires the preparation and characterization of washed platelet suspensions. Various techniques have been developed for isolating platelets and for elution of plasma coagulation proteins including albumin density gradient centrifugation [Walsh, 1972c; Walsh et al., 1977], differential centrifugation utilizing a variety of inhibitors of platelet activation [Mustard et al., 1972], and finally gel-filtration [Tangen et al., 1971; Timmons and Hawiger, 1978]. Important considerations in the application of any technique for preparing suspensions of isolated platelets are: 1) the technique must be sufficiently gentle to remove coagulation proteins with minimal disruption or activation of platelets; 2) the technique must effectively remove plasma coagulation proteins although certain proteins stored in alpha granules (e.g., fibrinogen, von Willebrand factor, factor V, and high molecular weight kininogen) or present in the platelet plasma membrane (e.g., factor XI), or in the cytosol (e.g., factor XIII) remain closely associated with well-washed platelets; and 3) optimal recoveries of platelets in suspensions containing the required concentrations of platelets must be obtained.

In our laboratory, nine volumes of blood from apparently healthy donors not receiving medications are collected by clean venipuncture directly into one volume of 3.8% trisodium citrate utilizing plastic containers and equipment throughout. Platelet-rich plasma is obtained and platelet suspensions prepared either by albumin density gradient centrifugation or by gel-filtration on a Sepharose 2B column into calcium-free, Hepes-buffered Tyrode's solution, pH 7.4, containing bovine serum albumin (1 mg/ml), 138 mM NaC1, 2.7 mM KCl, 1 mM $MgCl_2.6\ H_2O$, 3.3 mM $NaH_2PO_4.H_2O$, 15 mM Hepes, and 5.5 mM dextrose as previously described [Walsh and Griffin, 1981; Sinha et al., 1984b]. Platelets are counted electronically, utilizing a model ZBI Particle Counter (Coulter Electronics, Inc., Hialeah, FL), or by phase contrast microscopy [Brecher and Cronkite, 1950]. The time required for platelet isolation must be minimal, since platelets lose sensitivity to various agonists when stored in vitro, and therefore experiments should be completed within 2 hours of blood collection. Platelet suspensions obtained either by albumin density gradient centrifugation or alternatively by gel-filtration in our laboratory contain no detectable coagulant activities of prothrombin or factors VII, VIII:C, IX, X, or XII [Walsh and Griffin, 1981; Walsh, 1972c; Walsh et al., 1977]. Experiments with ^{125}I-labeled bovine serum albumin have demonstrated that contamination of platelet suspensions with plasma proteins amounts to less than 0.06% [Walsh and Griffin, 1981; Sinha et al., 1984b]. Ultrastructural, metabolic, and functional studies of human platelets washed by albumin density gradient centrifugation [Walsh, 1972c; Walsh et al., 1977; Timmons and Hawiger, 1978], by gel-filtration [Tangen et al., 1971; Timmons and Hawiger, 1978], or by differential centrifugation in the presence of inhibitors of platelet activation [Mustard et al., 1972] reveal maintenance of normal structural, functional, and biochemical characteristics.

Purification and Characterization of Coagulation Proteins

A prerequisite for studying the interaction between platelets and coagulant proteins is the preparation of highly purified coagulation proteins from human plasma. In our laboratory factor XI is purified to a specific activity of approximately 250 U/mg protein from human plasma by a modification [Sinha et al., 1984b] of the method of Bouma and Griffin or by immunoaffinity chromatography [Sinha et al., 1985], and appears as a single band at an apparent molecular weight of 160,000 on a nonreduced sodium dodecyl sulfate polyacrylamide gel and as a single 80,000 molecular weight band on reduced gels as previously reported [Sinha et al, 1984b; Kerbiriou et al., 1980]. Purified factor XI is activated to factor XIa by incubation with bovine factor XIIa as previously described [Sinha et al., 1984b]. High molecular weight kininogen is purified by the method of Kerbiriou and Griffin [1979] to a specific activity of approximately 15 U/mg protein. Prekallikrein (approximately 130 U/mg protein specific activity) is isolated by the method of Kerbiriou et al. [1980], and kallikrein is prepared from prekallikrein as reported by Bouma et al. [1980]. Human factor IX is purified in our laboratory to apparent homogeneity by alkaline gel electrophoresis, utilizing modifications [Walsh et al., 1984] of methods described by DiScipio et al. [1977] and by Miletich et al. [1980] to a specific activity of 185–200 U/mg protein and appears as a single band at a molecular weight of 57,000 by SDS gel electrophoresis [Walsh et al., 1984]. Factor XII is isolated from human plasma to a specific activity of approximately 80 U/mg protein as previously described [Griffin and Cochrane 1976]. Factor X (specific activity approximately 125 U/mg) and prothrombin are purified as previously reported [Tuszynski et al., 1984b] to at least 95% purity as judged by SDS gel electrophoresis. Factor Xa is prepared by incubation with purified Russell's viper venom as previously described [Tuszynski et al., 1984b].

Radiolabeling of proteins. Factor XI and factor XII have been radiolabeled with ^{125}I by a variety of methods including the insolubilized lactoperoxidase method [David and Reisfeld 1974], by the chloramine T method [McConahey and Dixon 1966], by the method of Bolton and Hunter [1973], and by the Iodogen procedure [Fraker and Speck, 1978] as previously described [Walsh and Griffin, 1981; Sinha et al., 1984b]. These proteins can be radiolabeled to specific radioactivities of $0.5 \times 10^6 - 5 \times 10^6$ cpm/μg without significant loss of biological activity. Factor IX and factor X are radiolabeled with tritium by modifications of methods originally described by Van Lenten and Ashwell, [1971] and adapted for bovine factor X by Silverberg et al. [1977] and further adapted for human factor IX in our laboratory [Walsh et al., 1984]. Removal of ^{125}I and other radioisotopes can be removed from the radiolabeled protein by passage over a 1 ml G-25 column [Tuszynski et al., 1980] and the proteins further dialyzed in the presence of ovalbumin (1 mg/ml) to remove any residual ^{125}I. Other coagulation proteins can be similarly radiolabeled and then characterized either by SDS gel electrophoresis and autoradiography [Tuszynski et al., 1984a] or fluorography [Bonner and Laskey 1974] as previously reported.

Assays. The coagulant activities of purified coagulation factors are assayed using minor modifications [Scott et al., 1984] of the kaolin-activated partial thromboplastin time [Proctor and Rapaport, 1961] using appropriate congenitally deficient substrate plasmas and results are quantified on double logarithmic plots of clotting times versus concentrations of pooled normal plasma. Coagulation zymogens converted to their active enzymatic forms by incubation with the appropriate enzyme can be assayed for amidolytic activity using the appropriate chromogenic substrate, for example PyrGlu-Pro-Arg-p-nitroanilide (S-2366) for factor XIa [Scott et al., 1984], H-D-Pro-Phe-Arg-p-nitroanilide (S-2302) for factor XIIa [Sinha et al., 1985], and N-Bz-Ile-Glu-Gly-Arg-p-nitroanilide (S-2222) for factor Xa [Tuszynski et al., 1984b]. Radioimmunoassay of factor XI and other coagulation proteins are carried out as previously described [Walsh et al., 1984; Scott et al., 1984]. Protein determinations are performed according to the method of Lowry et al. [1951], by the BioRad dye binding assay as described by Bradford [1976] or by adsorption at 280 nm utilizing the appropriate extinction coefficient for each protein. Polyacrylamide slab gel electrophoresis in SDS is carried out by the procedure of Laemmli [1970].

BINDING STUDIES

Utilizing methodology developed to examine the specific interaction of hormones with cells and to correlate ligand-receptor interactions with mechanisms of cell activation, numerous studies have now focused on the specific binding of coagulation proteins with platelets and with other cells. In some instances, such as the specific interaction of thrombin with platelets or the binding of fibrinogen to activated platelets, the results of ligand binding are observable as effects upon platelet activation or aggregation. In contrast, other studies have demonstrated the formation of coagulation enzyme, zymogen, or cofactor complex formation upon the platelet membrane with resultant effects observable not as cell activation but rather as acceleration of the proteolytic activation of various coagulation proteins. For example, the consequence of the assembly of the factor Xa-factor Va complex upon the platelet membrane is a 300,000-fold acceleration of the rate of prothrombin activation by factor Xa [Miletich et al., 1978; Kane et al., 1980; Tracy et al., 1981]. In this context it is important to correlate the results of ligand binding with the reaction rates of zymogen activation. For example, in our laboratory we have demonstrated that the specific, high-affinity, reversible binding of factor XIa to thrombin-activated platelets in the presence of high molecular weight kininogen is associated with no measurable acceleration of the rate of activation of the substrate, factor IX, by the bound enzyme, factor XIa [Sinha et al., 1984a; Walsh et al., 1986]. We have interpreted these results as suggesting that factor XIa binding may serve to localize factor IX activation to the platelet surface but not to accelerate the rate of the enzymatic reaction. Thus, it is imperative to examine the functional consequences of ligand-receptor interactions.

Binding Measurements and Their Validation

In our laboratory we have utilized a binding assay to examine the interaction of a variety of coagulation proteins with the platelet membrane including factor

XI [Greengard et al., 1986], factor XIa [Sinha et al., 1984b], high molecular weight kininogen [Greengard et al., 1986], factor IX [Ahmad et al., 1985], factor IXa [Ahmad et al., 1985], and factor Xa [Tuszynski et al., 1984b]. To measure the binding of a ^{125}I-labeled, purified coagulation protein to platelets over varying incubation times, at variable concentrations of added ligand or under different conditions, gel-filtered platelets, platelets isolated by albumin density gradient centrifugation or control cells (e.g., erythrocytes) are incubated at 37°C in 1.5 ml polypropylene centrifuge tubes (Sarstedt, Inc., Princeton, NJ) with the radiolabeled ligand. Determinations of the specificity of binding and measurements of nonspecific binding are made in the presence of 50–100-fold molar excesses of unlabeled ligand or other proteins. At specified incubation times, aliquots of the incubation mixture are layered over a mixture of silicon oils (1 volume of methyl silicon oil, DC200, to 5 volumes of "Hi Phenyl" silicon oil, DC550, William F. Nye, Inc., Fairhaven, MA), contained in microsediment tubes with narrow bore extended tips (Sarstedt, Inc., Princeton NJ). After centrifugation for 2 min in a microfuge (Model B, Beckman Instruments, Inc., Cedar Grove, NJ), the tips containing the platelet pellets are amputated and the sediments and supernatants counted separately in a gamma counter.

In order to validate the binding assay, it is necessary to determine that it is capable of separating bound from free ligand; that the radio-labeled ligand behaves in all respects, especially in its binding capacity, in a manner similar to the unlabeled protein; and finally to ascertain that the radioactivity recovered in the sediment in fact represents the ligand and not a contaminating protein. We have demonstrated that the fraction of cells sedimented in our binding assay is acceptably high by determining that more than 94% of platelets labeled with ^{51}Cr are recovered in the pellet [Sinha et al., 1984b]. Therefore, it can be assumed that any ligand bound to the platelets would be expected to appear in the sediment. It is also necessary to demonstrate that the "trapped volume" (i.e., the fraction of protein not specifically bound to platelets) is acceptably low. This has been demonstrated in our laboratory by incubating ^{125}I-labeled bovine serum albumin with platelets and determining the fraction of radioactivity appearing in the pellet, which in our laboratory is less than 0.005 [Sinha et al., 1984b].

To examine the binding affinity of radiolabeled vs. unlabeled ligand to platelets, we have incubated varying ratios of labeled and unlabeled ligand with platelets, maintaining the total concentration of ligand constant, and then determining the amount of radiolabeled ligand bound. For example, varying ratios of ^{125}I-labeled and unlabeled factor XIa were incubated for 5 min at 37°C with gel-filtered platelet (2.45×10^8/ml), thrombin (0.1 U/ml), and high molecular weight kininogen (12 μg/ml), which are optimal conditions for binding of factor XIa to platelets. Keeping the total concentration of factor XIa constant (0.10 μg/

ml), when the binding of ^{125}I-labeled factor XIa is plotted as a function of the fraction of ^{125}I-labeled factor XIa added, a straight line is obtained (Fig. 1). We have also determined that the coagulant activity and amidolytic activity of labeled and unlabeled factor XIa are the same, thus confirming that more than 85% of the functional activity of the ligand is retained after radiolabeling.

To examine the structural characteristics of the bound ligand in studies of the interaction of factor XIa with platelets, we have incubated gel-filtered platelets (4.5×10^8/ml) with ^{125}I-labeled factor XIa (2.5 μg/ml) in the presence of high molecular weight kininogen (20 μg/ml) and thrombin (0.1 U/ml) at 37°C for 8 min, conditions determined to be optimal for binding. The platelets were then centrifuged through 20% sucrose and the platelet pellet solubilized in 2.0% sodium dodecyl sulfate containing a mixture of protease inhibitors and EDTA (1 mM). The solubilized platelet pellet was then analyzed by sodium dodecyl sulfate polyacrylamide (7.5%) gel electrophoresis and subsequent autoradiography. As shown in Figure. 2, the radioactivity recovered in the pellet migrates on a reduced SDS gel in a manner indistinguishable from the factor XIa added to the incubation mixture and corresponds to polypeptides having molecular weights of 50,000 (the heavy chain of factor XIa) and 30,000 (the light chain). This experiment demonstrates that the bound and free proteins are structurally indis-

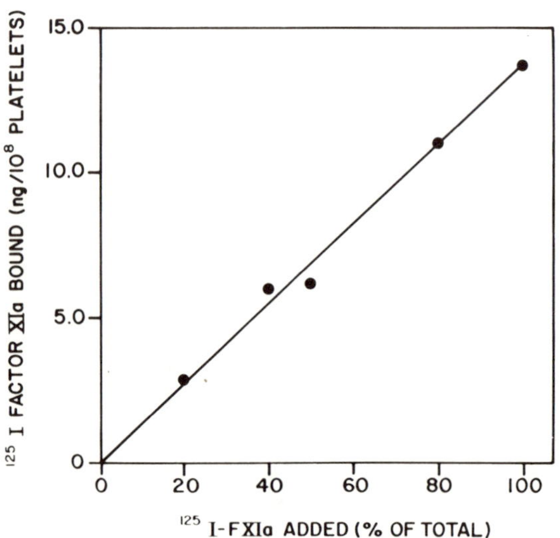

Fig. 1. Binding of ^{125}I-labeled factor XIa to thrombin-treated platelets in the presence of high Mr kininogen. Experimental details are given in the text. Figure reprinted with permission from Sinha et al. [1984b].

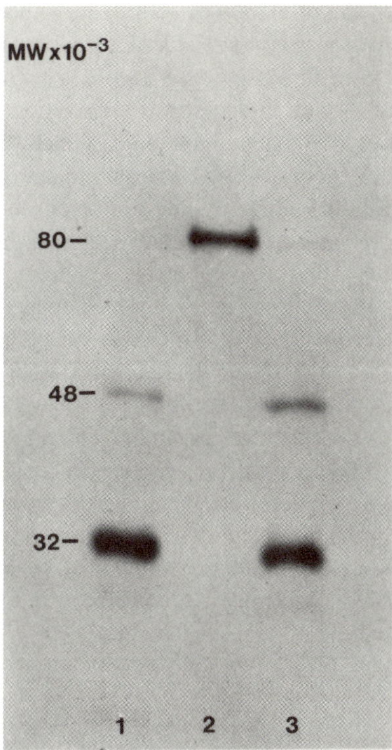

Fig. 2. Reduced SDS gel electrophoresis (7.5% polyacrylamide) and autoradiography of ^{125}I-labeled factor XIa (lane 1), ^{125}I-labeled factor XI (lane 2), and bound ^{125}I-labeled factor XIa (lane 3) after centrifugation through 20% sucrose. Experimental details are given in the text. Figure reprinted with permission from Sinha et al. [1984b].

tinguishable by SDS gel electrophoresis. From this experiment it can be concluded that the bound radioactivity represents factor XIa and not a contaminant and that the factor XIa has not been proteolytically degraded, nor has it formed a high molecular weight covalent complex with a platelet protein.

Characteristics and Analysis of Binding Data

A detailed study of the interaction between platelets and a coagulation protein involves an initial examination of the time course and requirements for binding of the ligand to the platelets, followed in turn by studies of specificity, saturability, reversibility, and finally quantitative analysis of the number of binding sites and affinity of binding. In designing experiments aimed at determining the binding requisites, it is important to consider the physiological relevance of conditions required for optimal binding. For example, in studying the binding of factor XI, factor XIa, and high molecular weight kininogen to platelets, we have carried out experiments at concentrations of added ligand encompassing a range around the concentration in plasma and have determined the requirements for cofactors for binding as well as the state of activation of platelets required for optimal binding. Thus, the optimal binding of factor XI to platelets requires platelet activation with agonists such as thrombin and the presence of zinc ions, calcium ions, and high molecular weight kininogen (the cofactor noncovalently bound to factor XI in plasma), at concentrations of these cofactors present in normal human plasma. The time course and requirements for binding of factor XIa to platelets are compared in Figure 3, which shows the results of a progress curve of binding of factor XIa to gel-filtered platelets incubated at 37°C in the presence or absence of high molecular weight kininogen and thrombin. From this experiment we conclude that the binding of factor XIa to platelets requires the presence of high molecular weight kininogen and that the rate and extent of binding are increased when platelets are stimulated with thrombin. Thus, the binding of factor XIa to platelets does not require the presence of divalent cations, since it also occurs in the presence of EDTA. Our studies suggest that factor XI and high molecular weight kininogen may bind to platelets as a coordinate complex, whereas factor XIa apparently binds to a site distinct from that for

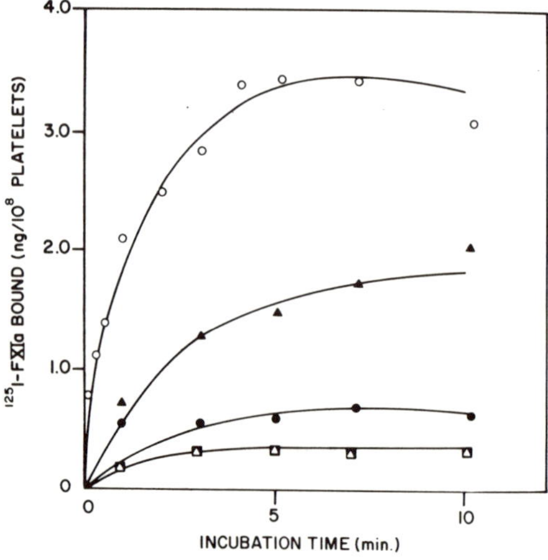

Fig. 3. Progress curves of binding of ^{125}I-labeled factor XIa to platelets or erythrocytes. Details are presented in the text. Figure is reprinted from Sinha et al. [1984b]. Incubation mixtures contained platelets + thrombin + high Mr kininogen (○); platelets + high Mr kininogen (▲); platelets + thrombin (●); platelets alone (△); or erythrocytes + thrombin + high Mr kininogen (■).

factor XI under conditions precluding the binding of high molecular weight kininogen [Sinha et al., 1984b].

We have examined the specificity of binding of these ligands to platelets both with respect to the ligand bound and with respect to the cell that binds it [Sinha et al., 1984b]. We have added a variety of proteins in 50–100-fold molar excess compared with the radiolabeled ligand in question under conditions shown to be optimal for binding. The results of such experiments, which have been previously published [Sinha et al., 1984b], indicate, for example, that factor XIa binding to platelets is unaffected by the presence of prothrombin, prekallikrein, factor XIIa, or even the zymogen, factor XI, whereas in contrast unlabeled factor XIa competes effectively for binding of the radiolabeled ligand. This exquisite specificity of binding for the ligand has also been demonstrated for the cell in question. Thus, when erythrocytes replace platelets in the binding assay, after incubation of factor XIa with high molecular weight kininogen and thrombin, only a low level of nonspecific, nonsaturable binding, unaffected by the presence of high molecular weight kininogen or thrombin, is observed (Fig. 3).

The mathematical analysis of binding data by equations, such as that developed by Scatchard [1949], requires the prior demonstration that the bound and free ligand exist in free equilibrium with one another, i.e., that the binding is freely reversible. We have examined reversibility of ligand binding to platelets by incubating reactants in a time course experiment similar to that depicted in Figure 3 until equilibrium is achieved, then adding a 50–100-fold excess of the unlabeled ligand and determining the amount of the radiolabeled ligand bound at subsequent time points. Results of such experiments demonstrate reversibility of the binding of factor XI, factor XIa, high molecular weight kininogen, factor IX, and factor IXa, thereby confirming that the ligand in solution exists in free equilibrium with that bound to the platelet surface [Sinha et al., 1984b].

To determine the number of binding sites and the affinity of binding of the ligand to its receptor, it is necessary to determine whether specific binding sites for the ligand are saturated under optimal conditions for binding when the ligand concentration is varied over a wide range. For example, to determine whether factor XIa binding to platelets is saturable, gel-filtered platelets were incubated for 5 min at 37°C with various concentrations of ^{125}I-labeled factor XIa in the presence of high molecular weight kininogen and thrombin (Fig. 4). "Nonspecific binding" was determined in the presence of excess, unlabeled factor XIa and was shown to be a small fraction of total binding and nonsaturable. Similar results were obtained when high molecular weight kininogen and thrombin were excluded from the incubation mixture or when red cells replaced platelets in the presence of high moleculear weight kininogen and thrombin. When "nonspecific binding" was subtracted from total binding, a hyperbolic curve, depicted by the

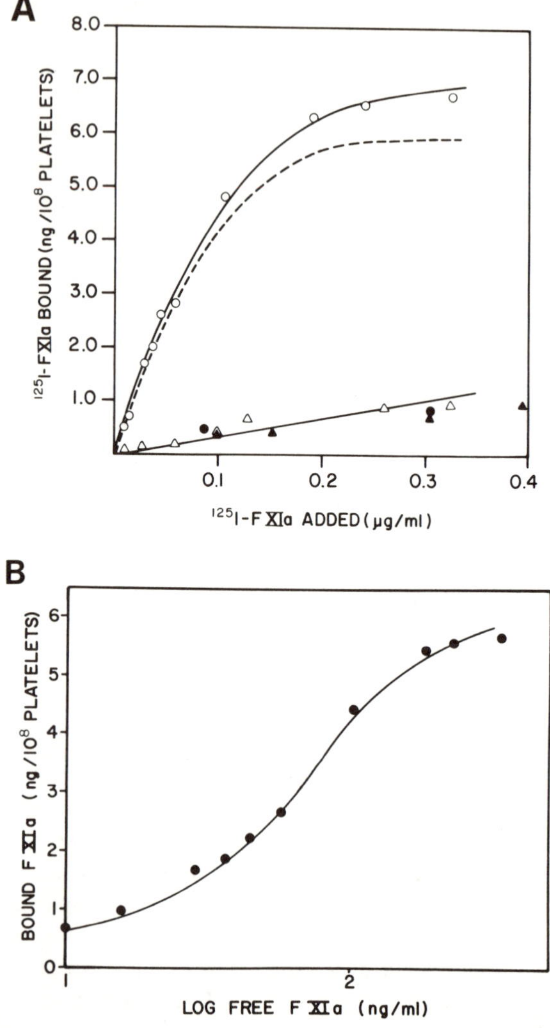

Fig. 4. Saturable binding of ^{125}I-labeled factor XIa to platelets in the presence of high Mr kininogen and thrombin. Experimental details are given in the text. Figure is reprinted with permission from Sinha et al. [1984b]. A. Data shown represent total binding (○) of ^{125}I-factor XIa to gel-filtered platelets (2.2 × 10^8/ml) incubated for 5 min at 37°C in the presence of thrombin (0.1 U/ml) and high Mr kininogen (12 μg/ml); nonspecific binding of ^{125}I-labeled factor XIa to platelets in the presence of high Mr kininogen + thrombin + a 50-fold excess of unlabeled factor XIa (●); platelets alone (△); or washed erythrocytes + thrombin + high Mr kininogen (▲). B. Specific binding data shown in Figure 4A, replotted as recommended by Klotz [1982]. C. Scatchard plot of same data.

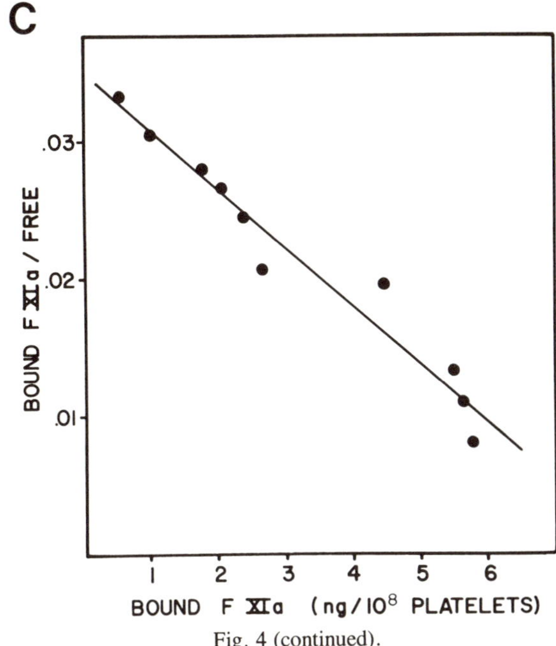

Fig. 4 (continued).

dashed line in Figure 4A, was the result, which was taken to represent specific binding.

Klotz [1982] has cautioned that many examples of apparently saturable ligand binding data have been published without fulfilling criteria for saturability and has suggested plotting the amount of ligand bound versus the logarithm of the amount of the ligand added as a means of determining whether or not a sufficient amount of ligand has been added in a binding experiment to approach saturation of binding sites. If saturation of binding sites has been approached, the results should describe a sigmoid curve, with the inflection point representing half-maximal binding. When the data representing specific binding of factor XIa to platelets (Figure 4A) are replotted according to the method of Klotz (Figure 4B), it is apparent that a sigmoid curve results and that approximately half the points plotted in this experiment represent data obtained at concentrations greater than those required to achieve half saturation. Since equilibrium between bound and free ligand has been demonstrated, these data justify Scatchard analysis [Scatchard, 1949] of the same data, which is represented in Figure 4C. On the basis of such analysis it can be estimated that the number of specific binding sites for factor XIa on activated platelets ranges from 130 to 500 molecules/platelet with a dissociation constant (Kd) of approximately 1 nM. Since the plasma concentration of factor XI is 25 nM and since saturation of receptors occurs when the concentration of added ligand is 2.5 nM (0.4 μg/ml) as shown in Figure 4, one can surmise that all the binding sites on activated platelets would be saturated when 10% of the factor XI in plasma is converted to factor XIa.

Interpretation of Binding Data

The rational interpretation of experiments examining ligand-receptor interaction requries a consideration of certain conceptual matters and answers to a variety of questions. First, it should be emphasized that in the strict sense the term receptor refers to the specific interaction of an agonist of cell activation with a binding site in the cell membrane that reacts biochemically and physiologically in a defined manner to activate the cell in question. In this chapter, we are dealing with interactions of coagulation ligands with platelet binding sites whose function is related to the assembly of coagulation complexes that regulate reaction rates leading to the generation of thrombin and the conversion of fibrinogen to fibrin. Thus, the results of these "ligand-receptor" interactions are realized in terms of their effects on plasma proteins rather than on the cell itself. Therefore, the term "receptor" is used in a generic and unrigorous sense to refer to any specific and saturable interaction between a ligand and a cell whose effects can be defined biochemically and functionally.

Answers to some of the following questions must be sought in considering interpretations of binding data. Are the conditions required for optimal binding physiological? Are concentrations of cofactors required similar to those that exist in vivo? Does binding of the ligand to the cell require cell activation by agonists whose effect is likely to be apparent in vivo? Does binding of the ligand to its receptor occur in a plasma milieu? Is the concentration of the ligand required for optimal binding and saturation of receptors (or half-saturation as reflected by the dissociation constant) comparable to the concentrations of ligand which might be present or generated in vivo? Is the time course required for optimal binding such that it is likely to be correlated with the time course of the reaction postulated to be a consequence of binding? Finally, and perhaps most importantly, what is the functional correlate of ligand-receptor interaction? For example, if the ligand is an enzyme, is the reaction rate catalyzed by that enzyme increased, decreased, or unaffected by binding of the enzyme to the receptor? The functional characterization of ligand-receptor interactions is the aim of methods developed to examine rates of zymogen activation by limited proteolysis as detailed in the following section.

ZYMOGEN ACTIVATION ASSAYS

Since it is important to define the functional consequences of binding of either an enzyme or a zymogen to the platelet surface, we have developed a variety of methods to examine the proteolytic activation of coagulation proteins, including factor XII, factor XI, factor IX, factor X, and prothrombin. These methods can be utilized to examine rates of activation of a zymogen under conditions of optimal binding to its platelet receptor. Alternatively, when the ligand in question is an enzyme, the rates of the reaction catalyzed by the platelet-bound enzyme can be compared with those occurring in free solution. The following section reviews some of the techniques utilized in our laboratory to address these questions, including coagulation assays, chromogenic assays, and assays of the proteolytic cleavage of coagulation substrates.

Coagulation Assays

In addition to their utility in characterizing purified coagulation proteins, coagulation assays help to measure the amounts of these coagulation proteins contained in suspensions of washed platelets, and to examine the capacity of platelets to promote the activation of coagulation proteins including factor XII, factor XI, factor IX, factor X, and prothrombin. In such studies we believe it is important to utilize coagulation assays as measures of zymogen activation. Such assays must be used in combination with other methods, such as radioimmunoassays, chromogenic assays, and methods to examine proteolytic cleavage of coagulation proteins, in order to avoid the problems of nonspecificity to which coagulation assays are subject. Thus, it is always important to recognize that since a whole cascade of reactions may influence the results of a coagulation assay that depends ultimately on the formation of fibrin, even carefully controlled experiments can be misinterpreted if one uncritically assumes that procoagulant activity observed in a particular substrate plasma reflects exclusively the activity or activation of the coagulation factor in question. However, when coagulation assays (described under General Methods) are used in combination with chromogenic assays, radioimmunoassays, and determinations of proteolysis of purified proteins, they can be useful if not essential in the definitive interpretation of the results of zymogen activation experiments.

Chromogenic Assays

Various chromogenic assays have been utilized in our laboratory for assessing either the activation of coagulation zymogens or the activity of coagulation enzymes, including factor XIIa, factor XIa, factor Xa, and thrombin. Some of the small peptide chromogenic substrates utilized in these assays have been alluded to in the section on General Methods. An example of such a method is an amidolytic assay for measuring the activation of factor XI [Scott et al., 1984], the utility of which is emphasized by the close correlations between factor XI amidolytic activity, coagulant activity, and radioimmunoassay, demonstrated in

Figure 5. This assay, which utilizes the chromogenic substrate S-2366 (PyrGlu-Pro-Arg-p-nitroanilide), can be employed to measure either factor XI in plasma or alternatively, in purified systems, to measure the generation or activity of factor XIa.

Assays of Proteolytic Cleavage

Coagulation proteins purified from human plasma can be radiolabeled with a variety of isotopes and examined for proteolytic cleavage by SDS gel electrophoresis and autoradiography or by other methods as described below. For example, we have examined the effects of platelets on the proteolytic activation of factor

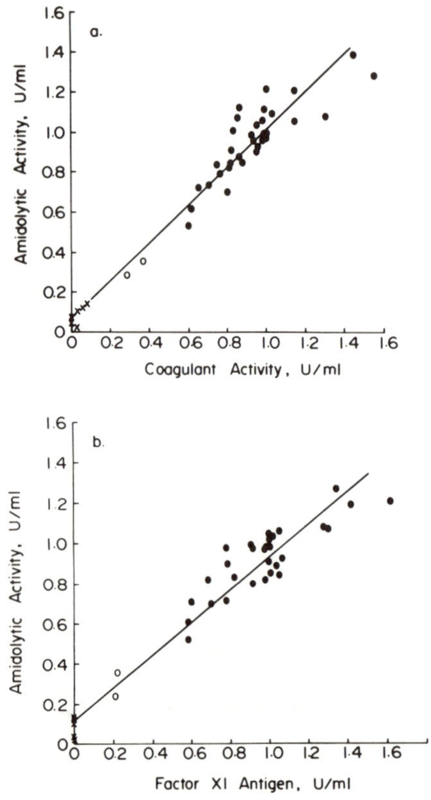

Fig. 5. Correlation of factor XI amidolytic and coagulant activity. Figure is reprinted with permission from Scott et al. [1984], and shows results of chromogenic and coagulation assays in plasma samples from 35 normal individuals (●), two patients with liver disease (○), and six patients with factor XI deficiency (X) (r = 0.95). Correlation of factor XI radioimmunoassay and amidolytic assay.

XI by factor XIIa in the presence of high molecular weight kininogen [Walsh and Griffin, 1981]. Purified human factor XI was radiolabeled to high specific activity with ^{125}I and incubated with factor XII, high molecular weight kininogen, and kallikrein in the presence or absence of collagen-treated or ADP-treated platelets (Fig. 6). The mixtures were then subjected to SDS gel electrophoresis on 7.5% polyacrylamide gels, which were sliced and counted in a gamma counter. The radioactive gel profiles demonstrate the cleavage of zymogen factor XI, which migrates at a molecular weight of 80,000 on reduced SDS gels and is cleaved by factor XIIa into proteolytic cleavage products of 50,000 and 30,000 molecular weight representing the heavy and light chains of factor XIa. This experiment demonstrates that collagen-treated platelets or ADP-treated platelets

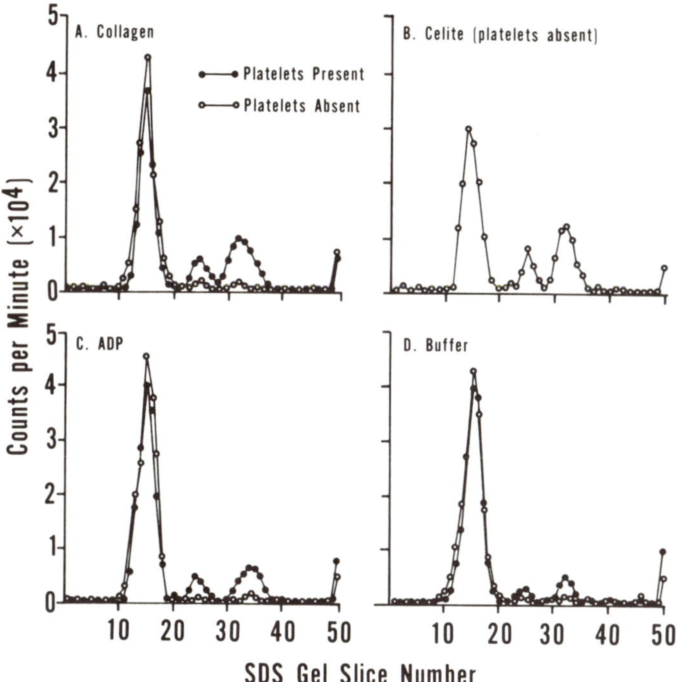

Fig. 6. Sodium dodecyl sulfate polyacrylamide (7.5%) gel electrophoresis of ^{125}I-labeled factor XI in mixtures incubated for 120 min at 37°C containing factor XII (3.6 μg/ml), kallikrein (5 μg/ml), and high Mr kininogen (5.4 μg/ml), in the presence (●) or absence (○) of platelets prepared by albumin density gradient centrifugation and gel-filtration and A. Collagen (15 μg/ml); B. Celite (0.08 mg/ml); C. ADP (2.5 μM); or Tris (50 mM), NaCl (150 mM), pH 7.4.; D. Buffer. Data shown are reproduced with permission from Walsh and Griffin [1981].

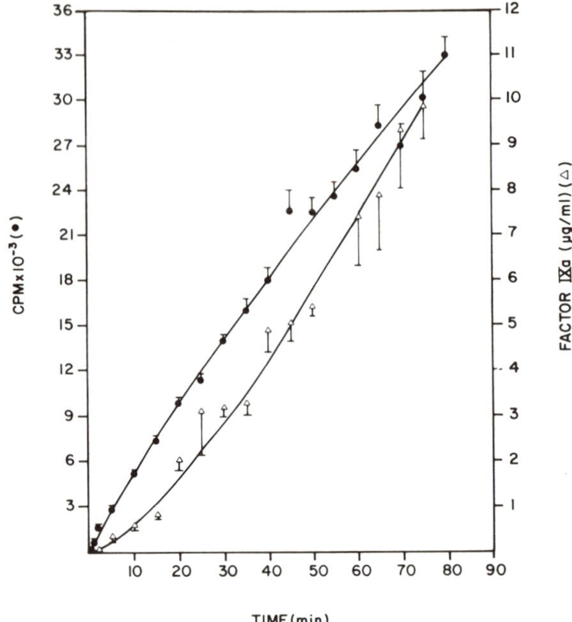

Fig. 7. Time course of activation peptide release (●) from [sialyl-^{3}H]-factor IX (0.35 μM) by factor XIa (6.2 nM) and the development of factor IX coagulant activity (△) in the presence of 5 mM $CaCl_2$. Data shown are reproduced with permission from Walsh et al. [1984] and show means ($\pm$ SEM) of triplicate determinations.

can promote the proteolytic activation of factor XI to factor XIa, since the results of proteolytic cleavage studies correlated well with the development of factor XIa activity as measured in a coagulation assay [Walsh and Griffin, 1981].

In order to examine the activation of blood coagulation factor IX by factor XIa we have developed an assay [Walsh et al., 1984] for factor IX activation by measuring the release of trichloroacetic acid-soluble, tritium-labeled activation peptide from factor IX by a modification of a method described by bovine factor IX activation by Zur and Nemerson [1980]. This assay takes advantage of the fact that factor IX is a single-chain glycoprotein containing 17% carbohydrate that is cleaved during activation at an arginine-alanine bond and at an arginine-valine bond to release a 10,000 dalton activation peptide that contains a majority of the carbohydrate residues in the molecule. The peptide is therefore heavily labeled with tritium when the molecule is oxidized and then reduced in the presence of ^{3}H-labeled sodium borohydride. Since the activation peptide remains soluble in 5% trichloroacetic acid, whereas the remainder of the molecule is

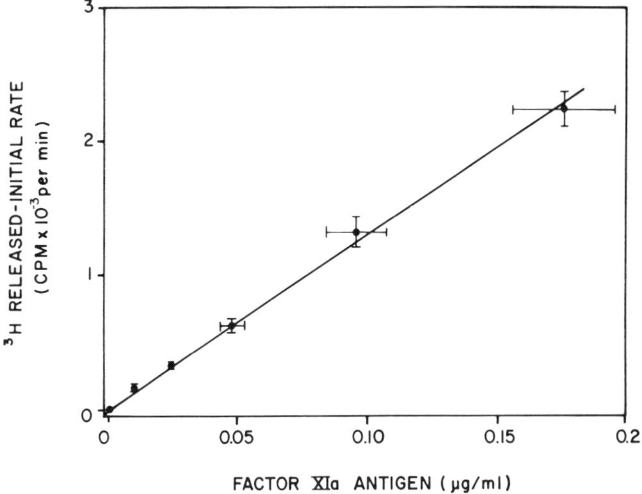

Fig. 8. Relationship between activation peptide released from [sialyl-^{3}H]-factor IX (88 nM) and amount of added factor XIa, measured by radioimmunoassay. Data are reproduced with permission from Walsh et al. [1984] and represent means (± SEM) of triplicate determinations.

insoluble in TCA, factor-IX activation can be assayed as release of the activation peptide. We have utilized this assay to measure initial rates of TCA-soluble tritium, which are linear over variable periods of incubation of purified factor IX with 5 mM $CaCl_2$ and catalytic concentrations of factor XIa. The time course of ^{3}H-labeled activation peptide release corresponds reasonably well with the development of factor IXa activity (Fig. 7), and the initial rates of activation peptide release are well correlated with the amount of factor XIa antigen added to the incubation mixture (Fig. 8). These observations established this procedure as a valid assay for factor-IX activation and for factor-XIa activity. We have utilized this method to determine the kinetics of the factor-XIa catalyzed activation of factor IX [Walsh et al., 1984] and to characterize platelet-bound factor XIa [Sinha et al., 1984a; Walsh et al., 1986]. It is clear that within the context of our experimental conditions the enzymatic activity of factor XIa as a factor IX activator is retained (neither enhanced nor inhibited) when it is bound to its platelet receptor [Sinha et al., 1984a]. Moreover, platelet bound factor XIa is protected from inactivation by its major inhibitor in plasma, alpha-1-protease inhibitor [Walsh, 1972b; Walsh and Biggs, 1972d; unpublished observations). We believe these observations suggest that factor XIa binding to platelets serves to localize factor-IX activation and subsequent coagulation reactions on the platelet membrane.

ACKNOWLEDGMENTS

This work was supported by NIH Grants HL25661 and HL14217, by Grant CTR1389 from the Council For Tobacco Research, Inc., by a grant from The W.W. Smith Charitable Trust, and by a grant from the American Heart Association Pennsylvania Affiliate. The authors are grateful to Patricia Pileggi for typing the manuscript.

REFERENCES

Ahmad SS, Sinha D, Babilon RW, Seaman FS, Walsh PN (1985). Binding of coagulation factors IX and IXa to washed human platelets. Blood 66:300a (Abstract).

Bennett JS, Vilaire G (1979). Exposure of platelet fibrinogen receptors by ADP and epinephrine. J Clin Invest 64:1393.

Bolton AE, Hunter WM (1973). A labelling of proteins to high specific radioactivities by conjugation to a ^{125}I-containing acylating agent. Biochem J 133:529.

Bonner WM, Laskey RA (1974). A film detection method for tritium-labeled proteins and nucleic acids in polyacrylamide gels. Eur J Biochem 46:83.

Bouma BN, Griffin JH (1977). Human blood coagulation factor XI. Purification, properties, and mechanism of activation by activated factor XII. J Biol Chem 252:6432.

Bouma BN, Miles LA, Berretta G, Griffin JH (1980). Human plasma prekallikrein. Studies of its activation by activated factor XII and of its inactivation by diisopropylphosphofluoridate. Biochemistry 18:1151.

Bradford MM (1976). A rapid and sensitive method for the quantitation of microgram quantities of protein utilizing the principle of protein-dye binding. Anal Biochem 72:248.

Brecher G, Cronkite EP (1950). Morphology and enumeration of human blood platelets. J Appl Physiol 3:365,

David GS, Reisfeld RA (1974). Protein iodination with solid state lactoperoxidase. Biochemistry 13:1014.

Detwiler TC, Feinman RD (1973). Kinetics of the thrombin-induced release of adenosine triphosphate by platelets. Comparison with release of calcium. Biochemistry 12:2462.

DiScipio RG, Hermodson MA, Yates SG, Davie EW (1977). A comparison of human prothrombin, factor IX (Christmas factor), factor X (Stuart factor) and protein S. Biochemistry 16:698.

Fraker PJ, Speck JC (1978). Protein and cell membrane iodinations with a sparingly soluble chloramide, 1,3,4,6-tetrachloro-3a,6a-diphenylglycoluril. Biochem Biophys Res Comm 80:849.

Greengard JS, Heeb MJ, Ersdal E, Walsh PN, Griffin JH (1986). Binding of blood coagulation factor XI to human platelets. Biochemistry 25:3884.

Griffin JH, Cochran CG (1976). Human factor XII (Hageman factor). Meth Enzymol 45:56.

Heeb MJ, Greengard J, Nova CP (1985). Binding of human factor IX and IXa to washed platelets. Thromb Haemost 54:131 (Abstract).

Hultin MB (1982) Role of human factor VIII in factor X activation. J Clin Invest 69:950.

Kane WH, Lindhout MJ, Jackson CW, Majerus PW (1980). Factor Va-dependent binding of factor Xa to human platelets. J Biol Chem 255:1170.

Kerbiriou DM, Griffin JH (1979). Human high molecular weight kininogen. Studies of structure-function relationships and of proteolysis of the molecule occurring during contact activation of plasma. J Biol Chem 254:12020.

Kerbiriou DM, Douma BN, Griffin JH (1980). Immunochemical studies of human high molecular weight kininogen and of its complexes with plasma prekallikrein or kallikrein. J Biol Chem. 255:3952.

Klotz IM (1982). Numbers of receptor sites from Scatchard graphs: Facts and fantasies. Science (Wash, DC) 217:1247.

Laemmli UK (1970). Cleavage of structural proteins during the assembly of the head of bacteriophage T. Nature (Lond) 227:680.

Lipscomb MS, Walsh PN (1979). Human platelets and factor XI. Localization in platelet membranes of factor-XI-like activity and its functional distinction from plasma factor XI. J Clin Invest 63:1006.

Lowry OH, Rosebrough NJ, Farr AL, Randall RJ (1951). Protein measurement with the Folin phenol reagent. J Biol Chem 193:265.

Lundblad RL, Davie EW (1965). The activation of Stuart factor (factor X) by activated antihemophilic factor (activated factor VIII). Biochemistry 4:113.

Majerus PW, Miletich JP (1978). Relationship between platelets and coagulation factors in Hemostasis. Annu Rev Med 29:41.

Marciniak E (1973). Factor-Xa inactivation by antithrombin III: Evidence for biological stabilization of factor Xa by factor V-phospholipid complex. Br J Haematol 24:391.

Marguerie GA, Plow EF, Edgington TS (1979). Human platelets possess an inducible and saturable receptor for fibrinogen. J Biol Chem 254:5357.

McConahey PJ, Dixon FJ (1966). A method of trace iodination of proteins for immunologic studies. Int Arch Allergy Appl Immunol 29:185.

Miletich JP, Jackson CM, Majerus PW (1977). Interaction of coagulation factor Xa with human platelets. Proc Natl Acad Sci USA 74:4033.

Miletich JP, Jackson CM, Majerus PW (1978). Properties of the factor Xa binding site on human platelets. J Biol Chem 253:6908.

Miletich JP, Broze GJ Jr, Majerus PW (1980). The synthesis of sulfated dextran beads for isolation of human plasma coagulation factors II, IX and X. Anal Biochem 195:304.

Mustard JF, Perry DW, Ardlie NG, Packham MA (1972). Preparation of suspensions of washed platelets from humans. Br. J Haematol 22:193.

Proctor RR, Rapaport SJ (1961). The partial thromboplastin time with kaolin. A simple screening test for first stage plasma clotting deficiencies. Am J Clin Pathol 36:212.

Rosing J, van Rijn JLML, Bevers EM, van Dieijen G, Comfurius P, Zwaal RFA (1985). The role of activated human platelets in prothrombin and factor X activation. Blood 65:319.

Scatchard G (1949). The attractions of proteins for small molecules and ions. Ann NY Acad Sci 51:660.

Schiffman S, Rapaport SI, Chong MMY (1966). The mandatory role of lipid in the interaction of factors VIII and IX. Proc Soc Exp Biol Med 123:736.

Scott CF, Sinha D, Seaman FS, Walsh PN, Colman RW (1984). Amidolytic assay of human factor XI in plasma: Comparison with a coagulant assay and a new rapid radioimmunoassay. Blood 63:42.

Silverberg SA, Nemerson Y, Zur M (1977). Kinetics of the activation of bovine coagulation factor X by components of the extrinsic pathway. Kinetic behavior of two-chain factor VII in the presence and absence of tissue factor. J Biol Chem 252:8481.

Sinha D, Koshy A, Bradford H, Seaman F, Walsh PN (1984a). Coagulation factor IX activation by platelet-bound factor XIa. Circulation 70:11.

Sinha D, Seaman FS, Koshy A, Knight LC, Walsh PN (1984b). Blood coagulation factor XIa binds specifically to a site on activated human platelets distinct from that for factor XI. J Clin Invest 73:1550.

Sinha D, Koshy A, Seaman FS, Walsh PN (1985). Functional characterization of human blood coagulation factor XIa using hybridoma antibodies. J Biol Chem 260:10714.

Tangen O, Berman HJ, Marfey P (1971). Gel filtration. A new technique for separation of blood platelets from plasma. Thromb Diath Haemorrh 25:268.

Timmons S, Hawiger (1978). Separation of human platelets from plasma proteins including factor VIII_{vwf} by a combined albumin gradient-gel filtration method using hepes buffer. Thromb Res 12:297.

Tollefsen DM, Feagler JR, Majerus PW (1975). Binding of thrombin to the surface of human platelets. J Biol Chem 249:2646.

Tracy PB, Nesheim ME, Mann KG (1981). Coordinate binding of factor Va and factor Xa to the unstimulated platelets. J Biol Chem 256:743.

Tuszynski GP, Knight L, Piperno JR, Walsh PN (1980). A rapid method for removal of ^{125}I-Iodide following iodination of protein solutions. Anal Biochem 106:118.

Tuszynski GP, Bevacqua SJ, Schmaier AH, Colman RW, Walsh PN (1982). Factor XI antigen and activity in human platelets. Blood 59:1148.

Tuszynski GP, Kornecki E, Cierniewski C, Knight LC, Koshy A, Srivastava S, Neiwiarowski S, Walsh PN (1984a). Association of fibrin with the platelet cytoskeleton. J Biol Chem 259:5247.

Tuszynski GP, Mauco GP, Koshy A, Schick PK, Walsh PN (1984). The platelet cytoskeleton contains elements of the prothrombinase complex. J Biol Chem 259:6947.

Van Lenten L, Ashwell G (1971). Studies on the chemical and enzymatic modification of glycoproteins. J Biol Chem 246:1889.

Walsh PN (1972a). The role of platelets in the contact phase of blood coagulation. Br J Haematol 22:237.

Walsh PN (1972b). The effects of collagen and kaolin on the intrinsic coagulant activity of platelets. Evidence for an alternative pathway in intrinsic coagulation not requiring factor XII. Br J Haematol 22:393.

Walsh PN (1972c). Albumin density gradient separation and washing of platelets and the study of platelet coagulant activities. Br J Haematol 22:205.

Walsh PN, Biggs R (1972d). The role of platelets in intrinsic factor Xa formation. Br J Haematol 22:743.

Walsh PN (1974). Platelet coagulant activities and hemostasis: An hypothesis. Blood 43:597.

Walsh PN, Mills DCB, White JG (1977). Metabolism and function of human platelets washed by albumin density gradient separation. Br J Haematol 36:281.

Walsh PN (1978). Different requirements of intrinsic factor Xa forming activity and platelet factor 3 activity and their relationship to platelet aggregation and release. Br J Haematol 40:311.

Walsh PN, Griffin JH (1981). Contributions of platelets to the proteolytic activation of blood coagulation factors XII and XI. Blood 57:106.

Walsh PN (1982). Platelet-coagulant protein interactions. In Colman RW, Hirsh J, Marder VJ, Salzman EW (eds): "Hemostasis and Thrombosis: Basic Principles and Clinical Practices." Philadelphia J.B. Lippincott Co., pp 404–420.

Walsh PN, Bradford H, Sinha D, Piperno JR, Tuszynski GP (1984). Kinetics of the factor XIa catalyzed activation of human blood coagulation factor IX. J Clin Invest 73:1392.

Walsh PN, Sinha D, Koshy A, Seaman FS, Bradford H (1986). Functional characterization of platelet-bound factor XIa: Retention of factor XIa activity on the platelet surface. Blood 68:225.

Zur M, Nemerson Y (1980). Kinetics of factor IX activation via the extrinsic pathway. Dependence of K_m on tissue factor. J Biol Chem 255:5703.

Modern Methods in Pharmacology, Volume 4
Methods for Studying Platelets and Megakaryocytes, pages 65–88

Methods for Studying the von Willebrand Factor–Platelet Interaction

EDWARD P. KIRBY and DAVID C.B. MILLS

INTRODUCTION

When flowing blood is exposed to areas of damaged endothelium, the blood platelets somehow recognize the damaged area, stick to it, and form aggregates on the surface. The exposed subendothelium is a matrix composed of collagen and elastin fibers, glycosaminoglycans, fibronectin, von Willebrand factor (vWF), and other proteins. The von Willebrand factor appears to be essential for this process of recognition and adhesion, since patients with von Willebrand's disease (vWD) who have defective or deficient vWF, have a bleeding syndrome due to ineffective platelet-mediated hemostasis [Zimmerman and Ruggeri, 1982]. Investigations on the mechanism of the vWF interaction with platelets, the platelet responses to these interactions, and the effects of different agonists on platelet responsiveness, may provide insight into early phases of the platelet response to damaged endothelium. In addition, the interaction of vWF with the platelets provides a convenient model for other cellular responses. The binding of vWF to platelets is followed by agglutination and a cascade of cellular responses similar to those induced by close cell contact. Cellular responses to other agents can in turn modulate the interaction with vWF.

VON WILLEBRAND FACTOR

Von Willebrand factor is a very large plasma glycoprotein. (See reviews by Hoyer [1981] and by Zimmerman and Ruggeri [1982] for general discussion of vWF structure and function.) It circulates in the plasma as polymers of a subunit with molecular weight approximately 230,000. The vWF is associated by disulfide bonding into multimers composed of from 2 to more than 50 subunits. It

From the Departments of Biochemistry and Pharmacology and the Thrombosis Research Center, Temple University School of Medicine, Philadelphia, Pennsylvania 19140.

appears that the highest molecular weight multimers are the most active physiologically, since bleeding syndromes are also seen in patients with variants of von Willebrand's disease in which the vWF, although present in near normal amounts, is less highly polymerized.

Clinical concentrates containing the highest proportion of large multimers are hemostatically most effective when infused into patients with vWD [Chediak et al., 1977]. VWF is synthesized and secreted primarily by vascular endothelial cells, but is also synthesized by megakaryocytes and is stored in platelet α-granules, whence it can be released upon appropriate stimulation. VWF circulates freely in the blood where it functions as a carrier for blood coagulation factor VIII:c (antihemophilic factor), but it can also adsorb to fibers in the subendothelial matrix [Sussman and Rand, 1982].

Our current model for the structure of vWF, which is based on studies by several groups [Fowler et al., 1985; Hamilton et al., 1985; Chopek et al., 1986; Girma et al., 1986; Titani et al., 1986; Bockenstedt et al., 1986] including our own [Mascelli and Kirby, 1987] indicates that the individual subunits of vWF are joined in a head-to-head fashion (see Fig. 1). Individual subunits are joined by multiple disulfide bonds in their C-terminal regions, and by only a small number (perhaps one or two) near the N-terminal. Platelet binding domains are located in the N-terminal half of the subunit. Fujimura et al. [1986] have identified a 50 kD peptide in proteolytic digests of vWF that binds to platelets in the presence of ristocetin. Partial sequence analysis shows this peptide to be composed of amino acids 449-729 of the vWF molecule. VWF also contains a site that is responsible for binding to ADP-stimulated or thrombin-stimulated platelets. This site contains an RGDS sequence (see below) located near the C-terminus [Titani

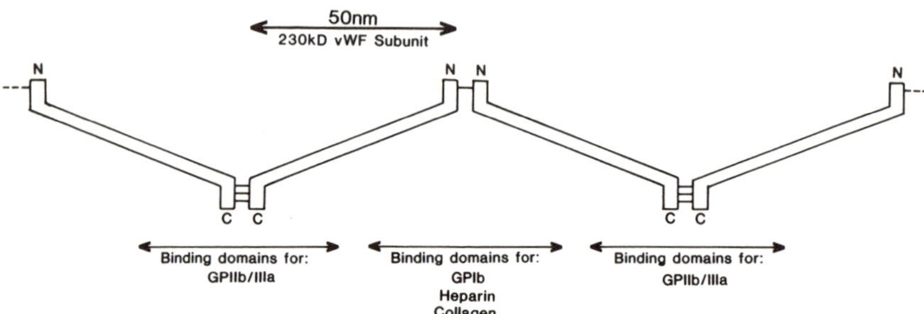

Fig. 1. Proposed structure of vWF. The subunits of vWF are linked near their C-terminal ends by multiple disulfide bonds to form dimeric protomers. These dimers are linked by only one or two disulfide bonds near the N-terminus of each subunit. Domains for binding to the platelet GPIb-associated receptor, to heparin, and to collagen are located in the N-terminal portion of the subunits, domains for binding to the GPIb/IIa-associated receptor are in the C-terminal region.

et al., 1986]. VWF binds to collagen [Kessler et al., 1984] and also to glycosaminoglycans such as heparin. The heparin- and collagen-binding domains also appear to be in the N-terminal portion of the molecule.

PLATELET RESPONSES TO VWF

Several in vitro models have been developed to help study the interaction of platelets and vWF. Those most frequently used are based on the observation of Howard and Firkin [1971] that vWF induces aggregation of platelets in the presence of the antibiotic ristocetin. Ristocetin promotes the binding of vWF to platelets, and the polymeric nature of vWF allows it to form bridges between one platelet and another [Coller, 1985]. This causes them to clump together—a response that is readily observed by eye and quantified in an aggregometer.

Bovine or porcine vWF binds directly to human platelets, without the need for ristocetin, and causes an agglutination of the platelets that is strikingly similar to that seen with ristocetin and human vWF [Kirby and Mills, 1975]. Bovine or porcine platelets, exposed to bovine or porcine vWF, agglutinate in the presence of ristocetin but not in its absence [Brinkhous et al., 1977]. This implies that ristocetin does not act simply by modifying human vWF to make it behave as bovine vWF does, or by making human platelets behave as bovine platelets. The explanation of these observations may lie in actions of ristocetin on both platelets and on vWF.

The response of platelets to vWF is multifaceted. Initial binding of vWF to the surface appears to be a relatively simple process. Stirring the suspension causes clumping of the platelets. This clumping is referred to as agglutination, since it does not require platelet metabolic activity and occurs with fixed platelets. These initial processes of vWF binding and platelet agglutination can be conveniently studied using platelets which have been fixed with formaldehyde, prepared from either a formalin solution [Kirby and Mills, 1975] or paraformaldehyde [Allain et al., 1975]. Extracellular Ca^{2+} is not required for agglutination. When unfixed platelets are used, however, and when Ca^{2+} is present, the response to vWF can be more complex. Although vWF binding does not induce platelet shape change, the cell-cell contact which occurs when platelets are agglutinated by vWF leads to the release of the constituents of platelet dense granules—including ADP, ATP, and serotonin. This process is associated with activation of platelet phospholipases and production of prostanoids, and involves stimulation of phosphoinositide turnover, release of inositol 1,4,5 trisphosphate, and mobilization of intracellular Ca^{2+}. The thromboxane A_2 produced and the released ADP can cause other platelet responses such as shape change and binding of other plasma proteins, e.g., fibrinogen and fibronectin, and the release of α granule constituents, including vWF.

One platelet response unique to vWF-associated platelet aggregation is a phenomenon called superaggregation, in which all of the small platelet aggregates formed initially are gathered into one or two very large clumps [Kirby et al., 1982]. This response is not seen with other agonists, such as ADP, prostaglandins, or the ionophore A23187, and it is blocked by fixation of the platelets. It does not require Ca^{2+} ions but may require lateral mobility of the receptors for vWF on the platelet surface.

Two distinct binding sites for vWF on the platelet surface have been identified. One is associated with the platelet membrane glycoprotein GPIb, the other with a complex of two membrane glycoproteins—GPIIb and GPIIIa. The GPIb-associated site is required for platelet adhesion to exposed subendothelium and for ristocetin-induced aggregation. GPIb is missing in patients with Bernard-Soulier syndrome [Jamieson et al., 1979], who have long bleeding times associated with defective platelet adhesion. Their platelets are not aggregated by bovine vWF or by human vWF in the presence of ristocetin. Antibodies to GPIb inhibit platelet adhesion and the agglutination induced by bovine vWF or by ristocetin. GPIb is associated with agglutination of platelets by wheat germ lectin [Okumura et al., 1976] and can also bind thrombin [Okumura and Jamieson, 1976].

The second binding site for vWF is associated with the glycoprotein IIb/IIIa complex, which is also responsible for binding of fibrinogen and fibronectin to platelets. VWF binding to GPIIb/IIIa requires Ca^{2+} ions and prior activation of the platelets. GPIIb and GPIIIa are defective in patients with Glanzmann's thrombasthenia, and these individuals' platelets do not aggregate in response to ADP or thrombin. As patients with thrombasthenia have prolonged bleeding times [Ruggeri et al., 1982a], though platelet adhesion and ristocetin-induced aggregation are normal, it appears that both GPIIb/IIIa and GPIb are important for the normal platelet response to damaged endothelial surfaces.

Binding of vWF to GPIIb/IIIa seems to be directly analogous to the binding of fibrinogen and fibronectin to this receptor. ADP stimulates the binding of both vWF and fibrinogen to GPIIb/IIIa, and fibrinogen competes directly with vWF for binding [Timmons et al., 1984]. Platelets first stimulated with ADP or thrombin, then fixed with formaldehyde and washed, still bind vWF [Plow et al., 1984]. Binding to this receptor involves a specific region in each of these proteins that contains the sequence arg-gly-asp-ser (RGDS). Synthetic peptides containing this sequence inhibit binding [Haverstick et al., 1985].

Monoclonal antibodies have also been prepared that are specific for either GPIb or the GPIIb/IIIa complex [Coller et al., 1983a,b]. Specific inhibition by these antibodies can provide evidence for linkage of a process to one or the other of the sites. GPIb is also very sensitive to proteolytic attack by enzymes including platelet calcium-activated protease [Kunicki et al., 1985], the metalloprotease from *Serratia marcescens* [Cooper et al., 1981], and neutrophil elastase [Wicki and Clemetson, 1985]. Incubation with these enzymes can often specifically inhibit responses associated with binding to GBIb, without affecting responses associated with GPIIb/IIIa.

An example in which it has been useful to distinguish between responses associated with the two types of binding sites comes from studies on the aggregation of platelets by desialated vWF. Treatment of human vWF with neuraminidase removes 90% of its sialic acid residues and causes it to bind to platelets and to aggregate them, without the need for ristocetin [Vermylen et al., 1976; DeMarco and Shapiro, 1981]. Aggregation is inhibited by EDTA, though some binding of vWF occurs in the absence of Ca^{2+}. The initial binding of asialo-vWF to the GPIb receptor (which can be blocked by monoclonal antibodies to GPIb) leads to the platelet release reaction and subsequent appearance of the GPIIb/IIIa site. Platelet aggregation induced by asialo-vWF occurs principally as a result of fibrinogen binding to GPIIb/IIIa and is blocked by antibodies to the GPIIb/IIIa complex [DeMarco et al., 1985; Gralnick et al., 1985]. Fibrinogen and vWF compete for the GPIIb/IIIa site, and since the plasma concentration of fibrinogen is much higher than that of vWF, platelet activation in plasma leads to saturation of these sites with fibrinogen and subsequent aggregation.

TYPES OF VON WILLEBRAND'S DISEASE

Several different conditions have been grouped together under the general term of von Willebrand's disease (vWD) (see reviews by Zimmerman and Ruggeri [1982] and by George et al. [1984]). The different types of vWD have been distinguished on the basis of the bleeding time, clinical symptoms, family history, vWF antigen levels, and multimer patterns. Distinction between types is sometimes complicated by variabilities in the assays [Abildgaard et al., 1980]. A simplified comparison of the major types of vWD is presented in Table I.

In type I vWD the amount of vWF measurable in plasma is decreased and all of the multimeric species of vWF are decreased proportionately. Patients with this disorder usually have some bleeding symptoms, especially those patients with a severe deficiency in which the vWF concentration is less than 10% of normal. Plasma levels of factor VIII:c are also decreased, presumably because of the role of vWF as a carrier for VIII:c in the plasma. The amount and multimeric composition of platelet vWF is normal in these individuals [Zimmerman and Ruggeri, 1982]. Administration of 1-deamino-[8-D-arginine]-vasopressin (DDAVP), which promotes secretion of vWF from endothelial cells, often restores vWF levels toward normal, with a parallel increase in all of the multimeric forms of vWF and a decrease in the bleeding time. The defect in type I

TABLE I. Types of von Willebrand's Disease

	Type I	Type IIA	Type IIB	Type III
Bleeding time	Prolonged	Prolonged	Prolonged	Prolonged
VWF antigen concentration in:				
Plasma	Decreased	Decreased	Decreased	Decreased
Platelets	Normal	Decreased	Normal	Decreased
VWF multimer distribution in:				
Plasma	Normal	Decreased large multimers	Decreased large multimers	—
Platelets	Normal	Decreased large multimers	Normal	—
Plasma ristocetin cofactor activity	Decreased	Decreased	Decreased	Decreased
Plasma factor VIII:C activity	Decreased	Decreased or normal	Decreased or normal	Decreased
Mode of inheritance	Autosomal dominant	Autosomal dominant	Autosomal dominant	Autosomal recessive

vWD appears to be in the production of vWF by endothelial cells, but not by megakaryocytes. Another protein—initially termed von Willebrand antigen II (vWAgII)—is also missing from the plasma of these individuals [Montgomery and Zimmerman, 1978]. Recent studies [Fay et al., 1986] have shown that vWAgII is the propeptide portion of vWF that is removed after vWF synthesis, and that is secreted along with vWF.

In type II vWD there is a decrease in the higher molecular weight multimers of vWF. This can have two causes. In type IIA, there appears to be a defect in vWF polymerization; vWF is synthesized normally but is not subsequently converted to the very high molecular weight multimers that are physiologically most active. Total amounts of vWF (measured immunologically) may be normal, but since the high molecular weight forms are absent, the responsiveness to ristocetin is very low and bleeding times are prolonged. Platelet vWF also has an abnormal multimeric composition in type IIA. Plasma vWF concentrations increase on administration of DDAVP, but the bleeding time remains prolonged [Ruggeri et al., 1982b].

In type IIB the higher molecular weight multimers are absent from plasma, but are present in platelets [Ruggeri and Zimmerman, 1980]. The platelet-rich plasma of these individuals is more than usually responsive to ristocetin. Much lower concentrations of ristocetin than normal are required to induce agglutination. Their vWF has an increased affinity for platelets and binds even in the absence of ristocetin. Preferential spontaneous binding of the more highly multivalent forms of the abnormal vWF to platelets may explain the depletion of these forms from plasma. On infusion of DDAVP, large multimers of vWF appear in the plasma, but then rapidly disappear as platelet aggregates containing vWF are trapped and removed from circulation. The bleeding time is usually not corrected [Ruggeri and Zimmerman, 1980]. Because the induced thrombocytopenia would make bleeding worse, DDAVP is contraindicated in patients with type IIB vWD [Holmberg et al., 1983].

In type III vWD the vWF in both plasma and platelets is either very low (1–5% of normal) or undetectable [Zimmerman and Ruggeri, 1982]. The bleeding times are very long, and the condition is inherited as an autosomal recessive, in contrast to the autosomal dominant inheritance of types I and II. All cells that synthesize vWF are affected. The synthesis and release of plasminogen activator from endothelial cells is also defective in some cases of type III vWD.

Careful differentiation between the different types of von Willebrand's disease requires not only the measurement of ristocetin cofactor activity (see below) and an immunological determination of the amount of von Willebrand factor in plasma, but also a measurement of the multimeric composition of the plasma vWF. This latter test is particularly helpful in distinguishing type II vWD from other conditions in which the vWF concentration is only marginally below the normal range.

A related syndrome, which has been termed "pseudo-von Willebrand's disease" or "platelet-type vWD," has recently been described [Weiss et al., 1982; Miller and Castella, 1982]. As in type IIB vWD the patient's platelet-rich plasma is more than usually sensitive to ristocetin; in this case the primary abnormality lies in the platelets, which show increased affinity for vWF. Higher molecular weight multimers of vWF are missing from the plasma. Spontaneous aggregation of platelets is often observed on stirring of the platelet-rich plasma and is promoted by addition of normal vWF containing large multimers. Normal vWF binds to these platelets in the absence of ristocetin [Weiss et al., 1982]. Spontaneous aggregation is inhibited by the presence of EDTA, suggesting some involvement of GPIIb/IIIa in these processes.

ASSAYS FOR STUDYING THE VWF-PLATELET INTERACTION

Several experimental models have been developed to study the function of vWF in platelet-mediated hemostasis. The first to be used was the bleeding time, which measures the time required for cessation of bleeding from a small standardized wound in the skin [Mielke et al., 1969]. The bleeding time is usually prolonged in vWD and in many other types of disorder in which platelets are involved. The test cannot discriminate between different types of disorders but is useful as an accurate monitor of the physiological effects of transfused platelets or of drugs used to enhance or suppress platelet mediated hemostasis.

One of the earliest in vitro tests for vWD was the adhesion of platelets to glass beads [Bowie et al., 1969]. In this assay whole blood is passed through a column of small glass beads. Platelet counts made before and after this procedure reveal the number of platelets removed. Patients with vWD have decreased adhesion, as do thrombasthenics. The test does not distinguish between adhesion and the subsequent formation of aggregates on the beads, so defects in platelet aggregation and secretion could influence the number of platelets removed by the column. The test is technically difficult, requires special apparatus, and is not easy to apply to large numbers of samples; consequently its current use is limited.

The in vitro test which most closely mimics the in vivo response of platelets to damaged endothelium is that developed by Weiss et al. [1978]. In this technique, segments of rabbit aorta are stripped free of endothelium, everted, and placed in a thermostated chamber. Whole blood or platelet-rich plasma is pumped over these segments at controlled rates of shear. The segments of aorta are fixed, sectioned, and examined microscopically. Adhesion of platelets, platelet spreading, and subsequent formation of platelet aggregates can be quantitated. At high shear rates, comparable to those present in small blood vessels, adhesion was blocked by antibodies to vWF [Baumgartner et al., 1980]. Again, however, the procedure is technically involved and not convenient for analysis of many samples.

Olson et al. [1983] have described a technique for measuring adhesion of platelets to dialysis membrane on which a layer of purified vWF is deposited by ultrafiltration. When these membranes are immersed in platelet suspensions, the platelet adherence can be determined by microscopic examination. Adhesion is prevented by antibodies to vWF and is not seen with platelets from patients with Bernard-Soulier syndrome.

Probably the most common assay used in studying the vWF-platelet interaction is the Ristocetin-Induced Platelet Aggregation (RIPA) assay. In this test, ristocetin (usually 1–2 mg/ml) is added to citrated platelet-rich plasma and the platelet aggregation measured optically in an aggregometer. The assay is convenient for measuring gross defects in the system, but it is sensitive to both the concentration and subunit composition of vWF in the patient's plasma, as well as to the responsiveness of the platelets. In addition, several plasma proteins, including albumin and fibrinogen, bind ristocetin nonspecifically and decrease its ability to induce platelet aggregation [Stibbe and Kirby, 1976]. Alterations in the levels of these nonrelated proteins in different patients may influence the RIPA assay.

A closely related assay that has been used extensively to measure functionally active vWF is the Ristocetin-Cofactor (RCF) assay. In this test a standard suspension of washed normal platelets is mixed with dilutions of normal or patient's plasma and aggregation is induced by the addition of ristocetin. Usually the standard platelets are fixed with formaldehyde before washing, since fixed platelets remain responsive for several weeks when stored at 4°C and longer when stored frozen. Platelet aggregation can be measured either in an aggregometer or by the formation of macroscopic aggregates in a tube, detected visually [Brinkhous et al., 1975]. The reciprocal type of assay, where washed platelets from the patient are tested with a standard sample of vWF and a known concentration of ristocetin, is more difficult. Problems occur in reproducibly washing platelets and in the lack of a stable standard preparation of purified vWF. Pooled normal plasma can be used as a standard vWF, but the high content of albumin and fibrinogen in plasma may cause secondary effects.

A more convenient and reproducible assay for platelet sensitivity to vWF might be to use a standard preparation of bovine or porcine vWF to induce aggregation, thus eliminating the need for ristocetin. Highly purified bovine vWF is stable for many months when frozen, but is not yet commercially available. Some commercial preparations of bovine fibrinogen contain sufficient vWF to induce platelet aggregation and have been used in some studies [Coller, 1981]; pooled frozen normal bovine plasma would probably be adequate as a standard for most studies. Fifty microliters of bovine plasma in 0.5 ml of normal human PRP induces good agglutination, and this test can detect most platelet defects associated with this system.

In all of these assays, care must be taken to distinguish between effects due to the initial vWF-platelet interaction, and those associated with subsequent events such as the release reaction, prostanoid synthesis, binding of proteins to GPIIb-IIIa, or superaggregation. Some of these secondary effects can be prevented by incorporation of aspirin, an inhibitor of prostaglandin synthesis, in the platelet suspension medium or by the addition of EDTA immediately before induction of vWF-induced aggregation.These treatments generally decrease the sensitivity of the assay (because they inhibit the amplification effects of subsequent events, such as nucleotide release), but improve its specificity.

A new agent for studying the vWF–platelet interaction which has recently been introduced is botrocetin, isolated from the venom of *Bothrops atrox*, which induces the aggregation of human platelets in the presence of vWF [Brinkhous et al., 1983]. Unlike ristocetin, which is more effective with the higher molecular weight forms of vWF, botrocetin seems to induce aggregation in the presence of all forms of vWF. The effect of botrocetin is not blocked by vancomycin [Howard et al., 1984] an inhibitor of ristocetin-induced agglutination [Baugh et al., 1978]—suggesting that the two agents act by different mechanisms. Botrocetin-induced aggregation involves the interaction of vWF with GPIb and occurs with formaldehyde-fixed platelets [Brinkhous and Read, 1980].

SPECIFIC METHODS

Purification and Labeling of von Willebrand Factor

Von Willebrand factor has been purified to homogeneity from human, bovine, and porcine plasma in several laboratories. Most procedures involve an initial cryoprecipitation by freezing the plasma and then slowly thawing it. Cryoprecipitation is promoted by addition of ethanol or polyethylene glycol. Subsequent steps often use glycine precipitation and/or adsorption of impurities onto bentonite or aluminum hydroxide. Most purification procedures use molecular sieve chromatography on a large pore gel such as Sepharose as a central step. The very large size of vWF causes it to elute in the void volume, while most other plasma proteins are retained. In most cases the eluted vWF is homogeneous, giving a single band on reduced SDS-polyacrylamide gels, although it is composed of a population of disulfide-linked multimers of different sizes. Procedures such as cryoprecipitation, precipitation with polyethylene glycol, and chromatography on Sepharose generally select for the highest molecular weight species, and the multimeric composition of purified vWF, determined by electrophoresis on SDS-agarose gels [Ruggeri and Zimmerman, 1981], may not be representative of vWF in plasma.

Human vWF has frequently been purified from standard cryoprecipitate preparations used for the treatment of hemophilia or von Willebrand's disease. Other purifications have started with commercial lyophilized concentrates. The latter are a very convenient source, but generally contain more of the lower molecular weight multimers of vWF. Currently, most commercial concentrates are heated to destroy viruses. This may make them less suitable as starting material for purification of native vWF.

Our current procedure [Mascelli et al., 1986] for purification of bovine vWF involves cryoprecipitation at pH 6.3 in the presence of 2.5% polyethylene glycol. Some fibrinogen is removed by adsorption on bentonite, fibronectin is depleted by glycine precipitation; vWF is then isolated by chromatography on Sepharose 4-B. Protease inhibitors, including diisopropylfluorophosphate, soybean trypsin inhibitor, and phenylmethanesulfonyl fluoride, are used in the early stages of the procedure to prevent proteolytic degradation of the vWF. Remaining trace impurities, generally aggregates of partially degraded fibrinogen, are removed by chromatography on heparin-agarose. Highly purified bovine vWF is stable and can be stored frozen for several months without loss of platelet-agglutinating activity. Less pure fractions are sometimes less stable, perhaps due to the presence of traces of protease activity.

VWF can be radiolabeled by iodination of tyrosine residues either with lactoperoxidase [David and Reisfeld, 1974] or with Iodo-Gen [Fraker and Speck, 1978]. Incorporation of low levels of iodine (less than 2 atoms/mole of vWF subunits) does not alter the binding or platelet-agglutinating activity of the vWF [Kirby, 1982]. Labeling with reagents that modify amino groups, such as Bolton-Hunter reagent [Bolton and Hunter, 1973], should be avoided, as free amino groups are important for the binding and platelet-agglutinating activity of vWF [Santoro, 1982].

Preparation of Platelets

The interaction of platelets with bovine vWF or with human vWF in the presence of ristocetin can be studied in platelet-rich plasma (PRP), prepared with citrate as anticoagulant. Venous blood is drawn into 1/9 volume of 3.8% Na_3 citrate, giving about 22 mM citrate in the plasma—assuming a packed cell volume of 45%. Red cells are removed by centrifuging for 10–15 min at 900 rpm (110 × g). The platelet count can be adjusted to a standard value by suitable addition of homologous plasma prepared by centrifuging blood at 2,000 × g for 15 min. Platelet-rich plasma is prepared and handled at room temperature to avoid the deleterious effects of cooling, which causes platelets to lose their disk shape, and can cause aggregation when they are rewarmed. Heparin at 1–10 units/ml or hirudin can be used in place of citrate, though usually with a lower recovery of platelets in the platelet-rich plasma.

Washed platelets. The presence of plasma proteins in PRP can make this medium unsuitable for some type of experiments, and a number of techniques have been developed for isolating platelets into a defined medium. Of these, centrifugation and gel-filtration through Sepharose 2B-CL have been most widely used. Centrifugation of citrated platelet-rich plasma often leads to aggregation of the platelets, associated with release of ADP. Aggregation can be suppressed by reducing the pH, by raising the citrate concentration, or by adding apyrase to destroy released ADP. Because released ADP can alter the interaction between platelets and vWF, care should be taken to avoid ADP release or to counteract its effects. Addition of prostacyclin (0.1–1 μM) or PGE_1 (0.5–5 μM) raises platelet cAMP content and effectively inhibits ADP release induced either by centrifugation or gel-filtration; the platelets may take some time to regain their responsiveness to aggregating agents, but then remain usable for up to 48 hours when stored at 4°C [Vargas et al., 1982].

Addition of EDTA to chilled platelets prevents aggregation without causing some of the more profound effects that occur at room temperature or higher. However, the possibility that peripheral components of the plasma membrane may be modified by treatment with EDTA, which removes calcium from the membrane, must be considered.

The recovery and longevity of platelets washed by centrifugation or gel-filtration are enhanced by including bovine serum albumin (0.3–3%) in the buffers, although albumin should be omitted from the final suspension medium when platelets are to be surface-labeled.

A washing procedure that we use is based on the procedure of Mustard et al. [1972]. The pH of platelet-rich plasma is brought to 6.5 by addition of 1 M citric acid. The platelets are sedimented by centrifugation at 2,000 rpm (540 × g) for 15 min at room temperature in 50 ml round bottom polycarbonate centrifuge tubes. The plasma is decanted and the platelets resuspended in a small volume (3.5 ml) of a medium composed of Tyrode's solution containing 3.5% bovine serum albumin (Sigma type V) and 2 units/ml apyrase (Sigma grade VII #A6535) to which is added 1/5 volume of 3.8% Na_3 citrate and 1 M citric acid to pH 6.5. The resuspended platelets are diluted with the same medium to 1/2 the original volume of PRP and incubated for 20 min at 37°C to destroy any released ADP. The centrifugation is repeated at 1,800 × rpm, and the platelets resuspended in a medium containing Tyrode's solution without Ca^{2+} and containing 20 mM HEPES at pH 7.4. Albumin can be added to this medium if desired. In our experience, the resuspended platelets remain responsive for longer periods of time when albumin is present.

Fixed platelets. Formaldehyde-fixed platelets are useful and convenient for measuring the RCF activity of human plasma fractions and the vWF activity of bovine plasma fractions. Both paraformaldehyde [Allain et al., 1975] and formalin [Macfarlane et al., 1975] have been used to prepare the fixative. The inhibitory effect of ADP on the interaction of vWF with the platelet GPIb-associated receptor is preserved after fixation, so care must be taken to ensure that ADP is removed before the addition of formaldehyde. This is most easily done by incubating the platelets at 37°C with apyrase before addition of the formaldehyde solution. Alternatively, 1 μM PGI_2 could be added to suppress the platelet responsiveness to ADP. Clinical platelet concentrates can be used for the preparation of fixed platelets, but they should be less than 24 hours old, not outdated. Different bags of platelet concentrates often yield fixed platelets with markedly different responsiveness to vWF. A commercial preparation of lyophilized fixed platelets is also available.

In our current procedure for the preparation of formalin-fixed platelets, blood is collected from normal volunteers into 1/9 volume of 3.8% trisodium citrate. (It is not important whether the donors have consumed aspirin recently.) Platelet-rich plasma is prepared by centrifugation at 110 × g for 10 min and incubated at 37°C for 30 min to ensure that the platelets are disk-shaped. An equal volume of

0.15 M NaCl, 0.01 M Tris buffer, pH 7.4, containing 7.4 gm/liter of formaldehyde (a freshly made 1:50 dilution of a stock formalin solution in Tris-saline buffer) is added and the suspension stored overnight at 4°C. The platelets are then washed three times by centrifugation and resuspension in 0.15 M NaCl, 0.01 M phosphate, buffer, pH 6.5, care being taken to remove contaminating red cells. The fixed platelets are finally suspended in phosphate-saline buffer containing 20 mg bovine serum albumin/ml such that a 1:10 dilution of this suspension has an OD_{500} of approximately 1.2 (this yields a platelet concentration of 3-4 $\times$ 10^9 per ml). The platelet suspensions are stored in 2 ml aliquots at −85°C. For reconstitution they are thawed rapidly at 37°C then diluted 1:10 in phosphate-saline buffer.

One problem encountered in the preparation and storage of fixed platelets is a small amount of platelet lysis. This can cause release of platelet vWF, which interferes with subsequent vWF assays. Lysis is also associated with the release of calcium-activated protease from platelets, which can cleave platelet membrane GPIb and cause a reduction in the responsiveness of the platelets to vWF.

Agglutination and Aggregation Studies

The response of platelets to ristocetin and to vWF is conveniently measured in an aggregometer. Addition of bovine vWF (1–10 μg/ml) to stirred platelet suspensions results in prompt and rapid agglutination (Fig. 2). Similar aggregations are seen when ristocetin (0.5–2 mg/ml) is added to platelet suspensions containing human vWF. This response can be quantified by measuring either the rate of change of the optical signal at the steepest part of the trace, or by measuring the extent of the pen deflection after a fixed time. We use the former method. Shape change is not seen with vWF-induced aggregation, even under conditions of maximal agglutination [Kirby and Mills, 1975]. In the absence of EDTA, a second wave of aggregation often occurs due to ADP released by platelets that have been agglutinated by vWF. This release of platelet nucleotides induced by vWF requires cell-to-cell contact and is not observed in unstirred suspensions.

Fixed platelets are very convenient for the assay of human or bovine vWF (Fig. 3). At lower concentrations of vWF agglutination is often preceded by a lag. The length of the lag can sometimes be used to estimate the magnitude of a marginal response.

When ristocetin is added to fixed platelets, an unexplained increase in absorbance is observed [Allain et al., 1975; Stibbe and Kirby, 1976]. If ristocetin is added to suspensions of fixed platelets containing vWF, this artifact will partially counter the absorbance decrease associated with the agglutination response and so make measurements difficult. Consequently, ristocetin is added first, then vWF, when the absorbance has stabilized (Fig. 3B).

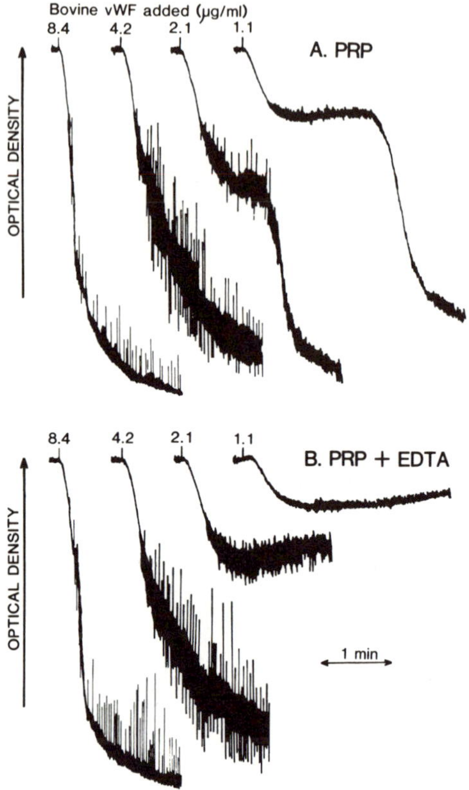

Fig. 2. Aggregation in platelet-rich plasma. Addition of purified bovine vWF to normal human platelet-rich plasma induces prompt aggregation both in the absence (A) or presence (B) of 5 mM EDTA to block the platelet release reaction. Superaggregation is seen with the highest doses of vWF and is distinguished by the diminution in size of the oscillations as platelets become clumped into only one or two large aggregates. The second phase of aggregation seen at lower concentrations of vWF, in the absence of EDTA, is due to release of platelet nucleotides and subsequent ADP-induced aggregation.

Ristocetin binds strongly to many proteins and can cause some to precipitate [Stibbe and Kirby, 1976]. This can be a problem in assays of ristocetin cofactor activity when the plasma is diluted extensively. To prevent the precipitation, which occurs at low protein concentrations, the fixed platelets are usually suspended in buffer containing albumin (2 mg/ml) and the plasma is diluted in buffer with 40 mg albumin/ml.

Agglutination assays using vWF proceed more efficiently at higher stirring speeds (1,200–1,500 rpm) and at 37°. Temperature control is not critical, but agglutination is slower at lower temperatures, and is not observed at all at 0–5°.

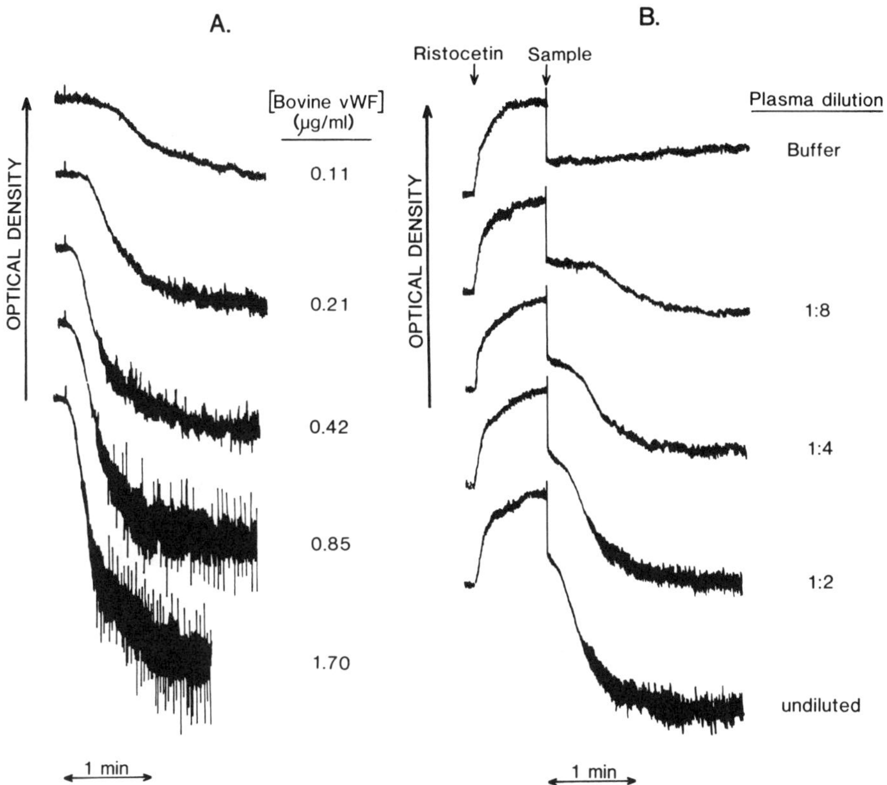

Fig. 3. Aggregation of fixed platelets. (A) Use of washed formalin-fixed platelets allows measurement of low concentrations of purified bovine vWF. (B) Addition of ristocetin (1 mg/ml) to fixed platelets (700 μl) induces an increase in the absorbance of the suspension. Subsequent addition of 100 μl of dilutions of normal human plasma in buffer containing albumin (40 mg/ml) induces an agglutination response proportional to the amount of vWF added.

Another way to quantitate vWF-induced agglutination is to measure the time required for the appearance of visible clumps of platelets after addition of ristocetin and/or vWF. This macroscopic agglutination test [Brinkhous et al., 1975] is simple, fast, reproducible, and convenient for testing many samples.

Binding Studies

Equilibrium binding of vWF to platelets is attained within 5–10 min at 37°C [Kirby, 1982]. Binding can be measured by adding vWF to washed platelet suspensions, incubating for short periods, centrifuging the platelets, and determining the vWF concentration in supernatant and platelet pellet. VWF concentration can be determined immunologically, or by measurement of the platelet-agglutinating activity in the supernatant, but it is more convenient to do binding studies with radiolabeled vWF.

Ristocetin-induced binding of human vWF or the binding of bovine vWF to human platelets is quite efficient (at 1–10 μg vWF/ml 20–50% of the vWF becomes bound to the platelets) so measurement of binding can be done simply by centrifuging the suspensions and counting the radioactivity of platelets and supernatants. Non-specific binding is determined in the absence of ristocetin or in the presence of a large excess of unlabeled vWF. Binding to formaldehyde-fixed platelets is readily reversible, but with metabolically intact platelets an irreversible component of binding has sometimes been observed.

Measurement of vWF binding to the GPIIb-IIIa site is more difficult because less is bound and nonspecific binding is relatively more significant. Incubation for 15–30 min is required to achieve equilibrium, and the test is frequently done at room temperature to decrease the extent of irreversible binding. After incubation the platelets are generally centrifuged through layers of silicone oil or sucrose to reduce the amounts of supernatant radioactivity trapped in the pellet.

Binding of vWF to GPIb can be distinguished from binding to GPIIb/IIIa in several ways. In platelet-rich plasma that has not been exposed to platelet agonists such as ADP or prostanoids, addition of 5 mM EDTA 30 sec before the addition of ristocetin or bovine vWF will ensure that essentially all vWF binding will be to GPIb. Binding of human vWF to GPIb essentially requires ristocetin (or botrocetin), so that binding measured in the absence of these agents will be almost entirely to GPIIb/IIIa. This can be confirmed by measuring competition for binding by an RGDS peptide or by fibrinogen, which bind only at the GPIIb/IIIa site. When testing binding induced by a new agonist, however, it would be preferable to determine the effects of monoclonal antibodies to GPIb or to GPIIb/IIIa on binding, since these are the best available discriminators between the two processes.

When binding isotherms to either GPIb or to GPIIb/IIIa are plotted according to Scatchard [1949], curved plots are often obtained, suggesting either cooperative binding or multiple classes of binding sites. Because the multimeric heterogeneity of vWF makes estimation of the molecular weight of the bound material difficult, the use of Scatchard plots to deduce the number and affinity of receptors is not straightforward, and the binding affinity may depend on the extent of vWF polymerization. Interpretation of binding isotherms should be limited to reporting variations in the extent of binding (μg vWF bound per 10^9 platelets) under different conditions and should always state the concentration of platelets and vWF. This limitation may eventually be overcome by the use of monomeric probes for vWF binding.

EFFECTS OF OTHER AGONISTS

Several drugs and hormones influence the interaction between platelets and vWF. We have already considered the effect of ADP, which can be released from the platelets themselves by slight injury such as may be caused by centrifugation or passage through a gel-filtration column, on promoting binding to GPIIb/IIIa. However, exposure of platelets to ADP inhibits the GPIb-associated agglutination by bovine vWF or by human vWF with ristocetin, and can cause a loss of reponsiveness during the washing procedure [Cohen et al., 1975; Grant et al., 1976; Mills et al., 1986]. This effect is also interesting as it represents a rare example of a negative interaction between platelet activators. Many platelet agonists, such as ADP, epinephrine, thrombin, prostanoids, and calcium ionophores, potentiate each other's actions. The mechanism of these effects is obscure. The inhibitory effect of ADP on vWF-associated agglutination is related to the ability of ADP to cause the transition from disk to irregular sphere that is known as platelet shape change. Shape change appears on the aggregometer tracing as a loss of the base line oscillations that are due to the alignment of discoid platelets in the planes of shear created by stirring, and as an increase in the optical density of the suspension. Other platelet agonists that induce a rapid and pronounced shape change, such as platelet activating factor (1-acyl-2-acetyl-glycerolphosphoryl choline, PAF) and prostanoid analogs of PGH_2 also inhibit the response to vWF.

Epinephrine causes aggregation of platelets in two phases. The second, more pronounced phase is associated with release of ADP and other contents of platelet storage organelles—dense bodies and α granule. The first phase occurs without shape change. Epinephrine does not inhibit the response of platelets to vWF.

Other agents that are weak inducers of shape change and aggregation, such as vasopressin and 5-HT, are much less able than ADP to inhibit the agglutination caused by vWF. The optical changes associated with shape change seen with these agents are either slower or less extensive than with ADP, which suggests that the shape change may reflect different processes—not all may be related to inhibition of the platelet interaction with vWF. ADP has little effect on the binding of labeled bovine vWF to platelets [Mills et al., 1986]; apparently binding of vWF to platelet receptors is only a part of the requirement for agglutination.

Many aggregating agents also inhibit adenylate cyclase, and an alternative explanation for their ability to interfere with vWF-induced agglutination is that they act through effects on cyclic AMP turnover. This is unlikely for several reasons. First, epinephrine, a powerful inhibitor of cyclic AMP formation, does not inhibit the platelet-vWF interaction. Second, platelet activating factor, although it inhibits adenylate cyclase in platelet membranes, has little effect in intact cells, while it inhibits vWF-induced agglutination strongly. Third, the nucleoside 2′,5′-dideoxyadenosine, which inhibits adenylate cyclase by interacting with the catalytic component of the cyclase system at the intracellular P- or purine-specific site, also has no effect on vWF-associated agglutination.

Dibutyryl cyclic AMP, and agents such as PGI_2 and PGE_1 that increase platelet cyclic AMP levels, inhibit vWF-induced platelet agglutination [Coller, 1981] although this effect is not seen in EDTA-treated PRP [Mills et al., 1986], suggesting that it may not be a direct effect of cyclic AMP. This is supported by the observation of Coller [1981] that the effects of these agents are prevented by cytoskeleton-disrupting agents, such as colchicine and vinblastine. Forskolin and PGD_2, which also increase platelet cAMP, inhibit both ADP-induced shape change and the inhibitory effect of ADP on vWF-induced agglutination [Mills et al., 1986].

The optical effects of the shape change induced by ADP are attenuated by incubation with 1–2 μM vincristine. This drug interferes with the reversible polymerization of tubulin and causes a slow loss of platelet disk shape, though it does not inhibit agglutination induced by vWF. Platelets that have been incubated with vincristine are unaffected in their sensitivity to the inhibitory effect of ADP on vWF-induced agglutination. This shows that the loss of the platelets' disk shape is not the only determinant of the inhibitory effect of ADP.

Evidence for the involvement of secondary membrane effects in vWF-induced platelet agglutination comes from the observation of Coller [1982] that local anesthetics, such as tetracaine and dibucaine, stimulate vWF-induced agglutination. These agents change the physical structure of membranes, and also disrupt microfilaments and microtubules. Their effects on vWF-associated platelet agglutination may be primarily due to their stimulation of platelet calcium-activated protease with subsequent effects on the association of glycoprotein Ib with actin binding protein and other components of the cytoskeleton [Solum and Olsen, 1985]. Fixed platelets with increased responsiveness can be obtained by fixation with formaldehyde after treatment with local anesthetic. Paradoxically, although the anesthetics increased the sensitivity of platelets to vWF, they decreased the amount of vWF that was bound to platelets [Coller, 1982].

USEFULNESS OF VWF IN PLATELET STUDIES

Assays of ristocetin-induced platelet agglutination in platelet-rich plasma and of the ristocetin cofactor activity of plasma can be done conveniently and reproducibly in most laboratories. This has led to the widespread use of these assays as screening tests for platelet disorders and for the diagnosis of different types of von Willebrand's disease.

Patients with Bernard-Soulier syndrome can be identified by their platelets' inability to agglutinate with bovine vWF or with ristocetin and a source of normal human vWF [Caen et al., 1976]. Of these tests the interaction with bovine vWF would be simpler to perform. These patients are rare and of value as a resource for the investigation of this aspect of platelet function.

Genetic deficiency of vWF has been identified in both dogs and pigs, and is associated with a bleeding syndrome, so that these animals may prove to be useful models for studying platelet adhesion. The observation of Fuster et al. [1978] that pigs with von Willebrand's disease given an atherogenic diet develop much less atherosclerosis than normal pigs on the same diet suggests that vWF-mediated platelet recognition of minimally damaged endothelium leads to the release of platelet growth factors and stimulation of intimal proliferation.

Investigation of the interaction between platelets and vWF is a tool for research into the roles of cell and protein in the interactions of platelets with damaged vessel walls. Already much is known about the involvement of membrane glycoproteins in the two types of platelet receptor for vWF. Are there other proteins involved in these receptors? The structure of vWF is unfolding in molecular terms, domains are being mapped for interactions with platelets and with heparin, and a head-to-head, tail-to-tail model has been proposed for the disulfide linkage in the polymeric form. This suggests that the smallest subunit with binding affinity would be the dimer, Mr 460,000, rather than the monomer. Development of a univalent ligand would facilitate the investigation of the pharmacologic properties of the receptor, and help identify the regions of the receptor protein involved in the interaction.

Monoclonal antibodies directed at different regions of the vWF molecule and of the receptors at which it binds have identified two types of receptor. Much is known about the vWF-receptor interaction, but much remains to be learned. Although in plasma the high concentration of fibrinogen would block vWF binding to the GPIIb/IIIa site, the situation could be different in a closely packed platelet aggregate. In this situation, platelet vWF released from its storage granules might play a role in mural thrombosis out of proportion to its ratio to vWF in plasma (about 1:4), especially since much of the "released" vWF remains associated with the platelet surface [Fernandez et al., 1982]. The mechanism of the inhibitory effect of ADP and other shape change-inducing agents is puzzling, as there is little reduction in the amount of vWF that binds to the platelets, although agglutination is greatly reduced. The inhibition survives fixation in formalin and so must be fixed into the structure of the membrane. What is happening to the receptor, and how? It is possible that mobility of the receptors may be involved, particularly to explain why superaggregation is inhibited by cross-linking aldehydes. In type IIB von Willebrand's disease the multimeric forms of vWF appear more than usually sticky. Nothing as yet is known of how this increased stickiness comes about. There are many intriguing puzzles left, and we hope that the methods we have described will help in solving some of them. The relevance of these problems to the behavior of a platelet encountering a damaged blood vessel is clear.

REFERENCES

Abildgaard CF, Suzuki Z, Harrison J, Jefcoat K, Zimmerman TS (1980). Serial studies in von Willebrand's disease: Variability versus "variants." Blood 56:712–716.

Allain JP, Cooper HA, Wagner RH, Brinkhous KM (1975). Platelets fixed with paraformaldehyde: A new reagent for assay of von Willebrand Factor and platelet aggregating factor. J Lab Clin Med 8:318–328.

Baugh RF, Jacoby C, Brown JE, Hougie C (1978). Effect of vancomycin on ristocetin and bovine PAF-induced agglutination of human platelets. Thromb Res 12:511–521.

Baumgartner HR, Tschoop TB, Meyer D (1980). Shear rate dependent inhibition of platelet adhesion and aggregation on collagenous surfaces by antibodies to human Factor VIII/von Willebrand factor. Br J Haem 44:127–139.

Bockenstedt P, Greenberg JM, Handin RI (1986). Structural basis of von Willebrand factor binding to platelet glycoprotein Ib and collagen. Effects of disulfide reduction and limited proteolysis of polymeric von Willebrand factor. J Clin Invest 77:743–749.

Bolton AE, Hunter WM (1973). The labeling of proteins to high specific radioactivities by conjugation to a ^{125}I-containing acylating agent. Biochem J 133:529–539.

Bowie EJW, Owen CA Jr, Thompson JH Jr, Didisheim P (1969). Platelet adhesiveness in von Willebrand's disease. Am J Clin Pathol 52:69–77.

Brinkhous KM, Graham JE, Cooper HA, Allain JP, Wagner RH (1975). Assay of von Willebrand factor in von Willebrand's disease and hemophilia: Use of a macroscopic aggregation test. Thromb Res 6:267–272.

Brinkhous KM, Thomas BD, Ibrahim SA, Read MS (1977). Plasma levels of platelet aggregating factor/von Willebrand factor in various species. Thromb Res 11:345–355.

Brinkhous KM, Read MS (1980). Use of venom coagglutinin and lyophilized platelets in testing for platelet-aggregating von Willebrand factor. Blood 55:517–520.

Brinkhous KM, Read MS, Fricke W-A, Wagner RA (1983). Botrocetin (venom coagglutinin): Reaction with a broad spectrum of multimeric forms of factor VIII macromolecular complex. Proc Natl Acad Sci USA 80:1463–1466.

Caen JP, Nurden AT, Jeanneau C, Michel H, Tobelem G, Levy-Toledano S, Sultan Y, Valensi F, Bernard J (1976). Bernard-Soulier syndrome: A new platelet glycoprotein abnormality. Its relationship with platelet adhesion to subendothelium and with the Factor VIII von Willebrand protein. J Lab Clin Med 87:586–596.

Chediak JR, Telfer MC, Green D (1977). Platelet function and immunologic parameters in von Willebrand's disease following cryoprecipitate and Factor VIII concentrate infusion. Am J Med 62:369–376.

Chopek MW, Girma JP, Fujikawa K, Davie EW, Titani K (1986). Human von Willebrand factor: a multivalent protein composed of identical subunits. Biochemistry 25:3146–3155.

Cohen I, Glaser T, Seligsohn U (1975). Effects of ADP and ATP on bovine fibrinogen- and ristocetin-induced platelet aggregation in Glanzmann's thrombasthenia. Br J Haem 31:343–347.

Coller BS (1981). Inhibition of von Willebrand Factor-dependent platelet function by increased platelet cyclic AMP and its prevention by cytoskeleton-disrupting agents. Blood 57:846–855.

Coller BS (1982). Effects of tertiary amine local anesthetics on von Willebrand Factor-dependent platelet function: Alteration of membrane reactivity and degradation of GPIb by a calcium-dependent protease(s). Blood 60:731–743.

Coller BS, Peerschke EI, Scudder LE, Sullivan CA (1983a). Studies with a murine monoclonal antibody that abolishes ristocetin-induced binding of von Willebrand factor to platelets: Additional evidence in support of GPIb as a platelet receptor for von Willebrand factor. Blood 61:99–110.

Coller BS, Peerschke EI, Scudder LE, Sullivan CA (1983b). A murine monoclonal antibody that completely blocks the binding of fibrinogen to platelets produces a thrombasthenia-like state in normal platelets and binds to glycoproteins IIb and/or IIIa. J Clin Invest 72:325–338.

Coller BS (1985). Platelet—von Willebrand factor interactions. In George JN, Nurden AT, Phillips DR (eds): "Platelet Membrane Glycoproteins." New York: Plenum Press, pp 215–244.

Cooper HA, Bennett WP, Kreger A, Lyerly D, Wagner RH (1981). The effect of extracellular proteases from gram-negative bacteria on the interaction of von Willebrand Factor with human platelets. J Lab Clin Med 97:379–389.

Davis GS, Reisfeld RA (1974). Protein iodination with solid-state lactoperoxidase. Biochemistry 13:1014–1021.

DeMarco L, Shapiro SS (1981). Properties of human asialo-factor VIII. A ristocetin-independent platelet-aggregating agent. J Clin Invest 68:321–328.

DeMarco L, Girolami A, Russell S, Ruggeri ZM (1985). Interaction of asialo von Willebrand factor with glycoprotein Ib induces fibrinogen binding to the glycoprotein IIb/IIIa complex and mediates platelet aggregation. J Clin Invest 75:1198–1203.

Fay PJ, Kawai Y, Wagner DD, Ginsburg D, Bonthron D, Ohlsson-Wilhelm BM, Chavin SI, Abraham GN, Handin RI, Orkin SH, Montgomery RR, Marder VJ (1986). Propolypeptide of von Willebrand factor circulates in blood and is identical to von Willebrand Antigen II. Science 232:995–998.

Fernandez MFL, Ginsberg MH, Ruggeri ZM, Batlle FJ, Zimmerman TS (1982). Multimeric structure of platelet factor VIII/von Willebrand factor: The presence of large multimers and their reassociation with thrombin-stimulated platelets. Blood 60:1132–1138.

Fowler WE, Fretto LJ, Hamilton KK, Erickson HP, McKee PA (1985). Substructure of human von Willebrand factor. J Clin Invest 76:1491–1500.

Fraker PJ, Speck JC Jr (1978). Protein and cell membrane iodinations with a sparingly soluble chloroamide, 1,3,4,6-tetrachloro-3α,6α-diphenylglycoluril. Biochem Biophys Res Commun 80:849–857.

Fujimoto T, Ohara S, Hawiger J (1982). Thrombin-induced exposure and prostacyclin inhibition of the receptor for Factor VIII/von Willebrand Factor on human platelets. J Clin Invest 69:1212–1222.

Fuster VF, Bowie EJW, Lewis JC, Fass DN, Owen CA Jr, Brown AL (1978). Resistance to arteriosclerosis in pigs with von Willebrand's disease. Spontaneous and high-cholesterol diet-induced arteriosclerosis. J Clin Invest 61:722–730.

George JN, Nurden AT, Phillips DR (1984). Molecular defects in interactions of platelets with the vessel wall. N Engl J Med 311:1084–1098.

Girma JP, Chopek MW, Titani K, Davie EW (1986). Limited proteolysis of human von Willebrand factor by *Staphylococcus aureus* V-8 protease: isolation and partial characterization of a platelet-binding domain. Biochemistry 25:3156–3163.

Gralnick HR, Williams SB, Coller BS (1985). Asialo von Willebrand factor interactions with platelets. Interdependency of glycoproteins Ib and IIb/IIIa for binding and aggregation. J Clin Invest 75:19–25.

Grant RA, Zucker MB, McPherson J (1976). ADP-induced inhibition of von Willebrand factor-mediated platelet agglutination. Am J Physiol 230:1406–1410.

Hamilton K, Fretto LJ, Grierson DS, McKee PA (1985). Effects of plasmin on von Willebrand factor multimers. Degradation in vitro and stimulation of release in vivo. J Clin Invest 76:261–270.

Haverstick DM, Cowan JR, Yamada KM, Santori SA (1985). Inhibition of platelet adhesion to fibronectin, fibrinogen, and von Willebrand factor substrates by a synthetic tetrapeptide derived from the cell-binding domain of fibronectin. Blood 66:946–952.

Holmberg L, Nilsson IM, Borge L, Gunnarson M, Sjorin E (1983). Platelet aggregation induced by 1-desamino-8-D-arginine vasopressin (DDAVP) in Type IIB von Willebrand's disease. N Engl J Med 309:816–821.

Howard MA, Firkin BG (1971). Ristocetin: A new tool in the investigation of platelet aggregation. Thromb Diath Haem 26:362.

Howard MA, Perkin J, Salem HH, Firkin BG (1984). The agglutination of human platelets by botrocetin: Evidence that botrocetin and ristocetin act at different sites on the factor VIII molecule and platelet membrane. Br J Haem 57:25–35.

Hoyer LW (1981). The factor VIII complex: Structure and function. Blood 58:1–13.

Jamieson GA, Okumura T, Fishback B, Johnson MM, Egan JJ, Weiss HJ (1979). Platelet membrane glycoproteins in thrombasthenia, Bernard-Soulier syndrome, and storage pool disease. J Lab Clin Med 93:652–660.

Kessler CM, Floyd CM, Rick ME, Krizek DM, Lee SL, Gralnick HR (1984). Collagen-Factor VIII/von Willebrand factor protein interaction. Blood 63:1291–1298.

Kirby EP (1982). The agglutination of human platelets by bovine factor VIII:R. J Lab Clin Med 100:963–976.

Kirby EP, Mills DCB (1975). The interaction of bovine factor VIII with human platelets. J Clin Invest 56:491–502.

Kirby EP, Mills DCB, Holmsen H, Russo M (1982). Factor VIII-induced superaggregation of human platelets. Blood 60:1359–1369.

Kunicki TJ, Montgomery RR, Schullek J (1985). Cleavage of human von Willebrand factor by platelet calcium-activated protease. Blood 65:352–356.

Macfarlane DE, Stibbe J, Kirby EP, Zucker MB, Grant RA, McPherson J (1975). A method for assaying von Willebrand factor (Ristocetin Cofactor). Thromb Diath Haem 34:306–307.

Mascelli MA, Kirby EP (1987). Proteolytic studies on the structure of bovine von Willebrand factor (in preparation).

Mascelli MA, Edgington TS, Kirby EP (1986). Characterization of a fragment of bovine von Willebrand factor that binds to platelets. Biochemistry 25:6325–6335.

Mielke CH, Kaneshiro MM, Maher IA, Weiner JM, Rapport SI (1969). The standardized normal Ivy bleeding time and its prolongation by aspirin. Blood 34:204–215.

Miller JL, Castella A (1982). Platelet-type von Willebrand's disease: Characterization of a new bleeding disorder. Blood 60:790–794.

Mills DC, Hunchak K, Karl DW, Kirby EP (1986). Induction of platelet shape change by ADP modulates vWF-associated platelet agglutination (in preparation).

Montgomery RR, Zimmerman TS (1978). Von Willebrand's disease antigen II. A new plasma and platelet antigen deficient in severe von Willebrand's disease. J Clin Invest 61:1498–1507.

Mustard JF, Perry DW, Ardlie NG, Packham MA (1972). Preparation of suspensions of washed platelets from humans. Br J Haem 22:193–204.

Okumura T, Jamieson GA (1976). Platelet glycocalicin: A single receptor for platelet aggregation induced by thrombin or ristocetin. Throm Res 8:701–706.

Okumura T, Lombart C, Jamieson GA (1976). Platelet glycocalicin. II. Purification and characterization. J Biol Chem 251:5950–5955.

Olson JD, Moake JL, Collin MF, Michael BS (1983). Adhesion of human platelets to purified solid-phase von Willebrand factor: Studies of normal and Bernard-Soulier platelets. Thromb Res 32:115–122.

Plow EF, Srouji AH, Meyer D, Marguerie G, Ginsberg MH (1984). Evidence that three adhesive proteins interact with a common recognition site on activated platelets. J Biol Chem 259:5388–5391.

Ruggeri ZM, Zimmerman TS (1980). Variant von Willebrand's disease: Characterization of two subtypes by analysis of multimeric composition of factor VIII/von Willebrand factor in plasma and platelets. J Clin Invest 65:1318–1325.

Ruggeri ZM, Zimmerman TS (1981). The complex multimeric composition of factor VIII/von Willebrand factor. Blood 57:1140–1143.

Ruggeri ZM, Bader R, deMarco L (1982a). Glanzmann thrombasthenia: Deficient binding of von Willebrand factor to thrombin-stimulated platelets. Proc Natl Acad Sci USA 79:6038–6041.

Ruggeri ZM, Mannucci PM, Lombardi R, Federici AB, Zimmerman TS (1982b). Multimeric composition of factor VIII/von Willebrand factor following administration of DDAVP: Implications for pathophysiology and therapy of von Willebrand's disease subtypes. Blood 59:1272–1278.

Santoro SA (1982). Amino group modification inhibits ristocetin cofactor activity of human von Willebrand factor. Biochem Biophys Commun 108:479–485.

Scatchard G (1949). The attractions of proteins for small molecules and ions. Ann NY Acad Sci 51:660–672.

Solum NO, Olsen TM (1985). Effects of diamids and dibucaine on platelet glycoprotein Ib, actin-binding protein and cytoskeleton. Biochim Biophys Acta 817:249–260.

Sussman II, Rand RH (1982). Subendothelial deposition of von Willebrand's factor requires the presence of endothelial cells. J Lab Clin Med 100:526–532.

Stibbe J, Kirby EP (1976). The influence of Haemaccel, fibrinogen and albumin on ristocetin-induced platelet aggregation. Relevance to the quantitative measurement of the ristocetin cofactor. Thromb Res 8:151–165.

Timmons S, Kloczewiak M, Hawiger J (1984). ADP-dependent common receptor mechanism for binding of von Willebrand factor and fibrinogen to human platelets. Proc Natl Acad Sci USA 81:4935–4939.

Titani K, Kumar S, Takio K, Ericsson LH, Wade RD, Ashida K, Walsh KA, Chopek MW, Sadler JE, Fujikawa K (1986). Amino acid sequence of human von Willebrand factor. Biochemistry 25:3171–3184.

Vargas JR, Radomski M, Moncada S (1982). The use of prostacyclin in the separation from plasma and washing of human platelets. Prostaglandins 23:929–945.

Vermylen J, Bottechia D, Szpilman H (1976). Factor VIII and human platelet aggregation. III. Further studies on aggregation of human platelets by neuraminidase-treated human Factor VIII. Br H Haem 34:321–330.

Weiss HJ, Turitto VT, Baumgartner HR (1978). Effect of shear rate of platelet interaction with subendothelium in citrated and native blood. I. Shear rate—dependent decrease of adhesion in von Willebrand's disease and the Bernard-Soulier syndrome. J Lab Clin Med 92:750–764.

Weiss HJ, Meyer D, Rabinowitz R, Pietu G, Girma JP, Vicic WJ, Rogers J (1982). Pseudo-von Willebrand's disease. An intrinsic platelet defect with aggregation by unmodified human factor VIII/von Willebrand factor and enhanced adsorption of its high-molecular-weight multimers. N Engl J Med 306:326–333.

Wicki KN, Clemetson KJ (1985). Structure and function of platelet membrane glycoproteins Ib and IV. Eur J Biochem 153:1–11.

Zimmerman TS, Ruggeri ZM (1982). Von Willebrand's disease. Prog Hemost Thromb 6:203–236.

Modern Methods in Pharmacology, Volume 4
Methods for Studying Platelets and Megakaryocytes, pages 89–108

Use of Monoclonal Antibodies to Probe Platelet Responses

JOEL S. BENNETT

The exquisite specificity of monoclonal antibodies makes them excellent custom-made reagents with which to probe platelet function. Thus, when presented with a potential application, the investigator's task is to produce, recognize, and isolate appropriate antibodies and design unambiguous experiments to exploit the antibodies' particular specificity. My laboratory has used monoclonal antibodies to examine the interaction of the platelet membrane glycoprotein IIb/IIa complex with fibrinogen and divalent cations. Recently, we have also employed monoclonal antibodies to study the molecular biology of the membrane complex. In this chapter I describe our approach to the production and use of monoclonal antibodies.

PREPARATION OF ANTIPLATELET MONOCLONAL ANTIBODIES

The production of hybridomas has become a standard laboratory procedure since the original description of the methodology of Kohler and Milstein [1975]. We have followed the technique as described in detail in the text *Monoclonal Antibodies Hybridomas: A New Dimension in Biological Analysis* edited by R.H. Kennett, T.J. McKearn, and K.B. Bechtol [1980]. Because the production of hybridomas is now standard, the issues in the production of monoclonal antibodies have been reduced to the presentation of antigen during immunization and the detection of the desired antibodies. Theoretically, the hybridoma technique permits one to use an impure or complex antigen for the immunization and obtain the desired antibodies by an appropriate screen of the population of successful hybridomas. However, we found that we could greatly facilitate our studies by limiting the number of extraneous antigens presented during the immunization.

From the Hematology/Oncology Section, Hospital of the University of Pennsylvania, Philadelphia, Pennsylvania 19104.

Production of Monoclonal Antibodies Against the Glycoprotein IIb/IIIa Complex

The goal of our initial experiments was to produce antibodies against the platelet membrane glycoprotein IIb/IIIa heterodimer complex that contains the platelet fibrinogren receptor [Bennett, 1985]. Therefore, C57BL/6 mice were immunized on three occasions with 10^8 washed normal human platelets. Five weeks after the initial immunization, plasma from the mice was found to contain antibodies against human platelets. The mice were then sacrificed and their splenic lymphocytes fused with the mouse myeloma cell line Sp2/0-Ag14 [Bennett et al., 1983]. Ten to fourteen days later, supernatants from cultures of the successful fusions were assayed for antiplatelet activity using an ELISA (enzyme-linked immunoassay). For this assay 5×10^7 washed normal human platelets or 5×10^5 human lymphocytes were fixed to the wells of polyvinylchloride microtiter plates. Sequential additions of 100 μl of 1% bovine serum albumin and 50–100 μl of hybridoma culture supernatant were then added to the wells. After a 1 hour incubation at 4°C, the wells were washed six times and the amount of bound antibody determined with ^{125}I-labeled rabbit antimurine F $(ab')_2$. Alternatively, 100 μl goat antimouse IgG conjugated with peroxidase was added to each well. After a 1 hour incubation at 25°C and thorough washing, 100 μl of substrate solution (10 ml 0.1 M sodium citrate, pH 4.5, 10 mg orthophenyl-diamine, 4 μl H_2O_2) was added and the amount of color developed at 30 min was measured in a microtiter plate reader. Hybridomas producing antibodies against platelets but not lymphocytes were selected and cloned by limiting dilution.

At this point, an arbitrary selection was necessary to limit the number of clones to those that could be physically characterized. The remainder were frozen in liquid nitrogen for subsequent examination. Two clones were chosen for further study because their culture supernatants inhibited platelet aggregation. One clone produced an IgM antibody and was not characterized further because of the potential difficulty of working with a large pentavalent antibody. The other antibody, an IgG2a named A2A9, was produced in quantity in mouse ascites and was purified by affinity chromatography on *Staphylococcal* Protein A-Sepharose [Bennett et al., 1983].

The production of A2A9 was the critical starting point for much of our subsequent research. Therefore, its characterization was important. A2A9 was removed from the mouse ascitic fluid by precipitation with 50% saturated ammonium sulfate and was redissolved in a minimum volume of 0.125 M sodium borate buffer, pH 8.4, containing 0.075 M sodium chloride. The pH of the solution was then adjusted to 6.0 with 0.1 M sodium citrate, pH 3.2, and it was applied to a column of *Staphylococcal* Protein A-Sepharose equilibrated with 0.1

M sodium citrate, pH 6.0 [Ey et al., 1978]. Chromatography was performed at 4°C. Fractions containing A2A9 were eluted with 0.1 M sodium citrate buffer, pH 4.5, and were immediately neutralized with 1 M Tris-HCl, pH 8.5. An alternative method was used to purify the monoclonal antibody AP-2 [Pidard et al., 1983]. Ammonium sulfate precipitation was followed by chromatography on DEAE-Sephadex equilibrated with 0.01 M potassium phosphate, pH 8.0, and antibody was eluted with a linear 0–0.5 M sodium chloride gradient in the phosphate buffer [Pidard et al., 1983]. The concentration of purified antibody was determined by its absorbance at 280 nm using an absorbance coefficient of 1.4 OD units/mg/ml. Aliquots of the purified antibody were stored at −70°C.

Identification of the Antigen Recognized by the Monoclonal Antibody A2A9

To identify the epitope recognized by A2A9, the antibody was coupled to cyanogen bromide-activated Sepharose 4B (Pharmacia) in a ratio of 1–2 mg of antibody per ml of Sepharose. Washed platelets were surface labeled with ^{125}I using lactoperoxidase/hydrogen peroxide [Phillips, 1972] and were extracted with 1% Triton X-100. The extracts were then centrifuged at 100,000 × g to remove undissolved debris and the supernatants applied to columns of uncoupled Sepharose 4B to remove material that might nonspecifically adsorb to Sepharose. Next, the flow-through fractions from these columns were applied to 3 ml columns of A2A9-Sepharose. The columns were extensively washed until a background level of ^{125}I was achieved in the wash buffer and retained antigen was eluted with buffer containing 0.05 M diethylamine, pH 11.5. The eluates were immediately neutralized with 2 M Tris, 1% Triton X-100, pH 7.4, and dialyzed extensively against 0.15 M sodium chloride, 0.01 M Tris-HCl, pH 6.8. To concentrate the eluted antigens and remove as much Triton X-100 as possible, the antigens were precipitated with 6 volumes of acetone overnight at −20°C. The precipitates were then dissolved in 0.01 M Tris-HCl, pH 6.8, containing 3% SDS with or without 0.2 M dithiothreitol and applied to 0.1% SDS-7.5% polyacrylamide slab gels prepared and run according to the method of Laemmli [1970]. As seen in Figure 1, two proteins were retained by and eluted from the A2A9-Sepharose when the chromatography was performed in the absence of divalent cation chelators. These proteins had apparent molecular weights unreduced of 140,000 and 90,000 that changed to 120,000 and 114,000, respectively following disulfide bond reduction. These unreduced molecular weights and the changes in molecular weight that follow disulfide bond reduction are characteristic for the platelet glycoproteins IIb and IIIa [Jennings and Phillips, 1982]. In addition, immunoblotting [Towbin, Staehelin, and Gordon, 1979] using antisera against the Pl^{A1} antigen found on glycoprotein IIIa [Kunicki and Aster, 1979]

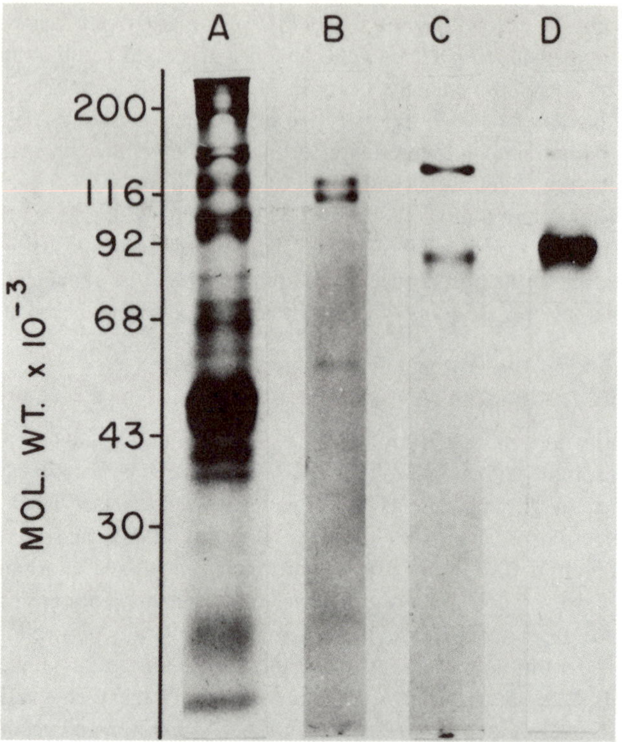

Fig. 1. Slab gel electrophoresis of platelet proteins isolated by affinity chromatography on immobilized A2A9. Washed human platelets dissolved in 1% Triton X-100 were applied to a column of A2A9-Sepharose. After extensively washing the column, adherent proteins were eluted with 0.05 M diethylamine, pH 11.5, and examined by 0.1% SDS-7.5% polyacrylamide gel electrophoresis. Proteins were visualized with 0.1% Coomassie brillant blue. Lane A, Triton X-100 solubilized platelets before application to the A2A9-Sepharose. Lane B, eluted polypeptides after reduction with 0.2 M dithiothreitol. Lane C, eluted polypeptides unreduced. Lane D, immunoblot of polypeptides in Lane C reacted with antiserum against the PI^{A1} antigen. ^{125}I-Staph A was used to identify sites of antibody binding. Lane D is an autoradiogram of the blot.

confirmed that the smaller protein was IIIa. Further experiments were performed to localize the A2A9 epitope to either IIb or IIIa. Because the IIb/IIIa heterodimer is calcium-dependent [Kunicki et al., 1981], we repeated the affinity chromatography in the presence of the calcium chelator EDTA. In the presence of EDTA neither IIb or IIIa was retained on the A2A9-Sepharose [Brass et al., 1985]. Moreover, ^{125}I-labeled A2A9 failed to interact with either IIb or IIIa on immunoblots or crossed immunoelectrophoreses of the dissolved platelet proteins. Thus,

A2A9 appears to interact with an epitope that requires an intact IIb/IIIa heterodimer for its expression.

Production of Antibodies Against Glycoprotein IIb and Glycoprotein IIIa

Our experience, and that of others, suggests that the intact human platelet IIb/IIIa heterodimer is highly immunogenic in mice. Thus, using intact platelets as an immunogen is likely to result in antibodies against the complex rather than against its components. To produce a library of monoclonals specifically against IIb and IIIa, we used A2A9 as an affinity reagent to purify the IIb/IIIa complex for use as an immunogen. C57BL/6 mice were immunized with the acetone precipitate of an eluate from an A2A9-Sepharose column dissolved in water and hybridomas were produced and screened as described above. Eight hybrids producing antiplatelet antibodies were selected and purified by cloning at limiting dilution. The specificity of the antibodies made by these hybrids was then determined by immunoblotting against membrane proteins separated by SDS-polyacrylamide gel electrophoresis. The antibodies made by seven of the eight hybrids reacted with proteins on the blots and were directed against glycoprotein IIIa. The eighth antibody did not react with a blotted protein but was subsequently also found to be directed against glycoprotein IIIa using affinity chromatography. Again, it appeared that platelet IIIa was highly immunogenic and that using our simple screening protocol, we preferentially selected for hybrids producing anti-IIIa antibodies.

To produce monoclonal antibodies against glycoprotein llb, it appeared that a third strategy would be required. The strategy we devised again depended on the ability of A2A9 to recognize the intact IIb/IIIa complex and has allowed us to prepare IIb and IIIa for a variety of purposes. Precipitated IIb/IIIa complexes from the A2A9-Sepharose eluates were dissolved in SDS and IIb was separated from IIIa by electrophoresis on unreduced SDS-polyacrylamide slab gels. The separated proteins were localized on the gels by staining one lane with Coomassie brillant blue and the regions of the gels containing the glycoproteins were existed with a razor blade. These gel slices were then placed in dialysis tubing and the tubing was suspended in an immunoblotting apparatus filled with Laemmli electrophoresis buffer. Following electrophoresis overnight, the buffer in the tubing, containing protein electroeluted from the gel slices, was aspirated and the protein was concentrated by acetone precipitation. As seen in Figure 2, we were able to prepare essentially pure preparations of either IIb or IIIa following this protocol. Mice were immunized with purified glycoprotein IIb in order to prepare monoclonal antibodies against this protein. IIb and IIIa purified in this manner have also been used to prepare monospecific polyclonal antisera in

Fig. 2. Purification of IIb and IIa using A2A9-Sepharose. Complexes of IIb and IIIa were isolated from Triton X-100 extracts of washed human platelets by affinity chromatography of A2A9-Sepharose as described in Figure 1. The IIb-IIIa complexes were then precipitated with six volumes of cold acetone, were dissolved in SDS, and IIb was separated from IIIa by electrophoresis on unreduced SDS-polyacrylamide slab gels. The separated proteins were localized on the gels by staining one lane with Coomassie brilliant blue. Regions of the gels containing the glycoproteins were excised with a razor blade. The gel slices were then placed in dialysis tubing, which was suspended in an immunoblotting apparatus filled with Laemmli electrophoresis buffer. Following electrophoresis overnight, buffer containing eluted protein was aspirated from the tubing and the protein was concentrated by acetone precipitation. The figure is a photograph of a Coomassie blue-stained SDS-polyacrylamide gel of the purified proteins. Lane A, IIIa; Lane B, IIb.

rabbits and have been fixed to the wells of microtiter platelets for a more specific ELISA. This ELISA has been used to screen for other IIb and IIIa monoclonals and to titer the polyclonal antisera.

USING MONOCLONAL ANTIBODIES TO PROBE PLATELET FUNCTION

Use of A2A9 to Study the Interaction of Fibrinogen With Activated Platelets

The effect of A2A9 on platelet function was tested by adding it either directly to platelet-rich plasma or to suspensions of gel-filtered platelets. The latter were prepared following the method of Tangen et al. [1982] except that the platelet elution buffer consisted of 137 mM sodium chloride, 2.7 mM potassium chloride, 1 mM magnesium chloride, 3.3 mM sodium dihydrogen phosphate, 4 mM HEPES (4-(2-hydroxyethyl)-1-piperazineethanesulfonic acid), 5.6 mM glucose, and 1 mg/ml bovine serum albumin, pH 7.8 [Brass et al., 1985]. Fibrinogen and calcium were both added to the suspensions when ADP and epinephrine-stimulated platelet aggregation was studied. However, exogenous fibrinogen and calcium were not required when thrombin was the platelet agonist, preventing distortion of thrombin-generated platelet aggregation tracings by fibrin clots. A disadvantage to the use of gel-filtered platelets is that the reactivity of these platelets tends to decline within 1–2 hours so that experiments using them must be performed quickly. In contrast, the reactivity of platelets in platelet-rich plasma remains stable for many hours if the platelet-rich plasma is maintained at room temperature. The result of adding A2A9 to suspensions of gel-filtered platelets prior to the addition of various aggregating agents is seen in Figure 3. A2A9 inhibited aggregation stimulated by all agonists in a concentration-dependent manner, but it had no effect on agonist-stimulated platelet shape change or on the aggregation-independent platelet secretion stimulated by strong platelet agonists like thrombin.

Because fibrinogen binding to activated platelets is a prerequisite for platelet aggregation, the effect of A2A9 on the binding of ^{125}I-fibrinogen to ADP-stimulated platelets was studied [Bennett and Vilaire, 1979]. Various concentrations of A2A9 were added to suspension of gel-filtered platelets containing both ^{125}I-fibrinogen and 0.5 mM $CaCl_2$. The platelets were then stimulated with 10 μM ADP and incubated without stirring for 3 min at 37°C. To separate platelet-bound from unbound fibrinogen, the suspensions of stimulated platelet were layered onto a mixture of silicone oils (Hi-phenyl silicone-DC550 and methyl silicone-DC200, manufactured by Dow-Corning and purchased through William F. Nye, Fairhaven, MA. The ratio of the two oils in the mixture was determined

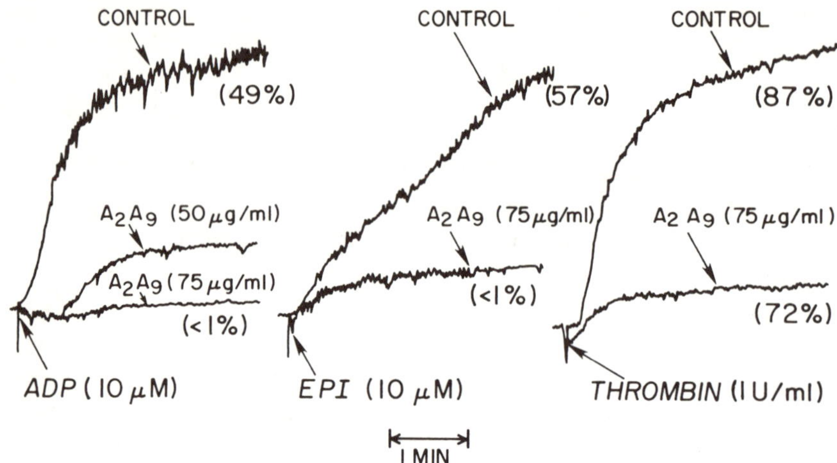

Fig. 3. Inhibition of platelet aggregation by the monoclonal antibody A2A9. 0.5 ml aliquots of suspensions of gel-filtered platelets ($\approx 5 \times 10^7$ platelets/ml) containing 100 μg/ml fibrinogen and 1 mM magnesium chloride were incubated with various concentrations of A2A9 for 2 min at 37°C in a platelet aggregometer. Platelet aggregation was then stimulated with either 10 μM ADP, 10 μM epinephrine, or 1 unit/ml thrombin. Exogenous fibrinogen was not required when thrombin was the platelet agonist. Platelet secretion was measured using platelets whose dense granules had been preloaded with ^{14}C-serotonin. The number in parentheses below each aggregation tracing indicates the percentage of the platelet content of ^{14}C-serotonin secreted under the particular conditions stated.

empirically but generally was 4:1). The platelets were sedimented through the oil mixture in an Eppendorf centrifuge (Brinkmann) and the tips of the centrifuge tubes, containing the pelleted platelets, were counted for ^{125}I in a gamma scintillation counter. The quantity of ^{125}I-fibrinogen nonspecifically associated with the pelleted platelets was determined by measuring ^{125}I-fibrinogen binding in the presence of a 15-fold excess of unlabeled fibrinogen, preventing labeled fibrinogen binding to the platelet fibrinogen receptor. As seen in Figure 4, A2A9 inhibited fibrinogen binding to ADP-stimulated platelets in a concentration-dependent manner. Fifty percent inhibition of fibrinogen binding (IC_{50}) occurred at an A2A9 concentration of 10 μg/ml (65 nM). By analyzing other experiments in which the concentration of A2A9 was held constant while the concentration of ^{125}I-fibrinogen was varied, we were able to demonstate that A2A9 was a competitive inhibitor of fibrinogen binding.

To compare the ability of A2A9 to bind to platelets with its ability to inhibit fibrinogen binding, direct A2A9 binding studies were performed using ^{125}I-labeled A2A9. A2A9 was radioiodinated for these studies using a modification of the chloramine-T/sodium metabisulfite technique. Because long exposures of

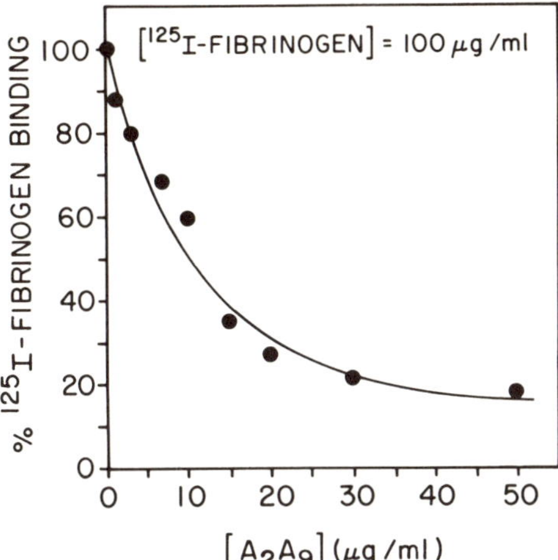

Fig. 4. Inhibition of fibrinogen binding to ADP-stimulated platelets by A2A9. Suspensions containing 5 × 10^7 platelets/ml were incubated with various concentrations of A2A9 for 2 min at 37°C. ^{125}I-fibrinogen (100 μg/ml) and 10 μM ADP were added and the incubations were continued for an additional 3 min at 37°C without stirring. To separate bound from free ^{125}I-fibrinogen, the platelets were sedimented through a mixture of silicone oils at 12,000 × g. The quantity of ^{125}I in the resulting platelet pellet was then measured in a gamma scintillation counter. Nonspecific fibrinogen binding was determined by performing the experiments in the presence of a 15-fold excess of unlabeled fibrinogen. Each point is the mean of triplicate determinations. Binding in the absence of A2A9 is set at 100%.

A2A9 to chloramine-T predictably destroyed its antibody activity, the exposure of the antibody to this oxidant was limited to 60 sec or less [Majerus and Brodie, 1972]. The labeled antibody was then incubated with 5 × 10^7 gel-filtered platelets for various time periods. To separate antibody-labeled platelets from unbound antibody, the platelets were sedimented through silicone oil mixtures as described for the fibrinogen binding studies. To determine the amount of unbound antibody trapped within the platelet pellet, platelets were incubated with the radioiodinated nonimmune mouse myeloma protein P3/X63-Ag8 and the amount of ^{125}I in the platelet pellet was measured. Trapped antibody amounted to 0.16% of the input radioactivity, equivalent to the extracellular space within the pellet measured with ^{3}H-sorbitol. An example of ^{125}I-A2A9 binding to normal platelets and to thrombasthenic platelets lacking IIb/IIIa is shown in Figure 5. Scatchard analysis of binding data from multiple normal subjects indicates that there are approximately 47,000 A2A9 binding sites/platelet and that 50% A2A9 binding (Kd) occurred at an antibody concentration of 60 μM. These experiments indicate that there is an excellent correspondence between the ability of A2A9 to bind to the

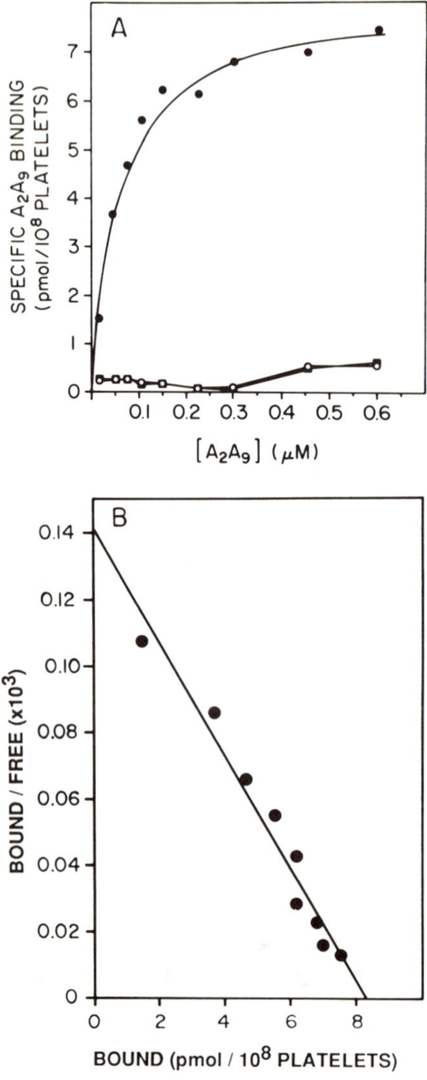

Fig. 5. A2A9 binding to normal and thrombasthenic human platelets. Suspensions containing 5×10^7 platelets/ml were incubated with various concentrations of ^{125}I-labeled A2A9 for 2 min at 37°C. Specific A2A9 binding was determined after sedimenting the platelets through a mixture of silicone oils. A. A2A9 binding isotherms: ●, normal subject; ○,■, thrombasthenic subjects. B. Scatchard analysis of the A2A9 binding data from the normal subject.

IIb/IIIa heterodimer (47,000 sites/platelet, Kd 60 nM) and its ability to inhibit fibrinogen binding to activated platelets (40,000 fibrinogen binding sites/platelet, IC_{50} 65 μM). When these data are combined with the observations that A2A9 does not bind to Glanzmann's thrombasthenic platelets [Bennett et al., 1983], that thrombasthenic platelets are deficient in IIb/IIIa complexes [Phillips and Agin, 1977], and that stimulated thrombasthenic platelets fail to bind fibrinogen [Bennett and Vilaire, 1979], they provide convincing evidence that the IIb/IIIa complex contains the platelet fibrinogen receptor.

Use of A2A9 to Study the Effect of Calcium on the Stability of the IIb/IIIa Complex

The ability of A2A9 to interact with the intact IIb/IIIa heterodimer complex, and not with either glycoprotein alone, provides a means to study factors involved in the maintenance of the integrity of the complex. The integrity of the IIb/IIIa heterodimer in platelets requires calcium ions [Kunicki et al., 1981]. However, it was not clear whether this calcium requirement was supplied by the platelet's external milieu or whether the calcium ions were provided when the concentration of calcium ions in the platelet cytosol increased following platelet stimulation [Rink et al., 1982]. We used A2A9 to examine this question [Brass et al., 1985]. Platelets surface-labeled with ^{125}I were extracted with Triton X-100 to solubilize membrane-associated IIb/IIIa, and the calcium concentration in these extracts was varied by adding specified amount of the calcium chelator EGTA. Then, affinity chromatography was performed on A2A9-Sepharose at the various calcium concentrations. The amount of IIb/IIIa retained by the columns was used as the indicator for the presence of intact IIb/IIIa heterodimers. We found that 50% of the applied IIb/IIIa was retained by the columns when the concentration of calcium ions was 0.4 μM. We also found that magnesium ions could substitute for calcium ions but were less effective in maintaining intact heterodimers.

Next, we studied the effect of external calcium on the integrity of membrane-associated IIb/IIIa complexes by measuring ^{125}I-A2A9 binding to intact, unactivated platelets as a function of the external calcium ion concentration. When these studies were performed at 25°C, much to our surprise, we found that A2A9 binding was independent of the calcium concentration (Fig. 6A). This suggests that the calcium ions responsible for maintaining the integrity of membrane-associated IIb/IIIa complexes were not accessible to the EGTA used to vary the external calcium concentration. However, Zucker and Grant [1978] had previously reported that incubation of platelets with EDTA at 37°C inhibited platelet aggregration without interfering with other platelet functions. Consequently, we repeated the A2A9 binding studies at 10^{-9}M calcium as a function of temperature. Under these conditions, we found that A2A9 binding was a linear

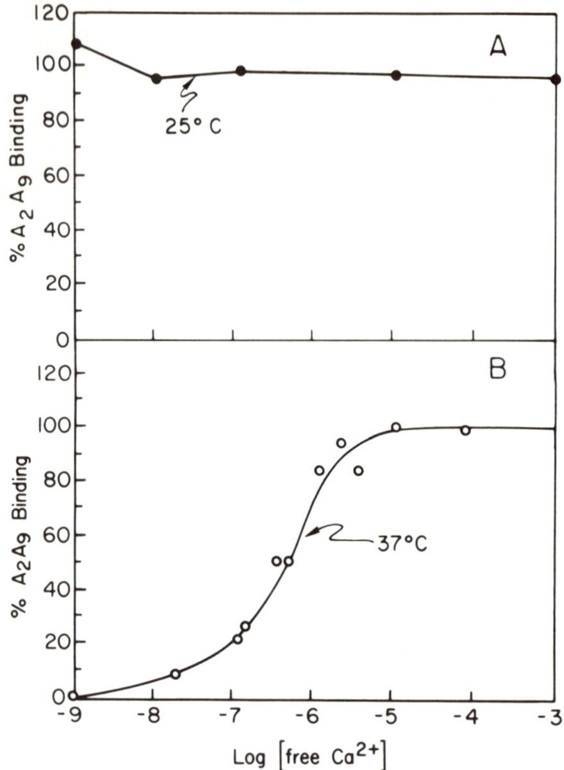

Fig. 6. Ca^{2+} dependence of ^{125}I-A2A9 binding to intact platelets at 25°C and 37°C. The Ca^{2+} concentration in aliquots of a suspension of gel-filtered platelets was buffered to the indicated values with EGTA. Specific ^{125}I-A2A9 binding to the platelets was then measured as described in Figure 5. Maximum A2A9 binding is 100% and corresponds to 32,000 molecules of A2A9/platelet. A, binding measurements performed at 25°C; B, binding measurements performed at 37°C.

function of temperature. Maximum A2A9 binding was seen at 25°C and essentially no binding was seen at 37°C. In view of these data, we repeated the measurements of A2A9 binding as a function of calcium concentration at 37°C. At this temperature, A2A9 binding was dependent on the concentration of calcium ions, and 50% A2A9 binding occurred at a calcium concentration of 0.4 μM (Fig. 6B). These experiments demonstrated that at physiologic temperature, the calcium ions responsible for the integrity of IIb/IIIa complexes in intact platelets are accessible to external chelators. Thus, these experiments indicate that the binding sites for these calcium ions are located on the external platelet surface. We also found a full complement of IIb/IIIa complexes on the surface of unactivated platelets. Because the affinity of the calcium binding sites responsible for the integrity of these complexes (0.4 μM) is lower than the cytosolic calcium ion concentration in unactivated platelets (0.1 μM), our data indicate that cytosolic calcium cannot be involved in the formation of IIb/IIIa complexes.

Use of Other Monoclonal Antibodies to Probe Platelet Function

Monoclonal antibodies have been used by a growing number of investigators to study platelet function. The goal of this section is to describe several of these studies to illustrate how others have made use of the hybridoma technology. Because the number of studies is large, I have limited this discussion to a few pertinent examples. These are listed in Table I.

Additional studies of the IIb/IIIa complex. Because of the critical role that the IIb/IIIa complex plays in platelet function, a number of anti-IIb/IIIa complex-specific monoclonal antibodies have been characterized and reported. Our observations using A2A9 were reported simultaneously by several other groups of investigators [Pidard et al., 1983; Coller et al., 1983; McEver et al., 1983; DiMinno et al., 1983]. Each of these reports confirmed that the IIb/IIIa complex contains the platelet fibrinogen receptor. However, each of the antibodies, including A2A9, bound to IIb/IIIa on unactivated platelets while fibrinogen binding to IIb/IIIa requires prior platelet activation. Thus, it is likely that none of the antibodies directly competes with fibrinogen for its binding site on IIb/IIIa. On the other hand, two antibodies have recently been produced that preferentially bind to IIb/IIIa on activated platelets. The antibody 7E3 was produced by immunizing BALB/c mice with washed platelets and was detected by a screening assay in which 7E3 hybridoma culture supernatant inhibited the agglutination of fibrinogen-coated beads by ADP-stimulated platelets [Coller, 1985]. As expected, purified 7E3 inhibited ^{125}I-fibrinogen binding to activated platelets and interacted with an epitope on the IIb/IIIa complex. However, 7E3 differed from the previously reported anti-IIb/IIIa monoclonal antibodies because its rate of binding to platelets was markedly accelerated when the platelets were activated. These experiments support the hypothesis that a change in the IIb/IIIa heterodimer is required to initiate its interaction with fibrinogen.

More direct evidence for this hypothesis was provided by studies using the monoclonal antibody PAC-1 [Shattil et al., 1985]. PAC-1 was produced by immunizing BALB/c mice with platelets from a patient with Glanzmann's thrombasthenia and was detected by a screening assay that selected for antibodies that preferentially bound to activated platelets. In this assay, aliquots of gel-filtered platelets were incubated with ADP, epinephrine, thrombin, or PGI_2 for 5 min. This was followed by a 30-min incubation with hybridoma supernatant. The

TABLE I. Monoclonal Antibodies As Probes of Platelet Function

Name	Specificity	Effect on platelet function	Reference
A2A9 AP-2 10E5 T10 B59.2	Ib/IIIa	Bind to unstimulated platelets, inhibit fibrinogen binding to stimulated platelets	Bennett et al., 1983 Pidard et al., 1983 Coller et al., 1983 McEver et al., 1983 DiMinno et al., 1983
PAC-1	IIb/IIIa	Binds only to stimulated platelets, inhibits fibrinogen binding	Shattil et al., 1985
7E3	IIb/IIIa	Binds more rapidly to activated platelets, inhibits fibrinogen binding	Coller, 1985
GTB's	IIbβ	Activates platelets	Jennings et al., 1985
TP82	23K protein	Activates platelets	Higashihara et al., 1985
AG-1	21K protein	Activates platelets	Miller et al., 1986
6D1 AP-1 LJIb1	Ibα	Inhibits vWf binding to ristocetin stimulated platelets	Coller et al., 1983 Montgomery et al., 1983 De Marco et al., 1985
LJP5	IIb/IIIa	Inhibits vWf, but not fibrinogen binding, to ADP and thrombin stimulated platelets	De Marco et al., 1985 Lombardo et al., 1985
LJP9	IIb/IIIa	Inhibits both vWf and fibrinogen binding to ADP and thrombin stimulated platelets	De Marco et al., 1985 Lombardo et al., 1985
S12	GMP-140	Binds to platelet α-granule protein bound to platelet plasma membrane after platelet secretion	McEver and Martin, 1984 Stenberg et al., 1985
KC4	PADGEM (140K protein)	Binds to platelet α-granule protein bound to platelet plasma membrane after platelet secretion	Hsu-Lin et al., 1984 Berman et al., 1986

platelet samples were then placed on a nitrocellulose filter in a dot blot apparatus and incubated with peroxidase-conjugated goat antimouse immunoglobin, hydrogen peroxide, and 1-chloro-4-naphthol. Color was generated if the platelets adsorbed to the filter contained mouse immunoglobulin. PAC-1 culture supernatant reacted with platelets that had been activated with ADP, epinephrine, and thrombin but did not react with platelets that had been exposed to the platelet inhibitor PGI_2. PAC-1 was subsequently purified and found to be an IgM antibody that only bound to IIb/IIIa complexes on activated platelets. The antibody was also found to inhibit the interaction of both A2A9 and fibrinogen with activated platelets, suggesting that it bound at the fibrinogen binding site. Further evidence for this suggestion was provided by studies using the tetrapeptide Arg-

Gly-Asp-Ser. This tetrapeptide sequence, found near the C-terminus of the fibrinogen α-chain, is a competitive inhibitor of fibrinogen binding to ADP-stimulated platelets [Gartner and Bennett, 1985]. In preliminary studies, Arg-Gly-Asp-Ser was also found to be a competitive inhibitor of PAC-1 binding to activated platelets [Gartner et al., 1985]. Thus, the behavior of PAC-1 with platelets is similar to that of fibrinogen, suggesting that the antibody binds to IIb/IIIa at or near the site that interacts with the fibrinogen α-chain.

In addition to containing a binding site for fibrinogen, the IIb/IIIa complex on activated platelets contains binding sites for von Willebrand factor (vWf) [Ruggeri et al., 1983] and fibronectin [Ginsberg et al., 1983]. Monoclonal antibodies have been used to study vWf and fibronectin binding to IIb/IIIa and to study the relationship of their binding sites to the binding site for fibrinogen. Four IIb/IIIa complex-specific monoclonal antibodies that inhibit fibrinogen binding to activated platelets also inhibit vWf and fibronectin binding to these platelets. This indicates that the binding sites for the three macromolecules on IIb/IIIa are in proximity [Plow et al., 1985; DeMarco et al., 1985; Lombardo et al., 1985]. Moreover, fibrinogen, vWf, and fibronectin each contain the Arg-Gly-Asp-Ser sequence [Pierschbacher and Ruoslahti, 1984; Sadler et al., 1985]. However, DeMarco et al. [1985] were able to produce a IIb/IIIa-specific monoclonal antibody, LJP5, that inhibited vWf binding to activated platelets without inhibiting fibrinogen binding [Lombardo et al., 1985]. These studies suggest that although the binding sites for fibrinogen and vWf are nearby on IIb/IIIa, differences exist between the sites that can be recognized by a monoclonal antibody.

To clarify the physiologic significance of fibrinogen and vWf binding to IIb/IIIa on activated platelets, Schullek et al. [1984] used a monoclonal antibody against vWf to detect platelet-bound vWf and monoclonal antibodies against platelet glycoprotein Ib and against the IIb/IIIa complex to differentiate between vWf bound to Ib or IIb/IIIa. They found that fibrinogen at physiologic concentration prevented vWf binding to activated platelets. However, when the fibrinogen concentration was decreased, either by heating normal plasma or by using plasma from afibrinogenemic individuals, vWf binding to activated platelets could now be detected. Subsequently, DeMarco et al. [1986], using the monoclonal antibody LJP5, found that IIb/IIIa-bound vWf could support platelet aggregation in afibrinogenemic plasma. This suggests that IIb/IIIa-bound vWf could be physiologically important if plasma fibrinogen is either depleted or abnormal.

Monoclonal antibodies that activate platelets. The processes that result in platelet activation are not well understood. Recently, there were three reports of monoclonal antibodies that activate platelets. Interestingly, each antibody recognized an epitope on a low molecular weight platelet protein. Higashihara et al. [1985] immunized mice with intact human platelets and detected the antibody

TP82 in a screening assay that selected for reactivity with washed platelets. Purified TP82 reacted equally well with normal platelets and with platelets from individuals with the Bernard-Soulier syndrome, lacking glycoprotein Ib, and platelets from individuals with Glanzmann's thrombasthenia, lacking IIb/IIIa. TP82 also immunoprecipitated an as yet unidentified 23,000 molecular weight surface protein from detergent-solubilized platelets. Jennings et al. [1985] immunized mice with purified glycoprotein IIb and detected anti-IIb monoclonal antibodies using a radioimmunoassay in which isolated membranes were fixed to the wells of microtiter plates. They detected a series of monoclonal antibodies, each of which immunoprecipitated a 23,000 molecular weight polypeptide thought to be glycoprotein IIbβ. The ability of these antibodies to activate thrombasthenic platelets was reduced, consistent with this conclusion. Miller et al. [1986] immunized mice with platelets from a patient with platelet-type von Willebrand disease and detected antiplatelet antibodies using a screening assay in which culture supernatants inhibited the agglutination of patient platelets by asialo-vWf. Paradoxically, several supernatants enhanced, rather than inhibited, agglutination. Subsequently, these antibodies were found to activate platelets independently. The monoclonal antibody chosen for further characterization, AG-1, immunoprecipitated a 21,000 molecular weight protein, plus several other proteins with molecular weights of 22,000 to 28,000. These proteins appeared to be distinct from the known platelet proteins in this molecular weight range: Ibβ, IIbβ, and glycoprotein IX. The AG-1 immunoprecipitate also contained Ib, suggesting that at least some of the Ib in the platelet membrane is associated with the proteins containing the AG-1 epitope. The physiologic significance of these reports is not clear but the similarity of the results is intriguing. Studies to confirm that the antibodies actually recognize epitopes on distinct structures would help to put these reports in perspective.

Studies of the interaction of von Willebrand factor with glycoprotein Ib. Platelet adhesion to substances in the vascular subendothelium exposed by trauma is mediated by the plasma protein vWF and represents the initial step in the formation of a hemostatic platelet plug [George et al., 1984]. The in vitro equivalent of this reaction occurs when the antibiotic ristocetin is added to platelet-rich plasma. Following the addition of ristocetin to platelet-rich plasma, vWF binds to the platelet surface, resulting in platelet agglutination. Because platelets from individuals with the Bernard-Soulier syndrome fail to respond in this way to ristocetin and because Bernard-Soulier platelets lack the platelet membrane glycoprotein Ib, it is likely that Ib represents the platelet binding site for the vWF involved in platelet adhesion. The interaction of Ib with vWF has been explored in detail using anti-Ib monoclonal antibodies. These studies have indicated that there are approximately 25,000 Ib molecules/platelet [Coller et al.,

1983a] and that vWF binds to a site on an externally located portion of Ibα that corresponds to glycocalicin [Coller et al., 1983a; Montgomery et al., 1983]. vWF binding to Ib is an entirely different process from vWF binding to IIb/IIIa and is unaffected by monoclonal antibodies to IIb/IIIa [Ruggeri et al., 1983a]. Therefore, these studies have unequivocally established that platelets contain two distinct and functionally separate binding sites for vWF.

Monoclonal antibodies that identify platelet granule proteins on the platelet surface. Two monoclonal antibodies have been reported that were produced by immunizing BALB/c mice with thrombin-stimulated platelets and are directed against a platelet α-granule protein that is expressed on the platelet surface following platelet secretion [McEver and Martin, 1984; Hsu-Lin et al., 1984]. One antibody, S-12, was selected for study because it did not appear to be directed against IIb/IIIa and its binding was substantially augmented by platelet stimulation with thrombin [McEver and Martin, 1984]. The other antibody, KC4, was selected during a screening assay devised to detect antibodies that bound to activated, rather than unactivated, platelets [Hsu-Lin et al., 1984]. Both S-12 and KC4 recognize epitopes on the same 140,000 molecular weight protein [Stenberg et al., 1984; Berman et al., 1985]. This protein is found in the α-granule membrane of resting platelets and is incorporated into the platelet surface membrane following platelet secretion. Although the function of this protein is not known, its presence on the platelet surface is an indication of prior platelet activation.

Monoclonal antibodies have proven to be extraordinarily useful reagents with which to probe platelet function. It is noteworthy that many of the most useful antibodies were found serendipitously from hybridomas originally produced for other purposes. Thus, one must be continuously alert for opportunities when they present themselves. More important, however, this experience indicates that a carefully crafted strategy for antigen presentation and hybridoma screening is essential to maximally utilize the power of the hybridoma technology.

ACKNOWLEDGMENTS

Dr. Bennett is supported by grant HL23809 from the National Institutes of Health, grant 1570M from The Council for Tobacco Research-U.S.A., and is an Established Investigator of the American Heart Association.

REFERENCES

Bennett J (1985). The platelet-fibrinogen interaction. In George JN, Nurden AT, Phillips DR (eds): "Platelet Membrane Glycoproteins." New York: Plenum Press, pp 193–214.

Bennett JS, Hoxie JA, Leitman SF, Vilaire G, Cines DB (1983). Inhibition of fibrinogen binding to stimulated human platelets by a monoclonal antibody. Proc Natl Acad Sci USA 80:2417–2421.

Bennett JS, Vilaire G (1979). Exposure of platelet fibrinogen receptors by ADP and epinephrine. J Clin Invest 74:1393–1401.

Berman CL, Yeo EL, Wencel-Drake JD, Furie BC, Ginsberg MH, Furie B (1985). A platelet alpha granule membrane protein that is associated with the plasma membrane after activation. J Clin Invest 78:130–137.

Brass LF, Shattil SJ, Kunicki TJ, Bennett JS (1985). Effect of calcium on the stability of the platelet membrane glycoprotein IIb-IIIa complex. J Biol Chem 260:7875–7881.

Coller BS (1985). A new murine monoclonal antibody reports an activation-dependent change in the conformation and/or microenvironment of the platelet glycoprotein IIb/IIIa complex. J Clin Invest 76:101–108.

Coller BS, Peerschke EI, Scudder LE, Sullivan CA (1983). A murine monclonal antibody that completely blocks the binding of fibrinogen to platelets produces a thrombasthenic-like state in normal platelets and binds to glycoproteins IIb and/or IIIa. J Clin Invest 72:325–338.

Coller BS, Peerschke EI, Scudder LE, Sullivan CA (1983a). Studies with a murine monoclonal antibody that abolishes ristocetin-induced binding of von Willebrand factor to platelets: Additional evidence is support of GPIb as a platelet receptor for von Willebrand factor. Blood 61:99–110.

DeMarco L, Giromlami A, Zimmerman TS, Ruggeri ZM (1985). Interaction of purified type IIB von Willebrand factor with the platelet membrane glycoprotein Ib induces fibrinogen binding to the glycoprotein IIb/IIIa complex and initiates aggregation. Proc Natl Acad Sci USA 82:7424–7428.

DeMarco L, Giromlami A, Zimmerman TS, Ruggeri ZM (1986). von Willebrand factor interaction with the glycoprotein IIb/IIIa complex. J Clin Invest 77:1272–1277.

DiMinno G, Thiagarajan P, Perussia B, Martinez J, Shapiro S, Trinchieri G, Murphy S (1983). Exposure of platelet fibrinogen binding sites by collagen, arachidonic acid, and ADP: Inhibition by a monoclonal antibody to the glycoprotein IIb-IIIa complex. Blood 61:140–148.

Ey PA, Prowse SJ, Jenkin CR (1978). Isolation of pure IgG_1, IgG_{2a}, and IgG_{2b} immunoglobulins from mouse serum using protein A-sepharose. Immunochemistry 15:429–436.

Gartner TK, Bennett JS (1985). The tetrapeptide analogue of the cell attachment site of fibronectin inhibits platelet aggregation and fibrinogen binding to activated platelets. J Biol Chem 260:11891–11894.

Gartner TK, Power JW, Beechey EH, Bennett JS, Shattil SJ (1985). The tetrapeptide analogue of the alpha chain and the decapeptide analogue of the gamma chain of fibrinogen bind to different sites on the platelet fibrinogen receptor. Blood (suppl. 1) 66:305a.

George JN, Nurden AT, Phillips DR (1984). Molecular defects in interactions of platelets with the vessel wall. N Engl J Med 311:1084–1098.

Ginsberg MH, Forsyth J, Lightsey A, Chediak J, Plow EF (1983). Reduced surface expression and binding of fibronectin by thrombin-stimulated thrombasthenic platelets. J Clin Invest 71:619–624.

Higashihara M, Maeda H, Shibata Y, Kume S, Ohashi T (1985). A monoclonal anti-human platelet antibody: A new platelet aggregation substance. Blood 65:382–391.

Hsu-Lin S-H, Berman CL, Furie BC, August D, Furie B (1984). A platelet membrane protein expressed during platelet activation and secretion. J Biol Chem 259:9121–9126.

Jennings LK, Phillips DR (1982). Purification of glycoprotein IIb and III from human platelet plasma membranes and charaterization of a calcium-dependent glycoprotein IIb-III complex. J Biol Chem 257:10458–10466.

Jennings LK, Phillips DR, Walker WS (1985). Monoclonal antibodies to human platelet glycoprotein IIbβ that initiate distinct platelet responses. Blood 65:1112–1119.

Kenneth RH, McKearn TJ, Bechtol KB (1980). "Monoclonal Antibodies Hybridomas: A New Dimension in Biological Analysis." New York: Plenum Press.

Kohler G, Milstein C (1975). Continuous cultures of fused cells secreting antibody of predetermined specificity. Nature (London) 256:495–497.

Kunicki TJ, Aster RH (1979). Isolation and immunologic characterization of the human platelet alloantigen PI^{A1}. Mol Immunol 16:353–360.

Kunicki TJ, Pidard D, Rosa J-P, Nurden AT (1981). The formation of Ca^{++}-dependent complexes of platelet membrane glycoproteins IIb and IIIa in solution as determined by cross-immunoelectrophoresis. Blood 58:268–278.

Laemmli UK (1970). Cleavage of structural proteins during the assembly of the head of the bacteriophage T4. Nature (London) 227:680–682.

Lombardo VT, Hodson E, Roberts JR, Kunicki TJ, Zimmerman TS, Ruggeri ZM (1985). Independent modulation of von Willebrand factor and fibrinogen binding to the platelet membrane glycoprotein IIb/IIIa complex as demonstrated by monoclonal antibody. J Clin Invest 76:1950–1958.

Majerus PW, Brodie GN (1972). The binding of phytohemagglutinins to human platelet plasma membranes. J Biol Chem 247:4253–4257.

McEver RP, Martin MN (1984). A monoclonal antibody to a membrane glycoprotein binds only to activated platelets. J Biol Chem 259:9799–9804.

McEver RP, Bennett EM, Martin MN (1983). Identification of two structurally and functionally distinct sites on human platelet membrane glycoprotein IIb-IIIa using monoclonal antibodies. J Biol Chem 258:5269–5273.

Miller JL, Kupinski JM, Hustad KO (1986). Characterization of a platelet membrane protein of low molecular weight associated with platelet activation following binding by monoclonal antibody AG-1. Blood 68:743–751.

Montgomery RR, Kunicki TJ, Taves C, Pidard D, Corcoran M (1983). Diagnosis of Bernard-Soulier syndrome and Glanzmann's thrombasthenia with a monoclonal assay on whole blood. J Clin Invest 71:385–389.

Phillips DR (1972). Effect of trypsin on the exposed polypeptides and glycoproteins in the platelet membrane. Biochemistry 11:4582–4588.

Phillips DR, Agin PP (1977). Platelet membrane defects in Glanzmann's thrombasthenia. Evidence for decreased amounts of two major glycoproteins. J Clin Invest 60:535–545.

Pidard D, Montgomery RR, Bennett JS, Kunicki TJ (1983). Interaction of AP-2, a monoclonal antibody specific for the human platelet glycoprotein IIb-IIIa complex, with intact platelets. J Biol Chem 258:12582–12586.

Pierschbacher MD, Ruoslahti E (1984). Cell attachment activity of fibronectin can be duplicated by small synthetic fragments of the molecule. Nature (London) 309:30–33.

Plow EF, McEver RP, Coller BS, Woods VL, Marguerie GA, Ginsberg MH (1985). Related binding mechanisms for fibrinogen, fibronectin, von Willebrand factor, and thrombospondin on thrombin-stimulated human platelets. Blood 66:724–727.

Rink TJ, Smith SW, Tsien RY (1982). Cytoplasmic free Ca^{2+} in human platelets: Ca^{2+} thresholds and Ca-independent activation for shape change and secretion. FEBS Lett 148:21–26.

Ruggeri ZM, Bader R, DeMarco L (1983). Glanzmann's thrombasthenia: Deficient binding of von Willebrand factor of thrombin-stimulated platelets. Proc Natl Acad Sci USA 79:6038–6041.

Ruggeri ZM, DeMarco L, Gatti L, Bader R, Montgomery RR (1983a). Platelets have more than one binding site for von Willebrand factor. J Clin Invest 72:1–12.

Sadler JE, Shelton-Inloes BB, Sorace JM, Harlan JM, Titani K, Davie EW (1985). Cloning and characterization of two cDNAs coding for human von Willebrand factor. Proc Natl Acad Sci USA 82:6394–6398.

Schullek J, Jordan J, Montgomery RR (1984) Interaction of von Willebrand factor with human platelets in the plasma milleu. J Clin Invest 73:421–428.

Shattil SJ, Hoxie JA, Cunningham M, Brass LF (1985). Changes in the platelet membrane glycoprotein IIb-IIIa complex during platelet activation. J Biol Chem 260:11107–11114.

Stenberg PE, McEver RP, Shuman MA, Jacques YV, Bainton DF (1985). A platelet alpha-granule membrane protein (GMP-140) is expressed on the plasma membrane after activation. J Cell Biol 101:880–886.

Towbin H, Staehelin T, Gordon J (1979). Electrophorectic transfer of proteins from polyacrylamide gels to nitrocellulose sheets: Procedure and some applications. Proc Natl Acad Sci USA 76:4350–4354.

Zucker MB, Grant RA (1978). Nonreversible loss of platelet aggregability induced by calcium deprivation. Blood 52:505–514.

Modern Methods in Pharmacology, Volume 4
Methods for Studying Platelets and Megakaryocytes, pages 109–131

Immunochemical Methods to Study Platelet-Associated Proteins

ALVIN H. SCHMAIER

INTRODUCTION

Investigations as to the function of platelets rely on assays that measure platelet adhesion, aggregation, and agglutination. These studies for the most part are global assays, testing the entire complex biological function of these cell particles. These types of assays are inadequate to identify and study the participation of a single platelet-associated protein in platelet function. Alternatively, enzymatic or coagulant assays designed to detect specific proteins associated with platelets usually have a high degree of sensitivity but often suffer from a low degree of specificity due to the complex array of enzymes and inhibitors found within platelets. Immunochemical assays offer a high degree of sensitivity and specificity. The following is a summary of various immunochemical techniques that can be applied to identify and determine the mechanisms of availability of platelet-associated proteins. Although these studies focus on one protein, platelet high molecular weight kininogen, they are applicable for study on any protein where specific antibodies to that protein are available.

The plasma kininogens (high and low molecular weight) are substrates from which the vasoactive peptide bradykinin is released. Recent studies also indicate that both plasma kininogens are inhibitors to tissue-derived cysteine proteinases: cathepsins, papains, and calpains [Muller-Esterl et al., 1985; Ohkubo et al., 1984; Sueyoshi et al., 1985; Schmaier et al., 1986a]. High molecular weight kininogen (HMWK) is also the procofactor for activation as well as a substrate of the plasma serine proteases, factor XIIa, kallikrein, and factor XIa. Plasma kallikrein cleaves HMWK in a three-step sequence pattern [Mori and Nagasawa, 1981] (Fig. 1). The first cleavage yields a "nicked" kininogen composed of two disulfide-linked 62,000 and 56,000 Mr chains on reduced SDS gels. The second

From the Department of Medicine, Hematology/Oncology Section, and the Thrombosis Research Center, Temple University School of Medicine, Philadelphia, Pennsylvania 19140.

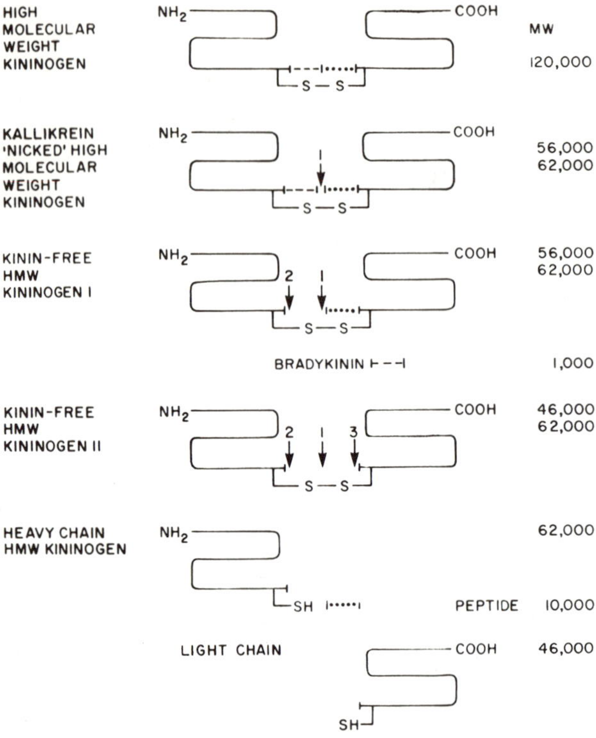

Fig. 1. Structure of plasma kininogens. Note that the heavy chains of LMWK and HMWK are identical and light chain of LMWK is not shown.

cleavage yields bradykinin and an intermediate kinin-free protein of equal molecular weight to nicked HMWK. A third cleavage results in a stable kinin-free protein composed of two disulfide-linked 62,000 and 46,000 Mr chains. Since one gene directs the synthesis of both plasma kininogens [Takagaki et al., 1985], the heavy chain of HMWK is indistinguishable from low molecular weight kininogen (LMWK). The molecules apparently differ, owing to gene splicing. The distinguishing feature between HMWK and LMWK is the presence of the Mr 56,000 light chain on the carboxy terminal end of HMWK compared to the Mr 5,000 light chain on LMWK. The light chain of HMWK contains unique antigenic sites and possesses coagulant activity due to its ability to bind to surfaces as well as prekallikrein and factor XII. Both these properties serve to distinguish it from LMWK.

Platelets have been proposed as an alternate pathway of intrinsic coagulation activation in the absence of factor XII [Walsh, 1972]. Platelets have associated factor XI-like activity and factor XI antigen [Tuszynski et al., 1982]. Factor XIa specifically binds to activated platelets in the presence of HMWK [Sinha et al., 1984]. The identification of a platelet form of HMWK [Schmaier et al., 1983] indicates that the platelet could participate in factor XI activation, as well as serve as a negatively charged surface for contact phase zymogen activation in vivo.

Preparation and Characterization of Antisera Antibodies to HMWK

HMWK is an alpha globulin with an isoelectric point of 4.7 [Kato et al., 1981]. Since the heavy chain of HMWK is identical to the heavy chain of LMWK, injection of purified HMWK into animals will usually result in antisera that recognizes both HMWK and LMWK. Polyclonal antisera to plasma kininogens is produced in goats by intramuscular injection of 500 μg purified HMWK in complete Freund's adjuvant followed by a 250 μg injection of HMWK in complete Freund's adjuvant 4 weeks later [Schmaier et al., 1984]. The specificity of the antisera to HMWK is tested by its ability to neutralize the coagulant activity of plasma HMWK. In order to perform a neutralization experiment, the crude antisera is precipitated with 50% ammonium sulfate followed by two successive kaolin adsorptions (40 mg/ml) for 30 min at 37°C so that the final crude antibody preparation has negligible HMWK, prekallikrein, factor XII, or factor XI coagulant activity.

Monospecific antisera to total plasma kininogen can most simply be produced by adsorption with total kininogen deficient plasma. Antitotal kininogen antisera results in a double precipitin arc against normal human plasma on immunoelectrophoresis (Fig. 2) [Schmaier et al., 1984]. Further adsorption of the antisera with Fitzgerald plasma (plasma deficient in HMWK but not LMWK), purified LMWK, or the heavy chain of HMWK will result in monospecific antisera to HMWK (Fig. 2) [Schmaier et al., 1983]. The most direct means to produce antisera that uniquely recognizes HMWK is to immunize with the purified light chain HMWK.

IMMUNOCHEMICAL ASSAYS

HMWK in plasma can be quantified and characterized by radial immunodiffusion, electroimmunodiffusion, and crossed immunoelectrophoresis. However, studies on platelets required the development of a more sensitive immunochemical assay.

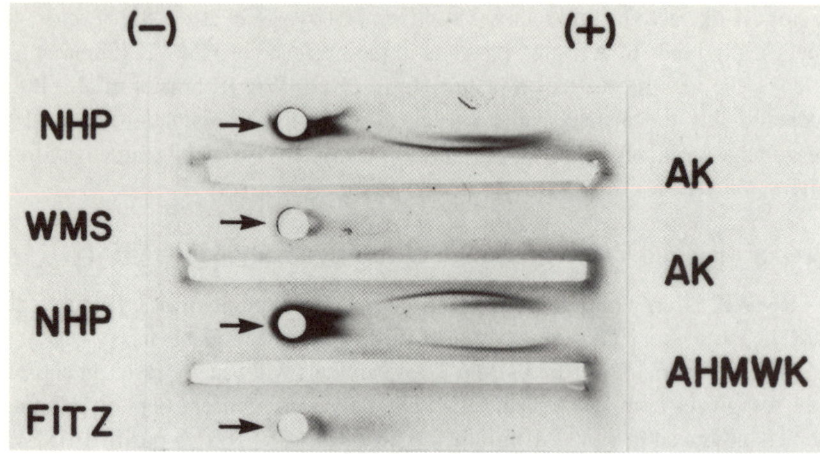

Fig. 2. Immunoelectrophoresis of antisera to plasma kininogens. Antisera to total kininogen (AK) (both HMWK and LMWK); NHP, normal human plasma; WMS, Williams plasma, i.e., plasma deficient in total kininogen; FITZ, Fitzgerald plasma, i.e., plasma deficient in only HMWK. Antisera to HMWK (AHMWK).

Competitive Enzyme Linked Immunosorbent Assay (CELISA) for HMWK

Reagents

Polystyrene cuvettes (Gilford Instr. Lab. Inc., Oberlin, OH)
Specific goat antisera or antibody to the light chain of HMWK
Rabbit antigoat whole immunoglobulin conjugated with alkaline phosphatase (Sigma Chemical Corp., St. Louis, MO)
Substrate: p-nitrophenylphosphate disodium (Sigma Chemical Corp., St. Louis, MO)
Radioimmunoassay grade bovine serum albumin (Sigma Chemical Corp., St. Louis, MO)
Coupling Buffer: 0.1 M Na_2CO_3 pH 9.8
Substrate Buffer: 0.05 M Na_2CO_3, 1 mM MgCl pH 9.8
PBS-Tween: 0.01 M sodium phosphate pH 7.4, 0.15 M NaCl containing 0.05% Tween 20

Procedure. This assay was based on a modification of the procedure of Engvall [1980]. A schematic of this competitive assay is shown in Figure 3. On day 1, 100–500 ng of purified HMWK diluted in 0.1 M Na_2CO_3 pH 9.6 is linked to the surface of polystyrene cuvette wells by overnight incubation at 37°C. On the same day, incubation mixtures in 1.5 ml conical polypropylene tubes precoated with 0.2% bovine serum albumin are made containing the following: 0.15 ml of

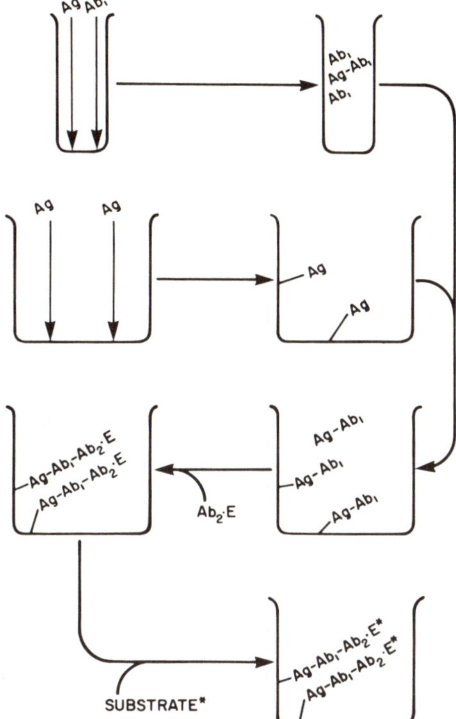

Fig. 3. Schematic of competitive enzyme-linked immunosorbent assay (CELISA) for HMWK. Ag, antigen linked to cuvettes; Ab_1, specific antibody or antisera; Ab_2-E, second antibody conjugated with enzyme. See text for method.

antigen (standards or test samples) diluted in PBS-Tween and 0.15 ml of a previously optimal titered specific goat antihuman HMWK antisera or antibody. These samples are incubated overnight at 37°C. On day 2, each antigen-linked cuvette well is washed three times with PBS-Tween and incubated with 0.2% bovine serum albumin in water for 1 hour at 37°C. After washing the cuvettes, 0.2 ml from each incubation mixture is added to each cuvette well and incubated for 2 hours at 37°C. At the conclusion of this incubation, the rewashed wells are exposed to a previous optimally titered second antibody (rabbit-antigoat whole immunoglobulin) conjugated with alkaline phosphatase diluted in PBS-Tween. After another 2.5-hour incubation at 37°C, the washed cuvettes receive sequentially timed additions of 0.4 ml of p-nitrophenylphosphate disodium (1 mg/ml) in substrate buffer. At precise time intervals (20–30 min) after the addition of the substrate to each well, the amount of hydrolysis of the substrate in each well is either stopped with sequential timed additions of 0.4 ml of 2 M NaOH (final concentration 1 M NaOH) or are sequentially measured spectrophotometrically in a PR 50 EIA Processor-Reader (Gilford Instr. Lab., Inc.) at 405 nm. Since this is a competitive assay, the amount of optical absorbance is inversely proportional to the amount of antigen.

The development of an assay such as this is dependent on the optimal titrations of linked-antigen, specific antibody, and enzyme-conjugated second antibody. The determinations of these optimal titrations can only be done empirically. In general, to obtain maximal sensitivity, the amount of antigen used for coating is decreased as far as practicable and the amount of antibody added should be limited. One approach is a checkerboard titration, as described by Engvall [1980], of dilutions of various amounts of linking antigen with one titer of specific antibody versus various titers of specific antibody with one concentration of linked-antigen. This titration approach presupposes that there is one optimal titer of enzyme-conjugated second antibody that is best for all amounts of specific antibody. Using commercial second antibody conjugates and different batches of specific antisera, this is often not the case. Another approach, which we use, is to decide in advance the range of sensitivity of the assay desired and then optimize the titration of the reagents at hand. For example, for design of an assay with a linear portion of the standard curve between 5 to 100 ng, antigen in 100–500 ng amounts will be linked to the cuvette. Specific antisera in multiple dilutions, followed by the enzyme-conjugated secondary antibody at various concentrations will be sequentially introduced (Fig. 4). The optical absorbance measured represents the total value (or the amount of absorbance if no antigen is preincubated with the antisera) to be obtained in the final CELISA. After comparison of the total absorbance of multiple specific antisera dilutions using a few different conjugated antibody titers, the titers of the two antibodies used, in sequence, that give the highest absorbance over the range of optical linearity of the spectrophotometer for a fixed reaction time (usually 20–30 min) are chosen. In Figure 4, using these principles we chose an initial dilution of the primary antibody at 1/500 with a dilution of the secondary antibody conjugated with alkaline phosphatase at 1/500. The final primary antibody dilution, if none were consumed in the overnight incubation, would be 1/1000. For this specific batch of primary antibody and conjugate, the total absorbance would be 2.0—the upper limit of linearity on our instrument and a value that would give the steepest slope on our competitive assay.

Although we use automated equipment, the entire assay can be performed in polystyrene test tubes and read manually in a spectrophotometer. A crucial feature for the success of this type of assay is that each reaction after the addition of substrate is read or stopped with NaOH at precisely the same time interval

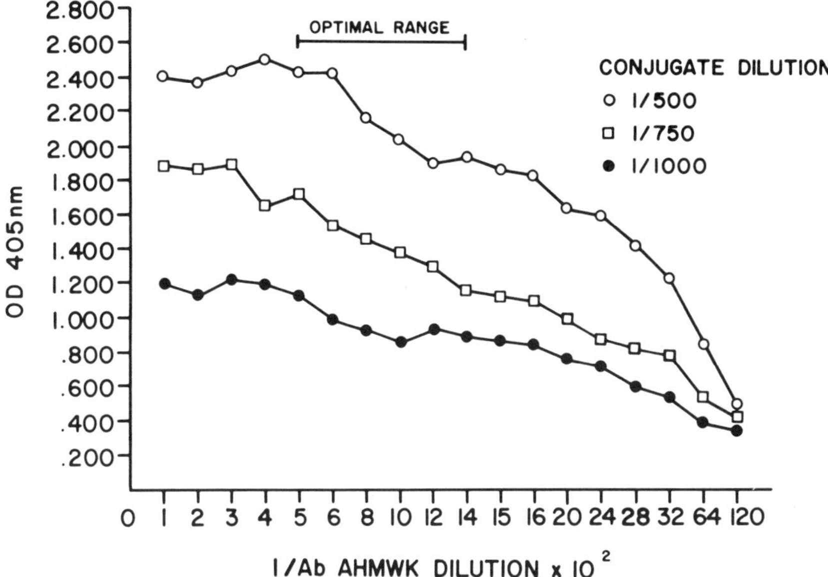

Fig. 4. Titering primary and secondary antibody for CELISA. The dilution of primary antibody (abscissa) is plotted aginst the optical density (OD) at 405 nm using three titers, 1/500 (○), 1/750 (□), 1/1000 (●) of second antibody conjugated with alkaline phosphatase. The optimal range of both primary and secondary antibody for use in the CELISA is given by the bar.

after beginning the enzyme hydrolysis. This manipulation requires some automated instrumentation. We have found it best to perform standard curves and test samples in triplicate at 10–15 different dilutions. In this laboratory, data for the standard curve and test sample determination are analyzed by a computer [Cannellas and Karu, 1981]. Antigen values are determined in absolute amounts and original concentration are calculated considering the dilutions of the standards and test samples.

Using the CELISA, HMWK antigen as a purified protein, as a purified protein reconstituted into total kininogen immunodeficient plasma, and as antigen in normal plasma gives superimposable, parallel competition inhibition curves (Fig. 5). On 20 individually obtained normal plasmas, HMWK antigen assayed as a concentration of 105 μg/ml. The interassay coefficient of variation of a single plasma sample assayed four times over a 1-month period is 3.0%. These values compare favorably as to sensitivity and precision with a previously reported radioimmunoassay for HMWK [Proud et al., 1980]. Using this radio-

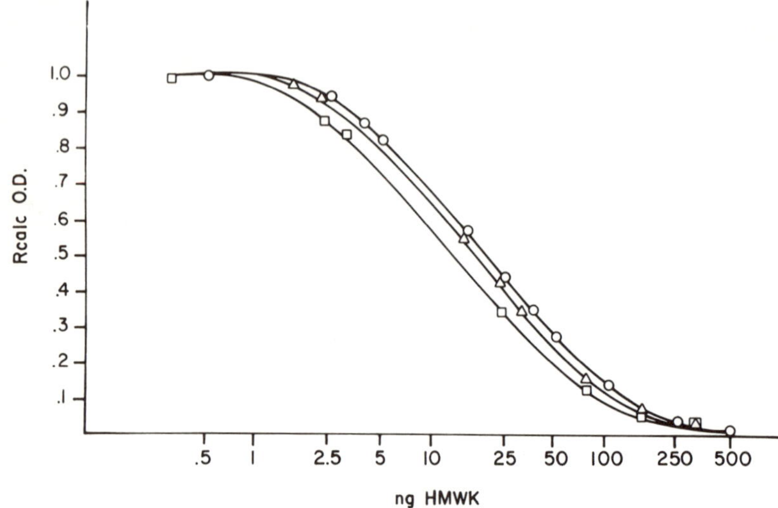

Fig. 5. Competitive inhibition curves of CELISA for HMWK. The ordinate is the relative absorbance (Rcalc O.D.) and the abscissa is the absolute amount of antigen incubated with antisera. Inhibition curve produced by purified HMWK (□); inhibition curve produced by pooled normal plasma (○); inhibition curve produced by total kininogen—immunodeficient plasma reconstituted with purified HMWK (△). From J Clin Invest 71:1477 [1983] by copyright permission of the American Society for Clinical Investigation.

immunoassay, the mean value of plasma HMWK in normal plasma by radioimmunoassay was 90 μg/ml.

PREPARATION OF PLATELETS

Albumin Density Gradient Centrifugation and Gel-Filtration (AGGF)

Platelets are washed by a modified combined technique of albumin density gradient centrifugation and gel-filtration [Timmons and Hawiger, 1978]. Eight ml of platelet-rich plasma is layered on a 2.5 ml discontinuous increasing albumin density gradient (10, 15, 20, 30, 40%) prepared according to the method of Walsh et al. [1977]. Forty percent stock solution of albumin (Sigma, bovine-serum albumin #4503) is prepared by the procedure of Walsh et al. [1977]. In preparation of the albumin gradient, it is diluted in Hepes buffered Tyrode's solution (3.5 g/l Hepes, 8 g/l NaCl, 0.2 g/l KCl, 1 g/l $NaCo_3$, 0.05 g/l NaH_2PO_4, 0.2 g/l $MgCl_2$, 3.5 g/l BSA, 1 g/l dextrose pH 7.35). After centrifugation for 20 min at 900g at 23°C, the platelet layer above the 40% albumin cushion is removed and 5 ml of resuspended platelets are applied to a 60 ml column of Sepharose 2B in Hepes buffered Tyrode's solution. Void volume fractions are pooled.

IDENTIFICATION OF PLATELET HMWK

Four issues were considered in the identification of platelet HMWK, which exists in trace quantities to the amount of HMWK in the surrounding plasma: 1) What was the degree of plasma contamination in the washed platelet aliquots that were studied for the total platelet HMWK content? 2) Was the HMWK antigen found with platelets really platelet-associated plasma HMWK? 3) Was plasma HMWK taken-up by platelets? and 4) What contribution did the suspension medium of washed platelets make to the total amount of platelet HMWK measured in platelet lysates?

^{125}I-HMWK is introduced in platelet-rich plasma (PRP) to be used as a tracer to determine the amount of the radiolabel recovered in the final washed platelets. HMWK was purified by a modified technique [Schmaier et al., 1986b] of Kerbiriou and Griffin [1979] and was radiolabeled with ^{125}I using Iodogen (Pierce) by a modified technique [Schmaier et al., 1983] of Fraker and Speck [1978]. The radiolabeled tracer technique is used to estimate the amount of plasma HMWK that might contaminate the washed platelet aliquot. Its use presupposes that the radiolabeled protein is in equilibrium with the unlabeled plasma HMWK. Whether the ^{125}I-HMWK was incubated 5 min or 3 hours with the PRP, the percentage of the tracer remaining with the washed platelets was the same. This study estimated that 0.028% or 2.24 ng HMWK/10^8 platelets could be due to plasma HMWK contaminating the washed platelet aliquot. At best, this technique is a lowest estimate of plasma contamination in washed platelets. Plasma antigen can be tightly bound and nonexchangeable with the platelet surface. In order to determine whether we are measuring platelet-associated plasma HMWK, a semiquantitative indirect antibody consumption assay using the CELISA was developed to estimate if plasma HMWK antigen was on the unstimulated platelet surface.

Indirect Antibody Consumption Assay Using the CELISA

7.5 ml of fresh platelets (1×10^9 plts/ml) pretreated with 1 μM PGE_1 (Sigma) and prepared by albumin density gradient centrifugation and gel-filtration are incubated at 37°C with an equal volume of anti-HMWK antisera. PGE_1 (1 μM) is also added to the resuspended platelets from the albumin gradient and to the gel-filtration buffer. Alternatively, platelets can be prepared by the technique of Mustard et al. [1972] without the addition of PGE_1. The antisera or antibody used was previously diluted to half its optimal titer for the CELISA in PBS-Tween and centrifuged at 100,000g for 30 min to remove aggregates. In addition, total kininogen-deficient plasma (1/250) was added to the diluted antisera to possibly prevent nonspecific absorbance of the antibody to platelet Fc receptors. One volume of intact washed platelets is incubated with antisera. A second 7.5 ml aliquot of identically washed platelets was centrifuged at 12,000g and its supernatant is also incubated 1:1 with anti-HMWK antisera prepared as above. After incubation of the antisera with platelets or its supernatant for 30–60 min, the platelets are removed by centrifugation at 12,000g and the adsorbed antisera is then incubated with known amounts of purified HMWK to generate a competition inhibition curve. Preliminary experiments with purified HMWK revealed that 90% of antigen-antibody interaction takes place within the first hour of incubation.

The principle of the indirect antibody consumption assay using the CELISA is illustrated in Figure 6. An optimal titer of antibody will give a certain slope. As the titer of antibody is decreased (e.g., 1/500 to 1/1500), the slope of the competitive inhibition curve will become flattened and shifted to the left, indicating a decreased slope. Thus, a change in the slope of the competitive curve indirectly indicates that antigen was available to adsorb and decrease the titer of

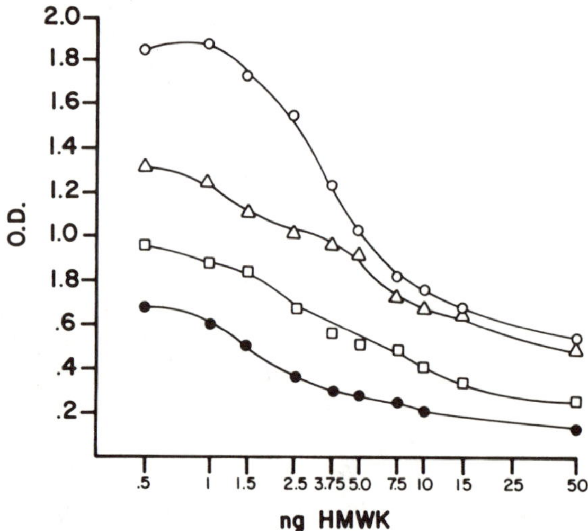

Fig. 6. Principle of indirect antibody consumption assay using the CELISA. Competition inhibition curves produced by antisera to HMWK from dilutions: 1:500 (○), 1:800 (▲), 1:1000 (□), 1:1500 (●), against the same amounts of purified HMWK. Curves are plotted with the actual optical density (O.D.) at 405 nm on the ordinate versus the absolute amount of HMWK antigen on the abscissa.

antibody that could subsequently react with known amounts of purified antigen. In our studies on platelet HMWK, unactivated platelets give a superimposable competition inhibition curve with the suspension medium of these platelets (Fig. 7) indicating that little ($\leqslant$ 3 ng/10^8 plts) platelet-associated plasma HMWK was tightly bound and nonexchangeable with the platelet surface.

Measurement of Total Platelet HMWK

Platelets for lysis to determine the total amount of platelet HMWK are prepared by AGGF. PEG_1 (1 μM) is included in the collection anticoagulant, resuspension buffer for the platelets from the albumin gradient, and the gel-filtration buffer. Without PGE_1, direct measurement of the platelet suspension buffer for HMWK antigen shows a two- to threefold increase in antigen levels suggesting that platelets were activated during the washing procedure. Platelets for assay for total HMWK antigen levels are then solubilized at 22°C for 30 min with 0.5% Triton X-100. In 15 normal donors, the mean platelet HMWK level was 55 ng $\pm$ 22/10^8 (mean $\pm$ SD) platelets (Fig. 8). Direct measurement on the suspension buffer of each aliquot of platelets revealed a mean value of 2.8 ng $\pm$

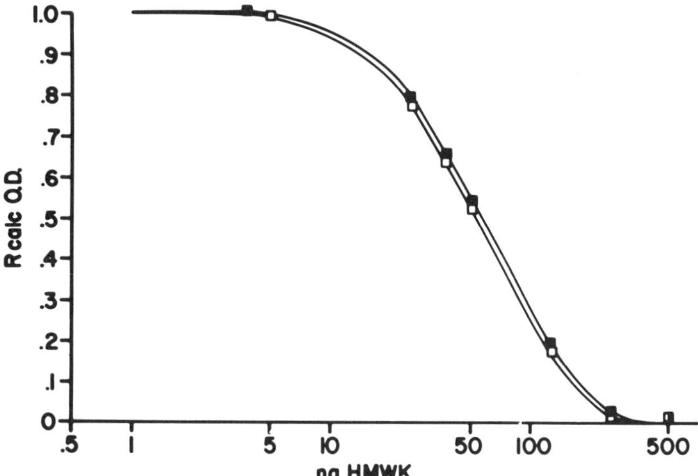

Fig. 7. Competition inhibition curves produced by purified HMWK with antiserum adsorbed with platelets and unadsorbed total kininogen antisera. Anti-total kininogen antisera were incubated with an equal volume of whole platelets or the supernatant of the platelet suspension. The platelet-adsorbed antisera and unadsorbed antisera were then incubated with equal amounts of purified HMWK to produce a standard curve using the CELISA. The standard curve produced by platelet-adsorbed antisera (□) is plotted along with the standard curve produced by unadsorbed antisera (■). From J Clin Invest 71:1477 [1983] by copyright permission of the American Society for Clinical Investigation.

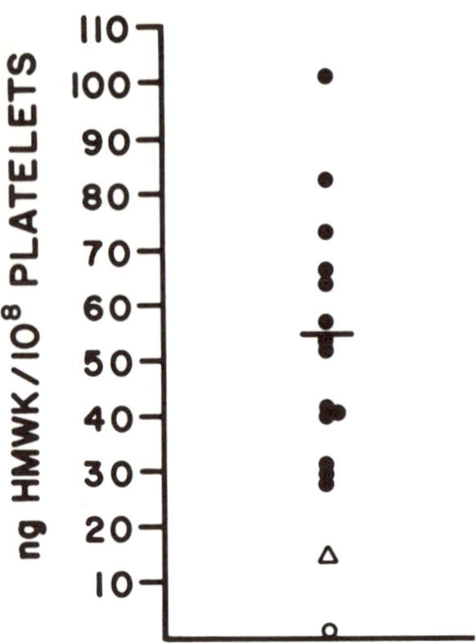

Fig. 8. Total platelet HMWK in normal (●), total kininogen-deficient platelets (○), and gray platelets (△).

2.1/10^8 platelets or 5% of the total. One individual with a congenital absence of platelet alpha granules (the gray platelet syndrome) had a total platelet HMWK level of 16 ng/10^8 platelets. Another individual with a plasma deficiency of both HMWK and LMWK was found to have a platelet HMWK level of less than 5 ng/10^9 platelets. The ability of platelets to take up plasma HMWK was studied by incubating washed total kininogen-deficient platelets in normal plasma for 1 hour at 37°C. After rewashing these platelets by AGGF, the level of platelet HMWK was still lower than 5 ng/10^9 platelets. This result indicated that the platelet and plasma pools of HMWK are separate. Lastly, platelet HMWK antigen from normal platelets was immunochemically identical to plasma HMWK as evidenced by the platelet antigen producing parallel competitive inhibition to plasma antigen (Fig. 9).

MECHANISMS OF AVAILABILITY

Secretion of Platelet HMWK

Platelet secretion studies were performed to determine whether platelet HMWK was made available from platelets by being released into the suspending platelet supernatant when platelets are activated. Secretion studies for platelet HMWK are performed on AGGF platelets. Values for the total content of platelet HMWK are obtained by lysing platelets by freezing and thawing, four times on

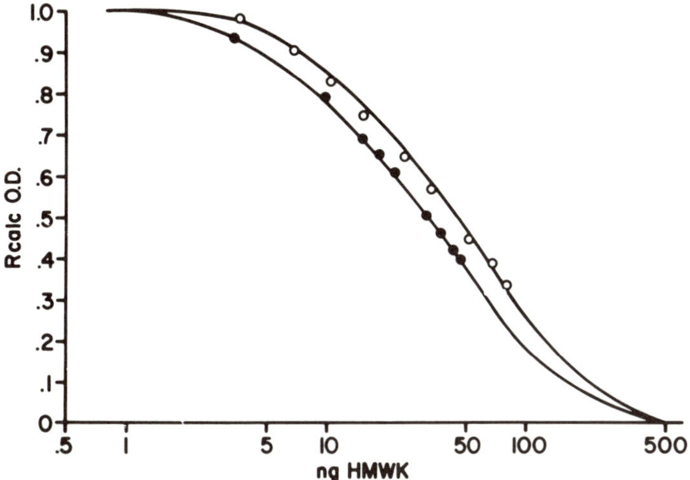

Fig. 9. Competition inhibition curve showing that platelet HMWK antigen is immunochemically indistinguishable from plasma HMWK antigen. Inhibition curve produced by pooled normal plasma (○); inhibition curve produced by solubilized platelets (●). From J Clin Invest 71:1477 [1983] by copyright permission of the American Society for Clinical Investigation.

dry ice and at 37°C after the platelets are diluted 1:3 with deionized water or by adding 0.2–0.5% Triton X-100 for 30 min at 22°C. By either technique, no difference in the amount of the total platelet HMWK is measured. A platelet dense granule marker for secretion studies was obtained by incubated platelets with ^{14}[C]5-hydroxytryptamine (New England Nuclear) and its secretion is assessed by the method of Jerushalmy and Zucker [1966]. Platelet lysis during agonist stimulation of platelets is determined by lactic dehydrogenase loss [Wroblewski and Ladue, 1955]. Platelet alpha granule secretion is assessed by the measurement of low affinity platelet factor 4 secretion [Rucinski et al., 1979]. Platelets to be used in secretion studies were also incubated the metabolic inhibitors, antimycin A (15 μg/ml), 2-deoxy-D-glucose (30 mM), and D-gluconic acid δ-lactone (10 mM) (all purchased from Sigma) to inhibit platelet aerobic and anaerobic glycolysis [Schmaier and Colman, 1980] as well as glycogenolysis [Dangelmaier and Holmsen, 1983]. The addition of D-gluconic acid δ-lactone is essential to block 95% of the platelets' ability to respond to platelet agonists.

For concentration-dependent reactions or fixed dose secretion experiments, platelets in glass or plastic cuvettes are incubated in an aluminum block or water bath at 37°C positioned over a magnetic stirrer (1,000 to 1,200 rpm). At precisely 10 min from the introduction of the stimulus, each cuvette is placed on ice. Aliquots of activated platelets used for ^{14}[C]5-hydroxytryptamine determination are centrifuged in a microcentrifuge tube at 12,000g containing 135 μM formaldehyde, 5 mM EDTA (4 parts platelets/1 part formaldehyde-EDTA). The addition of this mixture prevents artifactual loss of ^{14}[C]5-hydroxytryptamine during the centrifugation procedure [Dangelmaier and Holmsen, 1983]. Other platelet supernatants of activated platelets and controls for other studies are directly obtained after a 12,000g centrifugation in a microcentrifuge. All samples are then immediately frozen at −70°C till time of assay. All secretion studies are performed with a nonstimulated control. Percent secretion (or loss) is determined by the ratio of the supernatant of the agonist-treated specimen to the supernatant of the platelet lysates after the value of the control supernatant is subtracted from both. Lastly, the use of different platelet agonists requires special cautions. Soluble collagen has an acid pH so that each batch of collagen needs to be tested so that maximal doses are not producing artifactual platelet lysis from a drop in the pH of the reaction mixture to less than 7.3. Likewise, with doses of the calcium ionophore A23187 greater than 15 μM used on washed platelets, one may obtain cell lysis greater than 5%.

Platelet HMWK is secreted in a concentration-dependent manner using different agonists (Fig. 10). With both A23187 (CalBiochem Behring) and collagen (Worthington) at lower doses, secretion of platelet HMWK paralleled that of the alpha granule marker, low affinity platelet factor and appearing before the dense granule marker ^{14}[C]5-hydroxytryptamine. These functional data are consistent with an alpha granule location for platelet HMWK [Kaplan et al., 1979]. The alpha granule localization of platelet HMWK has been confirmed by studies on a patient with the gray platelet syndrome who had levels of total platelet HMWK 26% of normal (Fig. 8) and by formal platelet subcellular localization studies [Schmaier et al., 1986b] using the technique of Fukami et al. [1978]. The results of platelet secretion showed that at studies maximal doses of A23187 and collagen, 46% and 32%, respectively, of the total platelet HMWK was secreted. The extent of the total amount of secretion of HMWK with these agonists at maximal doses was less than that seen with the alpha granule marker, low affinity platelet factor four ($\geqslant$ 66% secretion). The secretion of only 25% to 40% of the total platelet content of a high molecular weight hemostatic cofactor contained within platelet alpha granules, in contrast to low affinity platelet factor 4 [Rucinski et al., 1979] has been noted previously for platelet fibronectin [Ginsberg et al., 1979], von Willebrand factor [Koutts et al., 1978], and C1 inhibitor [Schmaier et al., 1985]. This finding suggests that platelet alpha granules may differentially secrete their granule contents or that the proteins remain tightly bound to the external platelet membrane after secretion.

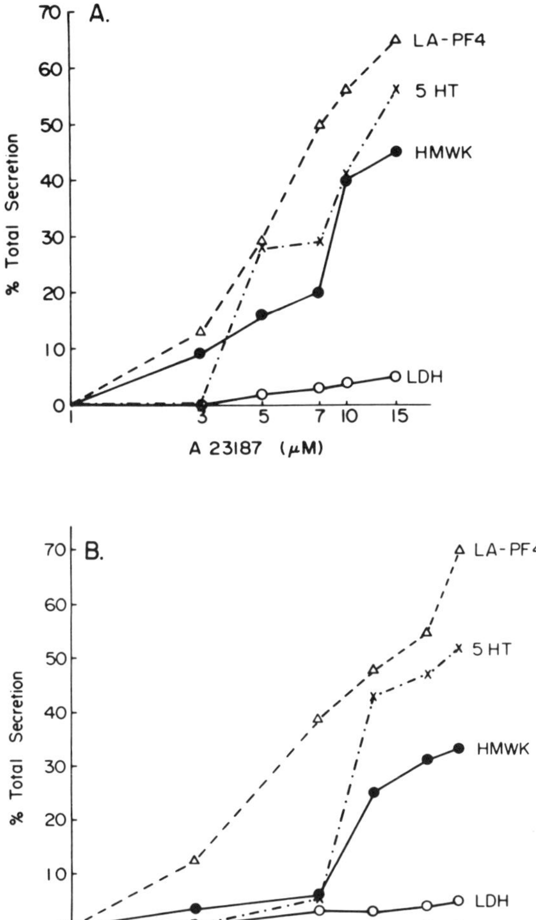

Fig. 10. Secretion of platelet HMWK by Ionophore A23187 (A) and collagen (B). Data plotted are one representative experiment with agonist. Final concentration is plotted on the abscissa of the dose-response of agonist to percentage of total secretion, plotted on the ordinate. LA-PF_4, low affinity platelet factor 4; 5HT, [^{14}C]5-hydroxytryptamine; LDH, lactic dehydrogenase. From J Clin Invest 71:1477 [1983] by copyright permission of the American Society for Clinical Investigation.

Expression of Platelet HMWK on the Activated Platelet Surface

Since platelets only secrete 40% of their total platelet HMWK, a study was performed to determine if some of the remaining platelet HMWK, not secreted, becomes localized on the external membrane of the activated platelets, using the CELISA in a quantitative indirect antibody consumption assay [Schmaier et al., 1986b]. Four hundred fifty ml of blood from two donors is collected (1:10) into 73 mM citric acid, 3 mM trisodium citrate, and 2% dextrose, and after adjusting the pH to 6.5 with the anticoagulant, the platelets are washed by the technique of Mustard et al. [1972]. Apyrase is prepared from potatoes by the method of Molnar and Lorand [1961] and is titered so that the minimal amount necessary to prevent second-wave platelet aggregation with ADP at a threshold dose is used. The final washed platelets are resuspended in HEPES buffered Tyrode's solution to a concentration from 3 to 9 $\times$ 10^9 platelets/ml. These washed platelets are used to prepare activated platelets.

A schematic for the preparation of activated platelets is shown in Figure 11. The washed platelets are divided into three aliquots. Two aliquots are treated with PGE_1 (1 μM) and incubated 40 min in a 37°C water bath. A third aliquot receives 0.4 mM Gly-Pro-Arg-Pro (Sigma). The Gly-Pro-Arg-Pro is to prevent fibrin polymerization and platelet aggregation of activated platelets [Harfenist et al., 1982]. After treating the platelets with Gly-Pro-Arg-Pro, thrombin (0.5 U/ml) is introduced and incubated for 10 min at 37°C without stirring. Following

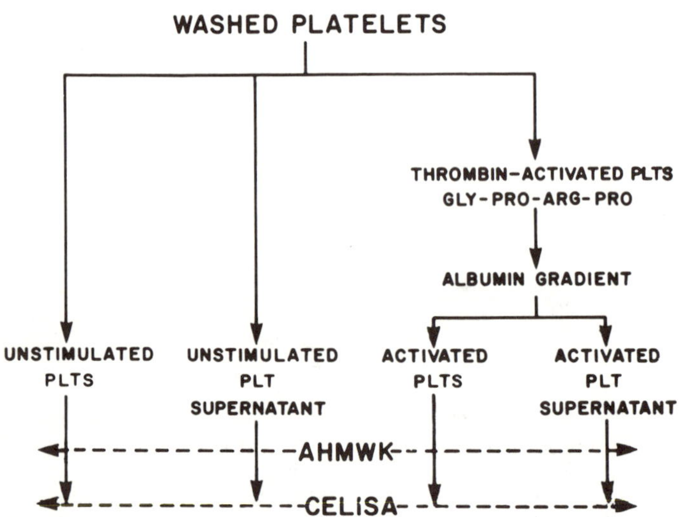

Fig. 11. Schematic for indirect antibody consumption assay to determine the expression of platelet HMWK antigen on the external platelet membrane. See text for method.

thrombin stimulation, the activated platelets are then layered on 2.5 ml discontinuous albumin density gradient and centrifuged at 900g for 20 min. The activated platelets form a layer over the 40% albumin cushion and the activated platelet supernatant—a platelet releasate—remains above the gradient. The activated platelets are then resuspended in HEPES buffered Tyrode's solution containing 0.4 mM Gly-Pro-Arg-Pro. A second platelet aliquot is centrifuged at 12,000g and the supernatant collected. Thus, four platelet specimens are collected: an aliquot of intact, unactivated platelets; supernatant from unactivated platelets; activated platelet supernatant; and activated platelets, themselves.

The platelet samples are prepared in order to be employed in a modified use of the CELISA for HMWK as an indirect antibody consumption assay. Since membrane-expressed platelet HMWK would not be soluble to allow for a direct determination of its presence and solubilization of activated platelets would liberate intracellular platelet HMWK, an experimental design was developed to determine if surface-expressed platelet HMWK could be detected when whole platelets were incubated with the antisera directed to HMWK. Conditions for this antibody consumption assay for surface-expressed platelet HMWK were developed so that intraplatelet HMWK (that which was neither secreted nor expressed on the external membrane) would not be interfering. The four platelet-derived specimens are then incubated with anti-HMWK antisera for 1 hour at 37°C in the indirect antibody consumption assay using CELISA for HMWK previously described. The objective of the assay is to determine the extent by which each of the four platelet specimens could reduce the titer of the starting anti-HMWK antibodies. After incubation with the four platelet specimens, four adsorbed anti-HMWK antibody aliquots are obtained for further analysis.

Four antibody samples per experiment are then compared by the CELISA assay for HMWK using known amounts of purified HMWK antigen to determine the slope of the competition inhibition curve produced by each batch of platelet-adsorbed or platelet supernatant-adsorbed antisera. The competition inhibition curves generated on the CELISA by the four aliquots of adsorbed antisera are produced by the method of incubation of samples indicated previously. However, since the aim of the assay is to determine whether the titer of the antisera would be decreased (consumed) by incubation with platelets or their supernatants, the final competition inhibition curves are analyzed by nonlinear regression to determine the slope of the competition inhibition curve produced by antisera adsorbed with each of the aliquots of platelet material. In all experiments the differently adsorbed aliquots of antisera are reacted with the same amounts of purified HMWK (1 to 125 ng). The data are plotted as the concentration of the purified HMWK used to determine the slope of the competition inhibition curve of the adsorbed antisera on the abscissa versus the optical density at 405 nm on the ordinate. The measured value of this assay is the slope of the competition inhibition curve (Fig. 13).

Quantification of the amount of platelet HMWK expressed on the surface of the platelet is obtained by comparing the values of the slopes produced by each sample of platelet—or platelet supernatant—adsorbed antisera with a standard curve of the anti-HMWK antisera adsorbed with known concentrations of purified HMWK (Fig. 12). In generation of this curve, the anti-HMWK antisera is adsorbed by purified HMWK at various concentrations (20–2,000 ng/ml) for 1 hour at 37°C. After incubation, the adsorbed antisera is then interacted with purified HMWK (1–125 ng) to determine the adsorbed antisera's competition inhibition curve. These slopes are also calculated by nonlinear regression. The data from these latter experiments are plotted as concentration of purified HMWK used to adsorb the antisera on the abscissa versus the slope of the resultant

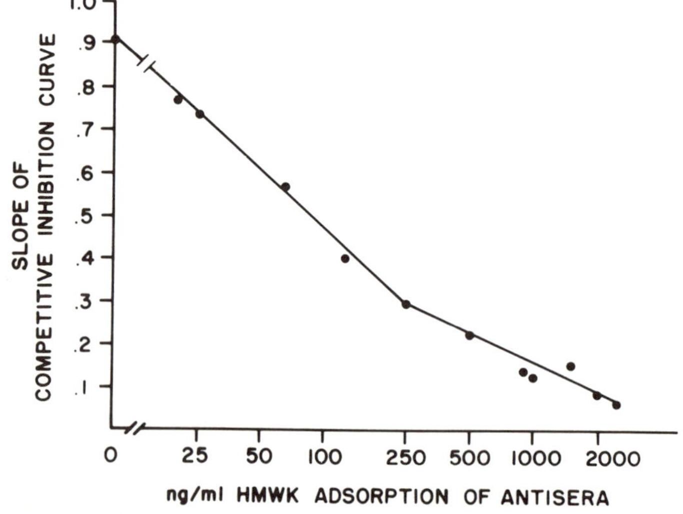

Fig. 12. The relationship of the slope of the competitive inhibition curve produced by anti-HMWK antisera versus the concentration of HMWK used to adsorb the antisera. Anti-HMWK antisera was prediluted 1:500 in PBS-Tween and incubated for 1 hour at 37°C in the absence or presence of purified HMWK at a concentration from 20 to 2,000 ng/ml in the suspending buffer. At the conclusion of the hour incubation, the adsorbed antisera was incubated overnight at 37°C with an equal volume of purified HMWK in an absolute amount from 1 to 125 ng. A CELISA assay was performed as indicated in text. The competitive inhibition curves produced by the unadsorbed and adsorbed antisera were calculated by nonlinear regression. In the figure the calculated slope of the adsorbed antisera was plotted on the ordinate and the concentration of purified HMWK used to adsorb the antisera for 1 hour was plotted on the abscissa. From Blood 67:119 [1986] by copyright permission of the American Society of Hematology.

competition inhibition curve on the ordinate. As can be seen in Figure 12, anti-HMWK antisera initially diluted 1:500 produced a competition inhibition curve with a calculated slope by nonlinear regression of 0.9. Incubating the anti-HMWK antisera initially diluted 1:500 in separate aliquots with increasing concentrations of purified HMWK (20–2,000 ng/ml) for 1 hour at 37°C resulted in competition inhibition curves with reduced calculated slopes (0.77–0.06).

In one representative experiment (Fig. 13), the competition inhibition curves produced by antisera adsorbed with the supernatant of unstimulated platelets (slope 0.34) and unstimulated platelets (slope 0.33) themselves gave parallel and almost superimposable curves. The competition inhibition curve produced by antisera adsorbed with the activated platelet supernatant was flattened with a decreased slope (0.20) when compared to that produced by the supernatant of unstimulated platelets (Fig. 13). Since platelet HMWK is secreted by thrombin-activated platelets this finding indicated that secreted platelet HMWK adsorbed and decreased the titer of the anti-HMWK antibody. The competition inhibition curve produced by activated platelets (slope 0.26) was similar to the curve that characterized the material released by platelets (Fig. 13). Antisera adsorbed with activated platelets showed a competition inhibition curve which had a reduced slope and left-shifted when compared to unstimulated platelets. Knowing the number of platelets in each experiment, the amount of HMWK (plasma or platelet) associated with the surface of the platelet or in its suspending medium is estimated by comparing the slopes of the competition inhibition curve produced by the antisera adsorbed with the platelet material with the slopes of the competition inhibition curves produced by known concentrations of purified HMWK. In the four experiments, unstimulated platelets and their supernatant had a mean of 4.9 ng HMWK/10^8 platelets and 4.2 ng HMWK/10^8 platelets, respectively, associated with the material. Alternatively, activated platelets and their supernatant had a mean of 17.3 ng HMWK/10^8 platelets and 17.2 ng HMWK/10^8 platelets, respectively, associated with the aliquots. The consumption of anti-HMWK antibody by activated platelets and their supernatant is specific for expressed platelet HMWK antigen because adsorption of the anti-HMWK antisera by unstimulated total kininogen-deficient platelets, thrombin-activated total kininogen-deficient platelets and activated deficient platelet supernatant produced competition inhibition curves with calculated slopes of 0.71, 0.78, and 0.77, respectively (Fig. 13, Inset). These slopes were similar to the competition inhibition curve produced by unadsorbed antisera and, when corrected for the number of platelets in the experiment, gave values for available HMWK less than 1 ng HMWK/10^8 platelets.

These combined results indicate that some of the platelet HMWK, in addition to being secreted, is also expressed on the external membrane of the activated

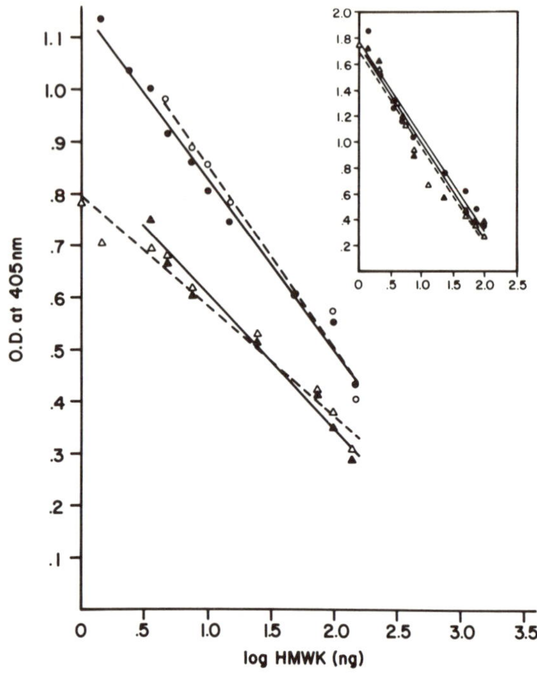

Fig. 13. Expression of platelet HMWK antigen on the activated platelet surface. The competitive inhibition curves produced by anti-HMWK antisera adsorbed with unstimulated platelet supernatant (○---○), unstimulated platelets (●—●), activated platelet supernatant (△—△), and activated platelets (▲—▲) are plotted. See methods for the preparation of each of the platelet samples. The ordinate is the observed optical density (O.D.) at 405 nm and the abscissa is the absolute amount (log HMWK in ng) of purified HMWK incubated with the prepared antisera. Inset Figure 13: The competitive inhibition curves produced by anti-HMWK antibody consumed by total kininogen-deficient platelets. The competition inhibition curves produced by anti-HMWK antisera adsorbed with unstimulated (●–●) and activated (△–△) total kininogen-deficient platelets as well as the activated platelet supernatant of total kininogen-deficient platelets (△---△) are plotted. All data in the Inset Figure 13 are plotted as above. In both plots, the competitive inhibition curves were calculated by nonlinear regression. From Blood 67:119 [1986] by copyright permission of the American Society of Hematology.

platelet. Platelets in addition to secreting their granule contents may also make these proteins available by expressing them on their external membrane upon activation. The expression of platelet HMWK on the activated platelet surface suggests that the platelet membrane has a receptor for this protein. This notion is supported by the recent findings that exogenous HMWK specifically binds to saturable sites on unstimulated [Gustafson et al., 1986] and activated [Greengard and Griffin, 1984] platelets. The possible presence of a receptor for HMWK on the platelet would suggest that the platelet could be a physiologic negatively charged surface for contact activation.

CONCLUSIONS

The methods contained in this review outline specific immunochemical techniques to identify and characterize the availability of proteins associated with platelets. These methods are applicable to any protein for which specific antibodies are available. Although these methods are sensitive and specific for the characterization of any protein associated with platelets, they do not address the specific role of a platelet-associated protein either in the regulation of platelet function or in the platelet contribution to plasma proteolysis. These further types of studies require other assays relating to the specific biologic function of the protein under study.

REFERENCES

Canellas PF, Karu AE (1981). Statistical package for analysis of competitive ELISA results. J Immunol Meth 47:375–385.

Dangelmaier CA, Holmsen H (1983). Measurement of platelet function. In Harker LA, Zimmerman TS (eds): "Methods in Haematology." Edinburgh and New York: Churchill Livingston, Vol 8, pp 92–114.

Engvall E (1980). Enzyme immunoassay ELISA and EMIT. Meth Enzymol 70:419–439.

Fraker PJ, Speck SC (1978). Protein and cell membrane iodinations with a sparing soluble chloroamide 1,3,4,6-tetrachloro-3a,6a-diphenylglycoluril. Biochem Biophys Res Commun 80:849–857.

Fukami MH, Bauer JS, Stewart GJ, Salganicoff L (1978). An improved method for the isolation of dense storage granules from human platelets. J Cell Biol 77:389–399.

Ginsberg MH, Painter RG, Birdwell C, Plow EF (1979). The detection, immunofluorescent localization and thrombin-induced release of human platelet-associated fibronectin antigen. J Supramol Struct 11:167–174.

Greengard JS, Griffin JH (1984). Receptors for high molecular weight kininogen on stimulated washed human platelets. Biochemistry 23:6863–6869.

Gustafson EJ, Schutsky D, Knight L, Schmaier AH (1986). High molecular weight kininogen binds to unactivated platelets. J Clin Invest 78:310–318.

Harfenist EJ, Guccione MA, Packham MA, Mustard JF (1982). The use of the synthetic peptide Gly-Pro-Arg-Pro, in the preparation of thrombin-degranulated rabbit platelets. Blood 59:952–955.

Jerushalmy Z, Zucker MB (1966). Some effect of fibrinogen degradation products (FDP) on blood platelets. Thromb Diath Haemorrh 15:413–419.

Kaplan KL, Brockman MJ, Chernoff A, Lesznik GR, Drillings M (1979). Platelet alpha-granule proteins: Studies on release and subcellular localization. Blood 53:604–618.

Kato H, Iwanaga S, Nagasawa S (1981). HMW and LMW Kininogens. Meth Enzymol 80:172–198.

Kerbiriou DM, Griffin JH (1979). Human high molecular weight kininogen. Studies of structure-function relationships and of proteolysis of the molecule occurring during contact phase activation in plasma. J Biol Chem 254:12020–12027.

Koutts J, Walsh PN, Plow EF, Fenton JW, Bouma BN, Zimmerman TS (1978). Active release of human platelet factor VIII-related antigen by adenosine diphosphate, collagen and thrombin. J Clin Invest 62:1255–1263.

Molnar J, Lorand L (1961). Studies of apyrase. Arch Biochem Biophys 93:353–363.

Mori K, Nagasawa S (1981). Studies in human high molecular weight (HMW) kininogen by the action of human plasma kallikrein. J Biochem 89:1465–1473.

Muller-Esterl W, Fritz H, Machleidt W, Ritonja A, Brzin J, Kotnik M, Turk V, Kellerman J, Lottspeich F (1985). Human plasma kininogens are identical with alpha-cysteine proteinase inhibitors. Evidence from immunological, enzymological and sequence data. Fed Eur Biochem Soc 182:310–314.

Mustard JF, Perry DW, Ardlie NM, Packham MA (1972). Preparations of suspensions of washed platelets from humans. Br J Haematol 22:193–204.

Ohkubo I, Kurachi K, Takasawa T, Shiokawa H, Sasaki M (1984). Isolation of human cDNA for alpha-2-thiol protease inhibitor and its identity with low molecular weight kininogen. Biochemistry 23:3891–3899.

Proud D, Pierce JV, Pisano JJ (1980). Radioimmunoassay of human high molecular weight kininogen in normal and deficient plasma. J Lab Clin Med 95:563–574.

Rucinski B, Niewiarowski S, James P, Waltz DA, Budzynski A (1979). Antiheparin proteins secreted by human platelets, purification, characterization, and radioimmunoassay. Blood 53:47–62.

Schmaier AH, Colman RW (1980). Crotalocytin: Characterization of the timber rattlesnake platelet activating protein. Blood 56:1020–1028.

Schmaier AH, Zuckerberg A, Silverman C, Kuchibhotla J, Tuszynski GP, Colman RW (1983). High-molecular weight kininogen. A secreted platelet protein. J Clin Invest 71:1477–1489.

Schmaier AH, Silver LD, Adams AL, Fischer GC, Munoz PC, Vroman L, Colman RW (1984). The effect of high molecular weight kininogen on surface-adsorbed fibrinogen. Thromb Res 33:51–67.

Schmaier AH, Smith PM, Colman RW (1985). Platelet Cl Inhibitor. A secreted alpha-granule protein. J Clin Invest 75:242–250.

Schmaier AH, Bradford H, Silver LD, Farber A, Scott CF, Schutsky D, Colman RW (1986a). High molecular weight kininogen is an inhibitor of platelet calpain. J Clin Invest 77:1565–1573.

Schmaier AH, Smith PM, Purdon AD, White JG, Colman RW (1986b). High molecular weight kininogen: Localization in the unstimulated and activated platelet and activation by a platelet calpain(s). Blood 67:119–130.

Sinha D, Seaman FS, Koshy A, Walsh PN (1984). Blood coagulation factor XIa binds specifically to a site on activated human platelets distinct from that for factor XI. J Clin Invest 73:1550–1556.

Sueyoshi T, Enjyoji K, Shimada T, Kato H, Iwanaga S, Bando Y, Kominami E, Katunuma N (1985). A new function of kininogens as thiol-proteinase inhibitors: Inhibition of papain and cathepsins B, H and L by bovine, rat and human plasma kininogens. Fed Eur Biochem Soc 182:193–195.

Takagaki Y, Kitamura N, Nakjanishi S (1985). Cloning and sequence analysis of cDNA for human high molecular weight and low molecular weight prekininogens. Primary structures of two human prekininogens. J Biol Chem 260:8601–8609.

Timmons S, Hawiger J (1978). Separation of human platelets from plasma proteins including factor VIII by a combined albumin gradient-gel filtration method using Hepes buffer. Thromb Res 12:297–306.

Tuszynski GP, Bevacqua SJ, Schmaier AH, Colman RW, Walsh PN (1982). Factor XI antigen and activity in human platelets. Blood 59:1148–1156.

Walsh PN (1972). The role of platelets in the contact phase of blood coagulation. Br J Haematol 22:237–253.

Walsh PN, Mills DCB, White JG (1977). Metabolism and function of human platelets washed by albumin density gradient separation. Br J Haematol 36:281–296.

Wroblewski F, Ladue JS (1955). Lactic dehydrogenase activity in blood. Proc Soc Exp Biol Med 90:210–213.

Modern Methods in Pharmacology, Volume 4
Methods for Studying Platelets and Megakaryocytes, pages 133–156

Methods of Studying Platelet Nucleotides

ADRIE J.M. VERHOEVEN and HOLM HOLMSEN

INTRODUCTION

From the early days of platelet research the nucleotides, notably the adenylates, have been extensively studied. This is first of all due to the recognition of ADP as a potent platelet agonist and the identification of ADP as one of the compounds that are secreted when platelets are activated, thus constituting an important cascade in primary hemostasis. Secondly, the platelet responses are dependent on the availability of metabolic energy, which is supplied through ATP. More recently, the important role of the cAMP second messenger system and of the GTP-binding proteins in receptor-coupled regulation of adenylate cyclase and polyphosphoinositide metabolism further raised the interest in nucleotides.

Of all nucleotides, the adenylates are the most abundant. In human platelets, total adenylates amount to 10.7–12.9 μmol/10^{11} platelets [Gordon and Drummond, 1974; D'Souza and Glueck, 1979], and constitute 78% of the acid-soluble nucleotide pool (Fig. 1). Guanine nucleotides are present in moderate quantities (13%), whereas levels of uracil and cytosine nucleotides are only minor (5% and 2%, respectively [D'Souza and Glueck, 1977]. In addition, low amounts of IMP (2%) are present. Since platelets are anucleate cells and contain only minor amounts of mitochondrial DNA and traces of RNA, the nucleotides are not used in nucleic acid metabolism. A substantial amount (64%) of the nucleotides is sequestered in the dense granules; once secreted, these become important in the propagation of the platelet activation process. The other nucleotides serve various roles in cellular metabolism; the adenylates are involved in energy metabolism

Abbreviations used: IMP, inosine monophosphate; NMR, nuclear magnetic resonance; HPLC, high-performance (high-pressure) liquid chromatography; PCA, perchloric acid; P_i, inorganic orthophosphate; PP_i, pyrophosphate; PRPP, phosphoribosyl pyrophosphate; TCA, trichloroacetic acid.

From the Department of Biochemistry, University of Bergen, N-5000 Bergen, Norway.

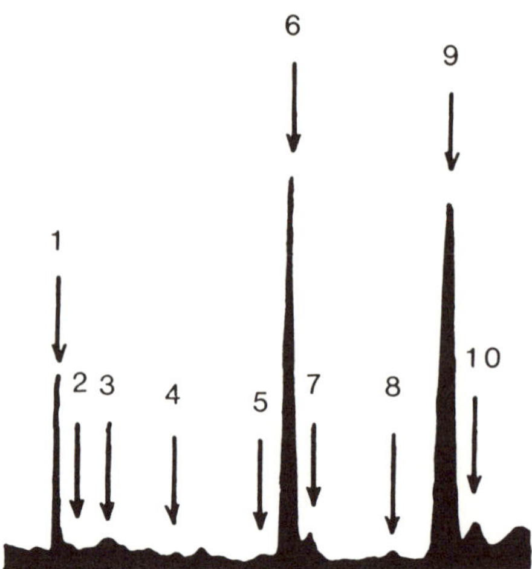

Fig. 1. Nucleotide profile of human platelets. The acid-soluble nucleotides were extracted from untreated human platelets with PCA, and separated by HPLC on an anion-exchange column. Nucleotides were eluted with a linear 10–700 mM NaH_2PO_4-gradient and detected by their extinction at 254 nm. The different fractions are identified as: (1) substances that are not absorbed on the column (e.g., hypoxanthine); (2) start of the gradient; (3) AMP; (4) IMP; (5) UDP; (6) ADP; (7) GDP; (8) UTP; (9) ATP; (10) GTP. (Redrawn after Daniel et al., 1980.)

and the guanylates in transmembrane signaling. cAMP, and possibly also cGMP, have second-messenger functions. The cytosine and uracil nucleotides are involved in phospholipid synthesis, and probably protein glycosylation and in vivo glycogen formation, respectively.

COMPARTMENTATION OF NUCLEOTIDES

The nucleotides exist in three physically distinct compartments: soluble in the cytosol including the mitochondria, bound to protein, and stored in the dense granules (Fig. 2). The cytosolic and mitochondrial nucleotides are commonly referred to as "metabolic" to designate that they participate in cellular metabolism and are readily labeled when platelets are incubated with isotopic precursors. The dense granule-stored nucleotides are secreted to the platelet environments upon proper stimulation of the cells and are absent in platelets from patients with storage pool deficiency [Holmsen and Weiss, 1979]. Most notably, these nucleotides exchange slowly with those in the metabolic pool and do not participate in metabolism. In addition, incubation of platelets with metabolic inhibitors results in an almost complete depletion of the cytosolic pool, whereas the dense granule

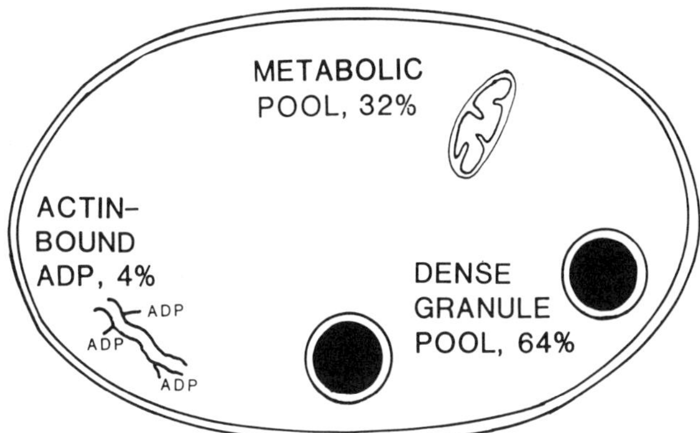

Fig. 2. Compartmentation of platelet adenine nucleotides. The percentages refer to the proportion of total adenylates in each compartment. Note that the metabolic pool includes the mitochondrial adenylates. Subcellular fractionation studies [Holmsen et al., 1969] yield an estimate of 3% for the contribution of the mitochondrial pool to the entire metabolic pool. The actual level of mitochondrial adenylates is probably higher, since the mitochondria may have lost some of the nucleotides during cell disruption and separation from the cytosol.

pool remains intact. The dense granules are the heaviest organelles of the platelet (1.21 g/cm^3) and can be separated from the soluble compounds by subcellular fractionation [Fukami et al, 1978]. Due to the aggregation of the nucleotides in these acidic granules, these nucleotides give NMR resonances in platelets from some species that are quite distinct from those of the cytosolic nucleotides [Ugurbil and Holmsen, 1981]. Substantial amounts of cytosolic ADP are tightly bound to F-actin. These protein-bound nucleotides are readily labeled when platelets are incubated with radioactive precursors [Daniel et al., 1980; 1986]. However, they are not readily available to the cytosolic enzymes [Daniel et al., 1979] and do not seem to give detectable NMR signals [Ugurbil et al., 1979]. These nucleotides are readily isolated from the others, since the tight binding to protein makes them insoluble in organic solvents such as ethanol or acetone.

In human platelets, 30% of ATP and GTP and 80% of ADP and GDP is sequestered in the granules. Ten percent of ADP (and possibly GDP) is protein bound. Of the uracil and cytosine nucleotides, more than 80% is present in the metabolic pool.

DENSE GRANULE-STORED NUCLEOTIDES

The identification of the dense granules as the storage site of the non-metabolic pool of nucleotides has been achieved by a combination of secretion and subcellular fractionation studies, by the study of storage pool-deficient platelets [Holmsen and Weiss, 1979], by NMR studies, and by electron microscopy using uranaffin staining [Richards and Da Prada, 1977]. Besides nucleotides, the granules also contain serotonin, divalent cations, P_i and PP_i [Holmsen and Weiss, 1979]. Platelets also contain diadenosine 5′, 5‴-P^1, P^4-tetraphosphate in a nonmetabolic, secretable form [Flodgaard and Klenow, 1982], which is absent in storage pool-deficient platelets [Kim et al., 1985], suggesting sole localization in the dense granules.

Dense granules from different species vary in the total amount of nucleotides, the ATP/ADP ratio, and the Ca^{2+}/Mg^{2+} ratio [Meyers et al., 1982]. In all species studied, however, the local concentration of nucleotides and divalent cations is extremely high, being in the molar range. Recent studies applying ^{31}P- and ^{1}H-NMR have revealed that the nucleotides are tightly packed in large aggregates [Ugurbil et al., 1984a,b]. These aggregates are probably stabilized by the divalent cations through their interaction with adjacent polyphosphate tails. Probably, serotonin is incorporated in these aggregates as well [Costa et al., 1979; Ugurbil et al., 1984b]. Depending on the type of cation the aggregates are free in solution (Mg^{2+}; pig; 37°C) or form an amorphous solid (Ca^{2+}; human; 4–37°C) or gel (Mg^{2+}; pig; $<20°C$). In the latter two structures the molecular mobility is severely restricted, resulting in the complete absence of NMR signals in the spectra of human platelets and pig platelets below 20°C, and the very distinct resonances in the spectrum of pig platelets above 30°C (Fig. 3).

Although the NMR studies give valuable information about the composition of the storage complexes of adenylates at high concentrations, little is known about the mechanism for concentration of the nucleotides in the granules. Nucleotide-containing granules are already present in the megakaryocyte [Richards and Da Prada, 1977], and concentration must, therefore, have taken place at this stage. In mature platelets, dense granule ATP and ADP are slowly labeled when the cells are incubated with radiolabeled adenine, adenosine, and P_i [Reimers et al., 1977]. Initially, the ratio of labeled ATP over ADP is identical to that in the metabolic pool, but after prolonged incubation it decreases toward the ratio of granule-stored amounts. This suggests that metabolic ATP is initally taken up by the granules and subsequently, part of it is coverted to ADP. Rabbit platelets that are made storage pool-deficient fail to regain their granule-stored nucleotides in vivo [Reimers et al., 1975]. Hence, net transport of nucleotides across the granule membrane does not seem to occur. Instead, uptake of metabolic ATP may occur through exchange with stored nucleotides. Studies on storage pool-deficient platelets lend additional support for the existence of a mutual relationship between the two compartments. Two studies on patient platelets [Akkerman et al., 1983c; Lages et al., 1983] and several studies on platelets from animals

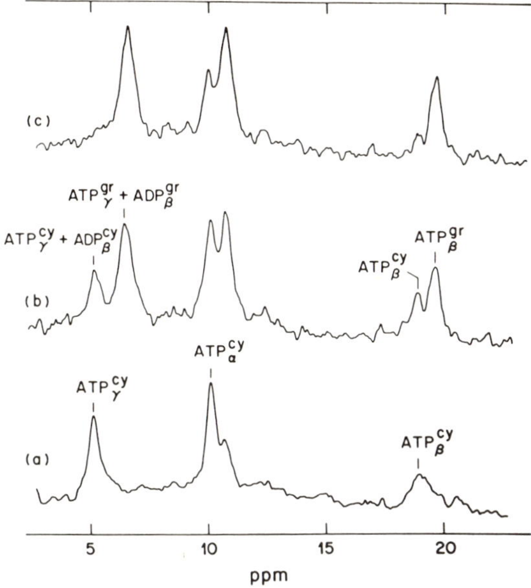

Fig. 3. ^{31}P NMR resonances of ATP and ADP in pig platelets. The nucleotide region of the 145.7 MHz ^{31}P-NMR spectrum of intact pig platelets at 4°C (a) and 37°C (b and c) is shown. At the low temperature, the spectrum shows three distinct resonances that are assigned to the three phosphoryl groups of metabolic ATP. At the elevated temperature, additional resonances appear, which originate from the granule-stored adenylates. The latter are not affected by incubation of platelets for 0.5–6 min (b) or 9–14.5 min (c) with 12.5 μM antimycin A plus 100 mM 2-deoxyglucose, in contrast to the resonances of metabolic ATP. Superscripts cy and gr denote cytosolic and granule-stored, respectively. (From Ugurbil et al., 1979.)

with Chediak-Higashi syndrome [Meyers et al., 1979a,b; 1981] show that the storage pool-deficiency is associated with a 20–40% reduction of metabolic adenylates. On the other hand, depletion of metabolic ATP by incubation with metabolic inhibitors leaves the total storage pool intact [Holmsen et al., 1974], but no data are available on the relative amounts of stored ATP and ADP. In platelets that have been treated for 15 min with H_2O_2 in the presence of cyanide, the total amount of stored adenylates was also unaffected despite a 45% reduction in metabolic ATP, but here a marked conversion of stored ATP to ADP was apparent, resulting in a decrease of ATP/ADP in the granules from 1.25 to 0.80 [Verhoeven et al., 1984a]. In another study, a reduction in the ATP/ADP ratio of the stored nucleotides to 0.45 took place upon treatment of platelets with N_3^- and H_2O_2 for 190 min [Ugurbil et al., 1979]. The mechanisms of this exchange of nucleotides and the marked intragranular conversion of ATP to ADP remain unclear. Since the distribution of the guanylates over the different pools is similar to that of the adenylates, it is likely that storage of these nucleotides occurs through the same mechanism(s). Although exchange of metabolic and granule-stored nucleotides is evident, this is very slow. In human platelets it amounts to about 1 nmol ATP/min/10^{11} cells [Reimers et al., 1977], which is 5,000 times slower than the turnover of ATP in the metabolic pool [Akkerman and Holmsen, 1980; Akkerman et al., 1983a]. Hence, the granule pool plays no part in general metabolism of the platelet. Walseth et al, [1983] recently reported that incubation of platelets with ^{18}O-enriched water results in a rapid incorporation of this label in the gamma-phosphate groups of all platelet ATP; no compartmentation of ATP was apparent, and the total ATP-pool was turning over in 2 min. This finding is in sharp contrast with all the above-mentioned studies. If the terminal phosphate of the ATP that is stored in the acidic granules was turning over at such a high rate, this would certainly have resulted in distinguishable ^{31}P-NMR resonances, but there is no evidence for such signals in the NMR spectra of intact platelets [Ugurbil and Holmsen, 1981]. The ^{18}O-labeling technique also gives an estimate for the fraction of ADP that is cytosolic (50%) that is more than twice the value found with all other methods. We feel, therefore, that this technique overestimates the contribution of the dense granule nucleotides in platelet metabolism.

METABOLIC NUCLEOTIDES

The metabolic compartment consists of both a soluble and a mitochondrial fraction. Platelets contain only a few tiny but active mitochondira. Probably less than 3% of total metabolic adenylates is present in these organelles [Holmsen et al., 1969].The metabolic nucleotides participate in cellular metabolism. Most is known of the adenylates, whereas only little is known of guanylate metabolism, and almost nothing of the metabolism of the other nucleotides. For the content of metabolic ATP a value of 3-3.5 μmol/10^{11} cells has long been used, but with the improvement in methodology this figure tends to increase. The most recent estimates vary between 4.4 [Akkerman et al., 1981] and 4.7 [Daniel et al., 1980] μmol/10^{11} cells. NMR studies have shown that 95–100% of the metabolic adenylates is complexed with Mg^{2+} [Ugurbil et al., 1979]. The amounts of $MgADP^-$ and MgAMP are set at one-tenth and one-hundredth, respectively, of $MgATP^{2-}$ through the adenylate kinase equilibrium. Metabolic ATP is crucial for platelet function, as illustrated by the inhibition of the different responses during a gradual fall of ATP availability during incubation of platelets with metabolic inhibitors [Holmsen et al., 1982]. A fall of the metabolic ATP concentration is *not* accompanied by a reduced responsivity if the value of the adenylate energy charge (AEC = (ATP + 1/2 ADP)/(ATP + ADP + AMP)) remains unaffected [Holmsen and Robkin, 1977; Murer et al., 1981; Akkerman et al.,

1983b], suggesting an important role of this ratio in the regulation of energy availability. The energy that is stored in ATP is made available through hydrolysis to ADP; the rate of hydrolysis, therefore, determines energy utilization. In unstimulated cells, ATP is hydrolyzed at a rate of 3.5–7 μmol/min/10^{11} cells [Akkerman and Holmsen, 1981; Akkerman et al., 1983a; Verhoeven et al., 1984b]. Upon stimulation of platelets with various agonists, this rate increases to up to 20 μmol/min, in parallel with stimulus-response coupling and execution of aggregation and secretion [Akkerman et al., 1983a; Verhoeven et al., 1984b, 1985a, 1986a].

In resting platelets the levels of ATP, ADP, and AMP remain fairly constant because ATP utilization is adequately balanced by its regeneration through glyco(geno)lysis and oxidative phosphorylation. Immediately upon stimulation, however, utilization exceeds regeneration and the steady-state ATP level falls [Fukami et al., 1976; Akkerman and Holmsen, 1981]. ATP is catabolized through AMP, IMP, and inosine to hypoxanthine, which diffuses out of the cell (Fig. 4). A similar ATP to hypoxanthine conversion is also seen in platelets that are incubated with metabolic inhibitors, or with H_2O_2, glyoxylate, or NaF [Holmsen, 1982; Holmsen and Robkin, 1977; Holmsen et al., 1982; Murer et al., 1981]. In contrast, when platelets are starved, the fall of ATP is accompanied by a much lesser formation of hypoxanthine and AMP accumulates [Akkerman and Gorter, 1980]; apparently, deamination of AMP to IMP is inhibited during starvation. The activity of the crucial enzyme, AMP deaminase, is mainly regulated by substrate AMP, activator ATP, and inhibitor P_i [Ashby and Holmsen, 1981, 1983]. Despite the detailed study on its regulation it is still not clear why this enzyme is turned on during platelet activation and metabolic stress, but not during starvation. Possibly, AMP deaminase is kept in the active state in the resting platelet, since the level of metabolic ATP exceeds that of P_i; its activity is, however, limited by the low rate of AMP generation. Upon platelet stimulation and during metabolic stress, AMP production is markedly increased and the enzyme is turned on. During starvation the level of P_i drastically increases concomitant with the fall in ATP, which results in the conversion of the enzyme to the inactive state (Verhoeven and Holmsen, unpubished).

The importance of the ATP to hypoxanthine conversion is unknown. The depletion of metabolic adenylates when energy consumption exceeds production would clearly help to stabilize the AEC value. However, this value is equally well maintained in platelets that have their AMP deaminase blocked by coformycin as in control platelets [Ashby et al., 1983]. Coformycin treatment also leaves secretion responses intact, and, hence, the ATP to hypoxanthine conversion is not coupled tightly to platelet activation to the stage of secretion. Lactate production is not affected by coformycin, which is held as evidence against the

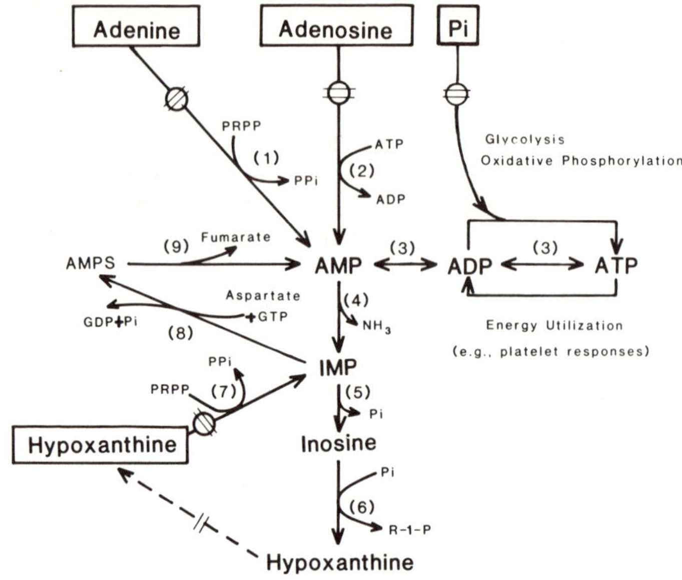

Fig. 4. Formation and degradation of adenine nucleotides in platelets. Under normal conditions, energy utilization and regeneration are balanced and the level of metabolic ATP and ADP remain stable. When utilization exceeds regeneration, however, ATP is catabolized to hypoxanthine, which diffuses out of the cell. The metabolic adenylates can be (re)synthesized from the precursors hypoxanthine, adenine, and adenosine, which each are transported across the plasma membrane through specific uptake mechanisms. Metabolic nucleotides can readily be studied when isotopically labeled precursors are used. In addition, the metabolic pool can also be labeled with ^{32}P-P$_i$, which is transported into the platelet through an as yet uncharacterized uptake system. The individual steps are catalyzed by: (1) adenine phosphoribosyl transferase; (2) adenosine kinase; (3) adenylate kinase; (4) AMP aminohydrolase; (5) 5′-nucleotidase; (6) purine riboside phosphorylase; (7) hypoxanthine-guanine phosphoribosyl transferase; (8) adenylosuccinate synthetase; and (9) adenylosuccinate lyase. Additional abbreviations: AMPS = adenylosuccinate; R-1-P = ribose 1-phosphate.

hypothesis that activation of AMP deaminase serves in the stimulation of ATP regeneration, for example, through ammonia activation of phosphofructokinase [Yoshino and Murakami, 1982]. The amount of ATP that is produced per mole of lactate depends on whether glycogen or glucose is the source; a shift from one to the other would markedly alter net ATP formation but leave lactate production unaffected. Although Ashby et al. [1983] did not find any effect of coformycin treatment on the rate of glycogenolysis, their figures are about 70 times higher than the maximal glycogen phosphorylase activity allows for [Chaiken et al., 1975]. It is still possible, therefore, that the ATP to hypoxanthine conversion which accompanies platelet stimulation contributes to the regulation of energy generation. Platelets have only limited ability to synthesize nucleotides de novo, but readily synthesize them from preformed bases and nucleosides [Holmsen, 1985]. Since only hypoxanthine is present in plasma at sufficiently high levels, this is probably the main in vivo source for adenylate synthesis. This may also explain why a defect in the hypoxanthine uptake system in Lesch-Nyhan syndrome leads to such a dramatic reduction in platelet adenylate content despite the presence of a normal adenine uptake system [Rivard et al., 1975a]. In light of this, it is surprising that only one report has appeared on the characterization of the hypoxanthine salvage pathway in platelets [Rivard et al., 1975b]. When hypoxanthine is taken up in the cell it is immediately converted to IMP by hypoxanthine-guanine phosphoribosyl transferase in the presence of PRPP (Fig. 4); guanine is converted to GMP by the same enzyme. IMP is slowly converted to AMP, probably through the purine nucleotide cycle. Adenine is also taken up, although through a different system, and it is immediately converted to AMP by adenine phosphoribosyl transferase [Sixma et al., 1973]. These phosphoribosylation steps appear so efficient that no free bases accumulate intracellularly. Moreover, an increase in available PRPP, for example by a H_2O_2-induced activation of the hexose monophosphate shunt, leads to an up to 2-fold increase in uptake of any of these purine bases [Holmsen et al., 1979]. It is possible, therefore, that uptake proceeds by a group translocation mechanism [French et al., 1974]. The incorporation of adenine is 100-times faster than that of hypoxanthine, probably through differences at the transport level. Adenosine enters the cell by two transport systems [Sixma et al., 1976]. Thus, at micromolar concentrations, adenosine is transported by a low K_m system which is inhibited by papaverine, and exclusively converted intracellularly to AMP by adenosine kinase in the presence of ATP. At millimolar concentrations uptake occurs mainly through a high K_m system which is inhibited by adenine; under this condition, the adenosine kinase is saturated, and the excess intracellular adenosine is immediately deaminated to inosine by adenosine deaminase.

The amount of metabolic guanine nucleotides is about one-eighth of that of the adenylates. The GTP/GDP ratio is similar to that of the adenylates in most conditions. However, treatment of platelets with substances that lower metabolic ATP, such as low doses of formaldehyde, leaves the level of GTP almost intact [Holmsen, 1985]. In platelets that are incubated with metabolic inhibitors, the consumption of GTP lags behind that of ATP (Verhoeven and Holmsen, manuscript in preparation). Apparently, the nucleoside diphosphate kinase (GTP + ADP $\rightleftharpoons$ GDP + ATP) does not favor the formation of ATP. This may be due to a different comparmentation, since GTP is bound to intramembrane proteins that couple receptor occupancy to adenylate cyclase and polyphosphoinositide phosphodiesterase activity [Berridge, 1985].

Platelets have large capacities for production of cAMP and cGMP. The significance of measurements of these cyclic nucleotides is described in chapter V.

PROTEIN-BOUND NUCLEOTIDES

About half of the nongranule ADP, i.e., 0.3–0.4 μmol/10^{11} platelets, is bound to a protein, which has recently been identified as F-actin [Daniel et al., 1986]. In platelets incubated with radioactive adenine the specific radioactivity of bound ADP is identical to that of the cytosolic adenylates [Daniel et al., 1980]. The rate of ^{14}C adenine incorporation into the actin-bound and metabolic pools is the same, but the incorporation into the actin-bound pool lags 5–10 sec behind [Daniel et al., 1986]. From this lag it was calculated that the actin-bound pool turns over once every 10 sec. Hence, the pools exchange at a rate of 1.8 μmol ADP/min/10^{11} cells. In spite of this rapid exchange, however, the actin-bound pool is not readily available to the cell's energy metabolism. For example, when platelets are incubated with metabolic inhibitors, this pool remains unaffected, whereas metabolic ATP and ADP are almost completely consumed [Holmsen et al., 1974; Daniel et al., 1979]. These phenomena may be explained by the treadmilling of F-actin. F-actin is constantly polymerized at one end by successive additions of G-actin-ATP units, and depolymerized at the opposite end to yield free G-actin and ADP without net growth of the F-actin oligomer [Wegner, 1976]. During polymerization ATP is hydrolyzed to ADP, which remains bound to F-actin. This treadmilling process acts, therefore, as an ATPase that accounts for 30–50% of total ATP utilization in the resting platelets.

At present, the possible role of this high rate of actin-treadmilling with its high ATP utilization is unknown. Upon stimulation of platelets, the actin state changes dramatically, but this is not accompanied by an enhanced exchange between the two metabolic adenylate pools (Daniel and Holmsen, unpublished). It has therefore been suggested that it relates to the high responsive state at which the platelets are maintained, so that the high rate of actin polymerization and depolymerization in the unstimulated platelet may enable it to change its morphological structure as rapidly as it does upon stimulation [Daniel et al., 1986]. The high cost of energy consumption associated with the treadmilling does therefore not represent an energy-wasting futile cycle, but is probably coupled to the maintenance of platelet responsivity. Besides ADP, GDP is also present in the ethanol-insoluble, protein-bound fraction (Daniel and Holmsen, unpublished). This GDP is labeled when platelets are incubated with ^{32}P-P_i, and is therefore also of a metabolic type. It is probably bound to tubulin, and may take part in a microtubule depolymerization-polymerization process analogous to F-actin treadmilling.

METHODOLOGY

Labeling

The metabolic nucleotide pool, and, hence, cellular metabolism, can easily be studied in platelets by incubating them with precursors that are labeled with either radioactive (^{3}H, ^{14}C, ^{32}P), heavy (^{18}O), or magnetic spin (^{13}C) isotopes (Fig. 4). Commonly, either ring-labeled ^{14}C- or ^{3}H-purines or ^{32}P-P$_i$ is used. Platelets are incubated for 1 hour with the precursor, and excess, nonincorporated radiolabel is removed by gel-filtering the platelets. When pulse-labeled with adenine, the specific radioactivity of all metabolic adenylates including protein-bound ADP and their derivatives is identical, and, hence, the radioactivity in each metabolite is directly proportional to its chemical amount [Daniel et al., 1980]. In addition, the radiolabel is only distributed among ATP, ADP, AMP, IMP, inosine, and hypoxanthine, which makes it possible to use total radioactivity in these compounds as an internal standard. This allows the measurement of the individual metabolites with less than $\pm$ 1% precision. In ^{32}P-P$_i$ pulse-labeled platelets, the radiolabel is distributed among virtually all phosphorylated acid-soluble intermediates, as well as some phosphoproteins and phospholipids. The specific radioactivity of each labeled phosphoryl group in nucleotides (the β- and γ-phosphoryls) and glycolytic intermediates is identical [Holmsen et al., 1983]. The phosphate-label is not incorporated into the γ-phosphoryls of nucleotides and cannot, therefore, be used in the study of cyclic nucleotide metabolism. The latter can be studied with the recently introduced technique of ^{18}O-labeling [Walseth et al., 1983] (see also chapter by Ashby and Grant).

Nucleotide metabolism can also be studied by labeling techniques employing non isotopic precursors. Agarwal and Parks [1975] incubated platelets with 2-fluoro-adenosine, which is readily converted intracellularly to 2-fluoro-ATP. This nucleotide accumulates to surprisingly high concentrations in the metabolic pool thereby replacing natural ATP. 2-Fluoro-ATP can be utilized by the energy-requiring processes of the cell, and is catabolized to fluorinated ADP and AMP. The latter is, however, not a good substrate for AMP deaminase and is, therefore, not metabolized any further. In HPLC, the fluorinated nucleotides separate cleanly from their natural counterparts and are readily measurable. Although some aspects of cellular nucleotide metabolism can be studied by ^{1}H- and ^{31}P-NMR techniques without the need of prior labeling, these methods are not very sensitive. Use of the fluor-label, however, has great potential as the ^{19}F-nucleus has a magnetogyric ratio similar to ^{1}H. It can therefore be detected at concentrations of 10^{-5} M or less, and gives very distinct spectra of 2-fluoro-adenine nucleotides [Costa et al., 1979]. The ^{13}C-nucleus also constitutes a potentially sensitive, but yet unexplored, label for studies of nucleotide metabolism by NMR.

Extraction

The most important step in the determination of nucleotides is their extraction from the platelet suspension. The great variation in reported nucleotide levels is probably due to differences in this step. The lower the AMP-level and the higher the ATP/ADP-ratio in the extracts are, the better is the efficacy of the methods used. Optimal values (ATP/ADP = 10-11 in the metabolic pool) are obtained when the platelet suspension is added to two volumes of EDTA-ethanol (10 mM EDTA, pH 7.4, in 86% ethanol) that is precooled at -40°C; this inhibits platelet ATPases instantaneously and preserves the F-actin-bound ADP pool [Holmsen, 1972; Daniel et al., 1979]. Extraction of nucleotides with 0.6 N perchloric acid (O°C) gives distinctly lower ATP/ADP-ratios (4-5 in the metabolic pool), due to the extraction of ADP that is bound to F-actin. When interested in this actin-bound pool, EDTA-ethanol extracts must first be prepared and subsequently, the nucleotides can be extracted from the washed, ethanol-insoluble material with 0.6 N perchloric acid [Daniel et al., 1980, 1986]. For the subsequent analysis of the extracts it is sometimes desirable to introduce a concentration step. Some investigators have isolated platelets from a suspension by centrifugation and then extracted the nucleotides from the pellet. However, this procedure gave extracts with up to fourfold higher AMP levels compared to extracts that were prepared directly from the platelet suspension [Holmsen, 1985], and is therefore not suitable. Whenever a concentration step is desired, this should be introduced at the stage of PRP preparation; platelet activation during this step can be prevented by decreasing the pH of PRP to 6.5, or by the addition of 1 μM prostacyclin [Vargas et al., 1982].

Separation of Nucleotides

High-voltage paper electrophoresis. Separation is based on the different number of charged groups of nucleotides and their derivatives under acidic conditions. For the separation of radioactive adenine nucleotides the electrophoresis buffer is 50 mM sodium citrate (pH 3.75–3.8) [Holmsen et al., 1972a], for guanine nucleotides both a 50 mM sodium citrate (pH 2.5) and a 20 mM sodium citrate/phosphate (pH 1.8) buffer are suitable (Holmsen, unpublished). In a 1-hour run at 60 V/cm the nucleotides and their derivatives are well separated except for hypoxanthine and inosine, which remain at the application point. Of this, invariably more than 80% is hypoxanthine [Sixma et al., 1976]. If wanted, these metabolites can be separated by eluting them from the paper with distilled water, and reelectrophoresing them in a 50 mM sodium borate buffer (pH 9) for 1 hour at 60 V/cm [Sixma et al., 1976]. The radioactive spots are visualized under UV (254 nm) by coelectrophoresis of a mixture of unlabeled nucleotides. Best results are obtained with ethanol-extracts. With PCA-extracts, separation of ATP and ADP is poor; here, one-dimensional paper chromatography with n-butanol/acetoned/acetic acid/concentrated ammonia/water (45:15:10:2:28, by volume) is a good alternative [Daniel et al., 1980]. Electrophoresis is not suitable for analysis of ^{32}P-P_i labeled metabolites, since radioactive adenine and guanine nucleotides, glycolytic intermediates, and P_i are not separated sufficiently.

Two-dimensional paper chromatography. All ^{32}P P_i-labeled intermediates are separable by this technique. Descending chromatography is performed at room temperature for 26 hours with isobutyric acid/concentrated ammonia/water/10 mM EDTA (500:21:279, by volume) in the first direction, and for 19 hours with n-butanol/n-propanol/acetone/formic acid/30% aqueous TCA/77 mM EDTA (200:100:125:125:75:10, by volume) in the second direction [Holmsen et al., 1983]. With these solvents UTP and GTP comigrate and come close to F-1,6-P_2, which is heavily labeled. To improve separation of these metabolites, t-butanol/0.5 N HC1 (2:1 by volume) may be used for the second dimension [Holmsen, 1965]. The position of the nucleotides can be detected under UV (254 nm) by cochromatography of unlabeled markers. Separation of nucleotides is equally well for PCA-, TCA- and ethanol-extracts.

High-pressure liquid chromatography. This method is based on the different affinity of nucleotides to charged groups on a resin. Scholar et al. [1973] first applied this method to platelets. Since then, the method has been optimalized, and at present all relevant nucleotides can be measured in a single 20-min run in extracts from a gel-filtered platelet suspension without the need of a prior concentration step (Fig. 1). Separation is achieved with an anion-exchange column using a linear sodium phosphate gradient (10–700mM). As little as 40 pmol of each individual nucleotide can be measured with a $\pm$ 5% precision. Separation on anion-exchange columns by FPLC is equally fast and excellent. An even faster separation (less than 10 min) is achieved by reversed-phase, isocratic HPLC on radially compressed columns [Rao et al., 1981]; moreover, these columns are immediately ready for a next analysis without prior regeneration, owing to the isocratic mode of elution. However, this also limits the sample volume that can be injected and, hence, necessitates a concentration step. HPLC on anion-exchange columns is ideally suited for analysis of PCA-extracts; since EDTA coelutes with ADP and GDP, this technique is not suited for the analysis of EDTA-ethanol extracts.

Other methods. Ion-exchange column [Rivard et al., 1975a; Witas et al., 1974] and thin-layer chromatography [Rivard et al., 1975b] are relatively simple techniques for the separation of purine-moiety labeled nucleotides. Both techniques can be performed without any sophisticated instrumentation; nevertheless, their application in platelet research is rare. Analysis by ion-exchange chromatography requires neutralized PCA- or TCA-extracts. Thin-layer chromatography can be performed on both acid- and ethanol-extracts. For a complete separation of all purine nucleotides, however, development in two directions is necessary [Rivard et al., 1975]. Thin-layer chromatography on PEI (polyethyleneimine)-cellulose combines tlc with ion-exchange chromatography [Honegger et al., 1977], and can be applied with both ethanol and neutralized PCA-extracts. Separation by this multistep chromatography is excellent, which makes this method especially suited for the measurement of radiolabeled cyclic nucleotides.

Quantification of Nucleotides

Firefly-assay. This is the current method for ATP microdetermination. In this assay ATP is allowed to react with luciferin in the presence of luciferase; the activated luciferin-AMP complex formed is immediately oxidized by O_2, which results in the emission of a photon and release of AMP. In the overall reaction, ATP is converted to AMP and pyrophosphate. The peak intensity of the corresponding light flash is directly proportional to the ATP concentration. ADP is measured with the same method by converting it to ATP with the pyruvate kinase system [Holmsen et al., 1972b; Steen and Holmsen, 1985]. In theory, other nucleotides can also be quantified by this method by conversion to ATP. Due to the specificity of the enzymes used, nucleotides can be measured directly without prior separation from each other. A mixture of luciferin-luciferase in a stabilizing buffer is commerically available. This technique is also employed in the lumiaggregometer for the continuous monitoring of dense granule secretion [Feinman et al., 1977].

NAD-linked enzymatic assays. The nucleotide to be measured is enzymatically converted in a reaction that is finally coupled to an oxido-reduction reaction involving NADH, which is then quantified spectrophotometrically or fluorometrically. The specificity of these assays depends entirely on that of the enzymes used; although prior separation of the nucleotides is not required, it may improve sensitivity for some minor nucleotides. Before the development of the firefly assay this was the method of choice [Karpatkin and Langer, 1968; Mills and Thomas, 1969], but it has hardly been employed thereafter.

Other methods. The total amount of nucleotides can simply be measured by their absorbance at 254 nm in acid extracts [Murer, 1969]. This method can be applied in the measurement of total nucleotide levels in extracts. Commonly, UV absorbance is used to quantify individual nucleotides after their separation by one of the above-mentioned techniques. Sensitivity is improved by measuring the difference in absorbance at 254 and 280 nm [Daniel et al., 1980].

APPLICATIONS

Determination of Cell Lysis

Cell lysis is monitored by the extracellular appearance of cytosolic markers, usually lactate dehydrogenase. In pulse-labeled platelets the radiolabeled adenylates are solely present in the cytosolic compartment; their extracellular appearance is therefore an excellent marker of lysis and can be detected far more accurately than lactate dehydrogenase, which tends to lose its activity under extreme dilutions. Moreover, these metabolites are much smaller than the protein, which makes them a more useful indicator of cell lysis under certain circumstances. The difference in molecular size between the adenylates and lactate dehydrogenase has got wide application in cell permeabilization studies. The main purpose of permeabilization is to generate holes in the plasma membrane that are just big enough to allow the entrance of small molecules, such as Ca^{2+} or inositol 1,4,5-trisphosphate, but leave the proteins inside the platelets [Haslam and Davidson, 1984; Auhti et al., 1986]. The efficacy of the permeabilization technique is easily monitored by the differential release of labeled nucleotides and lactate dehydrogenase.

Measurement of Dense Granule Secretion

Dense granule secretion can be monitored by the extracellular appearance of adenine nucleotides, either directly by NMR or the lumiaggregometer, or in extracts of the extracellular medium after the removal of the platelets. The lumiaggregometer has the advantage that secretion is monitored continuously and simultaneously with optical aggregation [Feinman et al., 1977]. It is obvious that the presence of the luciferin-luciferase reagent should not interfere with platelet function. However, both a potentiation and an inhibition of platelet aggregation has been described [Mehta et al., 1983; Thompson and Scrutton, 1985]. Huang and Detwiler [1980] made a note on the presence of a dialyzable inhibitor in the reagent. The inhibitory effect of the reagent has been extensively studied in suspensions of gel-filtered platelets by Thompson and Scrutton [1985]. They showed that the inhibitory effect could be overcome by decreasing Mg^{++} and albumin in the reagent, and by replacing EDTA by a low concentration of EGTA. These recommendations should be followed when using the lumiaggregometer.

These potential hazards are avoided by using the sampling mode of this assay. Moreover, secreted ADP (which is the major nucleotide secreted) can be measured in addition or together with ATP. In this technique, samples are withdrawn from the platelet suspension during aggregation, rapidly mixed with 135 mM formaldehyde-10 mM EDTA in saline (final concentration, O°C) and then centrifuged to remove the platelets from the medium. This fixation procedure is essential, since it instantaneously stops secretion and prevents centrifugation-induced secretion; it also inhibits plasma ATP- and ADPases [Holmsen and Setkowsky-Dangelmaier, 1977]. The amount of adenine nucleotides in the supernatant can then be measured by one of the above-mentioned methods.

Secretion of ATP and ADP can also be measured by NMR. Due to the time it takes to prepare a NMR spectrum, this technique is not suited for the continuous monitoring of the rapid secretion responses. Instead, a ^{31}P-NMR spectrum is made of a platelet suspension of 4°C before stimulation, and after the completion of secretion in the presence of EDTA [Ugurbil et al., 1979]. Secretion becomes evident by the appearance of new resonances, which is caused by the increase in molecular mobility of the secreted nucleotides, the pH-difference between the interior of the dense granules and the extracellular medium, and the virtual absence of divalent cations in the extracellular medium.

Quantification of Different Pool Sizes

The amount of nucleotides stored in the dense granules can easily be quantified by treating platelets under optimal conditions with a high dose of thrombin (5 units/ml, 5 min, 37°C), which results in their complete secretion into the suspending medium. Degradation of secreted nucleotides extracellularly can be prevented by EDTA. After removal of the platelets by centrifugation, the amounts of nucleotides are determined by one of the methods described above.

The cytosolic and dense granule nucleotides of gel-filtered platelets can also be rapidly separated by controlled digitonin-induced cell lysis followed by centrifigation through a phthalate layer, as described by Akkerman et al, [1980]. Again, EDTA is added to the platelet medium to prevent hydrolysis of ATP and ADP after cell disruption. Ethanol-soluble ATP and ADP is quantified in both the cytosol and granule fraction, thereby excluding actin-bound ADP. The nucleotides that are sequestered in the mitochondria are included in the dense granulefraction, but their quantity is negligible [Holmsen et al., 1969]. After appropriate corrections for the contribution of nonlyzed cells to the dense granule fraction (based on lactate dehydrogenase) and of nonspecific lysis of granules to the cytosol fraction (based on serotonin), data are obtained that agree well with those obtained with other methods. The method of correction for the leakage of dense granule-contents into the cytosolic compartment is not applicable with storage pool-deficient platelets, where a substantial fraction of cellular serotonin remains soluble [Akkerman et al., 1983c].

The observation of Daniel et al, [1980] that the specific radioactivity of actin-bound ADP is identical to that of the other metabolic adenylates in platelets that have been pulse-labeled with adenine is the basis for a simple, but very accurate method for the quantitation of the latter. Total adenine-radioactivity in each individual nucleotide is calculated into the actual concentration when the specific radioactivity of actin-bound ADP is known. This method does not require high platelet counts, which makes it especially useful in clinical situations where the amount of available platelets can be severely limited.

Determination of the Specific ^{32}P-Activity of ATP

Labeling of platelets with $^{32}P\text{-}P_i$ has proved a powerful tool in metabolic studies of phosphorylated compounds such as phosphoinositides, phosphoproteins, and glycolytic intermediates. It is often desirable to know the specific ^{32}P-activity of the γ-phosphoryl of metabolic ATP, which in most cases is the immediate phosphoryl donor. This is complicated by the presence of the large pool of nonmetabolic granule-stored nucleotides. This pool can be removed by treating the platelets with a high dose of thrombin and subsequently separating them from the suspending medium. Although the metabolic ATP pool is also reduced by 30–50% in this procedure [Fukami et al., 1976], its specific ^{32}P-activity remains unchanged, since in pulse-labeled platelets the specific ^{32}P-activity is identical for P_i, the β- and γ-phosphoryls of ATP and the major phosphorylated metabolites [Holmsen et al., 1983]. In platelets that are not labeled to equilibrium with $^{32}P\text{-}P_i$ (i.e., during uptake of $^{32}P\text{-}P_i$), however, thrombin-stimulation likely affects the specific ^{32}P-activity in ATP. Under those conditions, determination of the specific ^{32}P-activity of the β-phosphoryl in actin-bound ADP [Daniel et al., 1980] probably is a good alternative, although it has not been proven yet that this is identical to that of the β- and γ-phosphoryls of ATP. Due to the 5–10 sec delay in labeling between actin-ADP and cytosolic ATP [Daniel et al., 1986], this method is not suited for initial-incorporation studies. In that case, a double-labeling method may be used, in which platelets are first labeled to equilibrium with ^{3}H-adenine, and the incorporation of $^{32}P\text{-}P_i$ into metabolic ATP can then be monitored as the increase in $^{32}P/^{3}H$ ratio in ATP [Verhoeven et al., 1986b]. This method yields only relative data, but the $^{32}P/^{3}H$ ratio is highly sensitive indicator of changes in specific ^{32}P-activity of metabolic ATP.

Determination of Energy Consumption

For the assessment of ATP utilization in platelets during the rapid aggregatory and secretory responses, the conventional method of measuring lactate production and mitochondrial O_2-uptake is useless. Recently, a novel method was developed which allows the determination of energy consumption within 15–20 sec [Akkerman et al., 1983a]. In this method, energy consumption is derived from the initial changes in metabolic ATP and ADP following an abrupt, complete arrest of ATP regeneration. This is achieved by the addition of a mixture of metabolic inhibitors to platelets that have been pulse-labeled with radioactive adenine (Fig. 5). In the anaerobic protocol, platelets are incubated with KCN and glucose, and glycolysis and glycogenolysis are rapidly blocked with 30 mM 2-deoxyglucose and 10 mM gluconolactone, respectively [Akkerman et al., 1983a]. In the aerobic protocol, platelets are incubated without glucose, and an abrupt arrest of glycogenolysis and oxidative phosphorylation is induced with 10 mM gluconolactone and 15 μM antimycin A, respectively; to prevent antimycin-binding to the albumin in the platelet medium, this is replaced by gelatin [Verhoeven et al., 1984b]. The subsequent fall in ATP and ADP radioactivity is calculated into units of μmol/min/10^{11} cells on the basis of a metabolic ATP content of 4.5 μmol/min/10^{11} platelets, and the finding that immediately after gel-filtration 80% of total adenine radioactivity is present in ATP. In suspensions of unstimulated human platelets, both protocols of this method correlate well with the conventional methods. However, when applied to rat or rabbit platelets, which have a substantial creatine phosphokinase activity [Meltzer and Guschwan, 1972], the fall in creatine phosphate must also be quantified. In addition, when applied to platelets that have their pool of glycolytic intermediates artificially elevated, the contribution of these intermediates to ATP regeneration must also be accounted for [Verhoeven et al., 1985b].

CONCLUDING REMARKS AND SUMMARY

Platelets are rich in nucleotides, particularly adenylates, which participate in many aspects of metabolism and in the propagation of platelet activation. The adenylates are markedly compartmentalized in platelets, with 65% sequestered in the dense granules in a nonmetabolic form. The remainder is present in the cytosol in a metabolically active form, where a substantial portion of ADP (50%) is bound to F-actin. This marked compartmentalization is fundamental for the understanding of current methodology for determination of amounts and turnover of nucleotides. These methods include various combinations of isotopic labeling procedures, NMR, organic versus acid extractions, functional and detergent pool separation, nucleotide separation by electrophoresis, paper chromatography, and HPLC as well as direct determination of ATP and ADP by the bioluminescence technique. We have also described some specific uses of these methods in a selected number of common applications, such as the determination of cell lysis, secretion, pool sizes, specific radioactivity of ^{32}P-ATP, and energy consumption. The technique of noninvasive NMR has proven especially valuable in the study of nucleotide compartmentalization and the elucidation of the complex structure of the nucleotides stored in the dense granules. Developments within the field of NMR technology that make it possible to generate spectra of *diluted* platelet suspensions within *seconds* rather than minutes, will enable its application to the study of nucleotide metabolism and turnover.

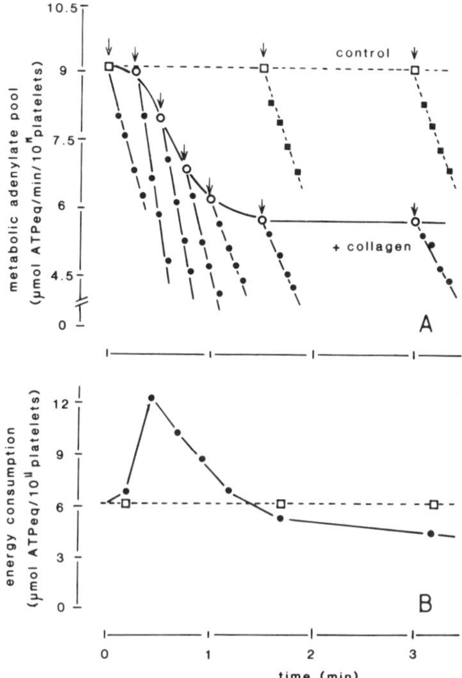

Fig. 5. Determination of energy consumption during collagen-induced responses. [^{3}H] Adenine labeled gel-filtered platelets were stimulated with 8 μg/ml of collagen (Hormon Chemie, Muchen, FRG: dialyzed for 20 hours against 1,000 vol of gel-filtration buffer in order to remove glucose) in the absence of extracellular glucose (○,●). This resulted in a 35% fall of the steady-state level of [^{3}H] ATP and [^{3}H] ADP, which started at 15 sec and was complete at 90 sec after addition of collagen (A). In a series of parallel incubations, a mixture of 15 μM antimycin A plus 10 mM glucono-δ-lactone was added to separate tubes, either simultaneously with collagen, or at 15, 30, 45, 60, 90, and 180 sec thereafter, as indicated by the arrows (●). From the subsequent fall of metabolic ATP and ADP, the rate of energy consumption during the initial 15-sec interval was determined and plotted at the midpoint of each interval (B;●). Similar studies were performed with unstimulated platelets (□;■). Collagen induced an increase in energy consumption between 15 and 90 sec. Under identical conditions, aggregation (monitored by the disappearance of single platelets) and secretion of serotonin and acid hydrolases started at 15 sec and were completed at 90 sec, in parallel with the increased energy consumption (data not shown). Moreover, rates of aggregation and secretion were highest between 15 and 30 sec after collagen addition, when also energy consumption is the highest. This illustrates the tight coupling between the collagen-induced responses and concomitant energy consumption. (ATPeq = ATP equivalent, which denotes the energy yield of the ATP to ADP conversion, with ATP corresponding to 2 ATPeq and ADP to 1 ATPeq.)

ACKNOWLEDGMENTS

A.J.M. Verhoeven was a NTNF (Royal Norwegian Council for Scientific and Industrial Research) Postdoctoral Fellow.

REFERENCES

Agarwal KC, Parks RE Jr (1975). Adenosine analogs and human platelets. Effects on nucleotide pools and the aggregation phenomenon. Biochem Pharmacol 24: 2239–2248.

Akkerman JWN, Gorter G (1980). Relation between energy production and adenine nucleotide metabolism in human blood platelets. Biochim Biophys Acta 501: 107–116.

Akkerman JWN, Holmsen H (1981). Interrelationships among platelet responses: Studies on the burst in proton liberation, lactate production, and oxygen uptake during platelet aggregation and Ca^{2+} secretion. Blood 57:956–966.

Akkerman JWN, Ebberink RHM, Lips JPM, Christiaens GCML (1980). Rapid separation of cytosol and particulate fraction of human platelets by digitonin-induced cell damage. Br J Haematol 44: 291–300.

Akkerman JWN, Gorter G, Schrama L, Holmsen H (1983a). A novel technique for rapid determination of energy consumption in platelets. Demonstration of different energy consumption associated with three secretory responses. Biochem J 210: 145–155.

Akkerman JWN, Gorter G, Soons H, Holmsen H (1983b). Close correlation between platelet responses and adenylate energy charge during transient substrate depletion. Biochim Biophys Acta 760: 34–41.

Akkerman JWN, Nieuwenhuis HK, Mommersteeg-Leautaud ME, Gorter G, Sixma JJ (1983c). ATP-ADP compartmentation in storage pool deficient platelets: Correlation between granule-bound ADP and the bleeding time. Br J Haematol 55: 135–143.

Ashby B, Holmsen H (1981). Platelet AMP deaminase. Purification and kinetic studies. J Biol Chem 256: 10519–10523.

Ashby B, Holmsen H (1983). Platelet AMP deaminase. Regulation by Mg-ATP^{2-} and inorganic phosphate and inhibition by the transition state analog coformycin. J Biol Chem 258: 3668–3672.

Ashby B, Wernick E, Holmsen H (1983). Coformycin inhibition of platelet AMP deaminase has no effect on thrombin-induced platelet secretion nor on glycolysis or glycogenolysis. J Biol Chem 258: 321–325.

Auhti KS, Evenden BJ, Crawford N (1986). Metabolic and functional consequences of introducing inositol 1,4,5-trisphosphate into saponin-permeabilized human platelets. Biochem J 233: 709–718.

Berridge MJ (1985). The molecular basis of communication within the cell. Sci Am 253: 124–135.

Chaiken R, Pagano D, Detwiler TC (1975). Regulation of platelet phosphorylase. Biochim Biophys Acta 403: 315.

Costa JL, Dobson CM, Kirk KL, Poulsen FM, Valeri CR, Vecchione JJ (1979). Studies of human platelets by ^{19}F and ^{31}P NMR. FEBS Lett 99: 141–146.

Daniel JL, Molish IR, Holmsen H (1980). Radioactive labeling of the adenine nucleotide pool of cells as a method to distinguish among intracellular compartments; studies on human platelets. Biochim Biophys Acta 632: 444–453.

Daniel JL, Molish IR, Robkin L, Holmsen H (1986). Nucleotide exchange between cytosolic ATP and F-actin-bound ADP my be a major energy-utilizing process in unstimulated platelets. Eur J Biochem 156: 677–684.

Daniel JL, Robkin L, Molish IR, Holmsen H (1979). Determination of the ADP concentration available to participate in energy metabolism in an actin-rich cell, the platelet. J Biol Chem 254: 7870–7873.

D'Souza L, Glueck HI (1979). Measurement of nucleotide pools in platelets using high pressure liquid chromatography. Thromb Haemost 38: 990–1001.

Feinman RD, Lubowsky J, Charo IF, Zabinski MP (1977). The lumi-aggregometer: A new instrument for simultaneous measurement of secretion and aggregation by platelets. J Lab Clin Med 90: 125–129.

Flodgaard H, Klenow H (1982). Abundant amounts of diadenosine 5′,5‴-P^1,P^4-tetraphosphate are present and releasable, but metabolically inactive, in human platelets. Biochem J 208: 737–742.

French PC, Sixma JJ, Holmsen H (1974). The uptake of adenine into isolated platelet membranes. Thromb Diathes Haemorrh 30: 57–64.

Fukami MH, Bauer JS, Stewart GJ, Salganicoff L (1978). An improved method for the isolation of dense storage granules from human platelets. J Cell Biol 77: 389–399.

Fukami MH, Holmsen H, Salganicoff L (1976). Adenine nucleotide metabolism of blood platelets. IX. Time course of secretion of changes in energy metabolism in thrombin-treated platelets. Biochim Biophys Acta 444: 633–643.

Gordon JL, Drummond AH (1974). A simple fluorimetric microassay for adenine compounds in platelets and plasma and its application to studies on the platelet release reaction. Biochem J 138: 165–169.

Haslam RJ, Davidson MML (1984). Potentiation by thrombin of the secretion of serotonin from permeabilized platelets equilibrated with Ca^{2+} buffers. Relationship to protein phosphorylation and diacylglycerol formation. Biochem J 222: 351–361.

Holmsen H (1965). Incorporation in vitro of P^{32} into blood platelet acid soluble organophosphates and their chromatographic identification. Scand J Clin Lab Invest 17: 230–238.

Holmsen H (1972). Ethanol-insoluble adenine nucleotides in platelets and their possible role in platelet function. Ann NY Acad Sci 201: 109–121.

Holmsen H (1982). Biochemistry of the platelet: Energy metabolism. In Colman RW, Hirsh J, Marder VJ, Salzman EW (eds): "Hemostasis and Thrombosis: Basic Concepts and Clinical Practice." Philadelphia: Lippincott, pp 431–443.

Holmsen H (1985). Nucleotide metabolism of platelets. Annu Rev Physiol 47: 677–690.

Holmsen H, Robkin L (1977). Hydrogen peroxide lowers ATP levels in platelets without altering adenylate energy charge and platelet function. J Biol Chem 252: 1752–1757.

Holmsen H , Setkowsky-Dangelmaier CA (1977). Adenine nucleotide metabolism of blood platelets . X. Formaldehyde stops centrifugation-induced secretion after A23187-stimulation and causes breakdown of metabolic ATP. Biochim Biophys Acta 497:46–61. 61.

Holmsen H, Weiss HJ (1979). Secretable storage pools in platelets. Annu Rev Med 30: 119–134.

Holmsen H, Dangelmaier CA, Akkerman JWN (1983). Determination of levels of glycolytic intermediates and nucleotides in platelets by pulse-labeling with ^{32}P orthophosphate. Anal Biochem 131: 266–272.

Holmsen H, Day HJ, Setkowsky CA (1972a). Behaviour of adenine nucleotides during the platelet release reaction induced by ADP and adrenaline. Biochem J 129: 67–82.

Holmsen H, Day HJ, Storm E (1969). Adenine nucleotide metabolism of blood platelets. VI. Subcellular localization of nucleotide pools with different functions in the platelet release reaction. Biochim Biophys Acta 186: 254–266.

Holmsen H, Kaplan KL, Dangelmaier CA (1982). Differential energy requirements for platelet responses. A simultaneous study of aggregation, three secretory responses, arachidonate liberation, phosphatidylinositol breakdown and phosphatidate production. Biochem J 208: 9–18.

Holmsen H, Robkin L, Driver H (1979). Reduction of the metabolic adenylate pool in platelets by hydroperoxides (HP): Studies on the mechanism. Fed Proc 38:826.

Holmsen H, Setkowsky CA, Day HJ (1974). Effects of antimycin and 2-deoxyglucose on adenine nucleotides in human platelets. Role of metabolic adenosine triphosphate in primary aggregation, secondary aggregation and shape change of platelets. Biochem J 144: 385–396.

Holmsen H, Storm E, Day HJ (1972b). Microdetermination of ADP and ATP in blood platelets: A modification of the plasma method. Anal Biochem 46: 489–501.

Honegger UE, Bogdanov SS, Bally PR (1977). Quantitative extraction, separation, and recovery of adenine-derived radioactivity in bases, nucleosides and nucleotides from blood platelets using PEI-cellulose thin-layer chromatography. Anal Biochem 82: 268–282.

Huang EM, Detwiler TC (1980). Reassessment of the evidence for the role of secreted ADP in biphasic platelet aggregation. J Lab Clin Med 95: 59–68.

Karpatkin S, Langer RM (1968). Biochemical energetics of simulated platelet plug formation. Effect of thrombin, adenosine diphosphate, and epinephrine on intra- and extracellular adenine nucleotide kinetics. J Clin Invest 47: 2158–2168.

Kim BK, Chao FC, Leavitt R, Fauci AS, Meyers KM, Zamecnik PC (1985). Diadenosine $5',5'''$-P^1,P^4-tetraphosphate deficiency in blood platelets of the Chediak-Higashi syndrome. Blood 66:735–737.

Lages B, Holmsen H, Weiss HJ, Dangelmaier C (1983). Thrombin and ionophore A23187-induced dense granule secretion in storage pool deficient platelets: Evidence for impaired nucleotide storage as the primary dense granule defect. Blood 61: 154–162.

Mehta P, Mehta I, Ostrowski N, Aguila E (1983). Potentiation of platelet aggregation by Chronolume^R. Thromb Res 32: 509–512.

Meltzer HY, Guschwan A (1972). Type I (brain type) creatine phosphokinase (CPK) activity in rat platelets. Life Sci 11: 121–130.

Meyers KM, Holmsen H, Seachord CL (1982). Comparative study of platelet dense granule constituents. Am J Physiol 243: R454–461.

Meyers KM, Holmsen H, Seachord CL, Hopkins GE, Borchard RE, Padgett GA (1979a). Storage pool deficiency in platelets from Chediak-Higashi cattle. Am J Physiol 237: R239–248.

Meyers KM, Holmsen H, Seachord CL, Hopkins GE, Gorham J (1979b). Characterization of platelets from normal mink and mink with the Chediak-Higashi syndrome. Am J Hematol 7: 137–146.

Meyers KM, Seachord CL, Holmsen H, Prieur DJ (1981). Evaluation of the platelet storage pool deficiency in the feline counterpart of the Chediak-Higashi syndrome. Am J Hematol 11: 241–253.

Mills DCB, Thomas DP (1969). Blood platelet nucleotides in man and other species. Nature 222: 991–992.

Murer EH (1969). A comparative study of the action of release inducers upon platelet release and phosphorus metabolism. Biochim Biophys Acta 192: 138–140.

Murer EH, Davenport K, Siojo E, Day HJ (1981). Metabolic aspects of the secretion of stored compounds from blood platelets. The effect of NaF at different pH on nucleotide metabolism and function of washed platelets. Biochem J 194: 187–192.

Rao GHR, Peller JD, White JG (1981). Rapid separation of platelet nucleotides by reversed-phase, isocratic, high-performance liquid chromatography with a radially compressed column. J Chromat 226: 446–470.

Reimers HJ, Mustard JF, Packham MA (1975). Transfer of adenine nucleotides between the releasable and nonreleasable compartments of rabbit blood platelets. J Cell Biol 67: 61–71.

Reimers HJ, Packham MA, Mustard JF (1977). Labeling of the releasable adenine nucleotides of washed human platelets. Blood 49: 89–99.

Richards JG, Da Prada M (1977). Uranaffin reaction: A new cytochemical technique for the localization of adenine nucleotides in organelles storing biogenic amines. J Histochem Cytochem 25: 1322–1336.

Rivard GE, Izadi P, Lazerson J, McLaren JD, Parker C, Fish CH (1975a). Functional and metabolic studies of platelets from patients with Lesch-Nyhan syndrome. Br J Haematol 31: 245–253.

Rivard GE, McLaren JD, Brunst RF (1975b). Incorporation of hypoxanthine into adenine and guanine nucleotides by human platelets. Biochim Biophys Acta 381: 144–156.

Scholar EM, Brown PR, Parks RE Jr, Calabresi P (1973). Nucleotide profiles of the formed elements of human blood determined by high-pressure liquid chromatography. Blood 41: 927–934.

Sixma JJ, Lips JPM, Trieschnigg AMC, Holmsen H (1976). Transport and metabolism of adenosine in human blood platelets. Biochim Biophys Acta 443: 33–48.

Sixma JJ, Trieschnigg AMC, Holmsen H (1973). Adenine nucleotide metabolism of blood platelets. VIII. Mechanism of adenine uptake by intact cells. Biochim Biophys Acta 298: 3–16.

Steen VM, Holmsen H (1985). Synergism between thrombin and epinephrine in human platelets: Different dose-response relationships for aggregation and dense granule secretion. Thromb Haemost 54: 680–683.

Thompson NT, Scrutton MC (1985). Inhibition by luciferin-luciferase reagents of aggregatory responses to excitatory agonists in washed platelet suspensions. Thromb Res 38: 109–119.

Ugurbil K, Holmsen H (1981). Nucleotide compartmentation: Radioisotopic and nuclear magnetic resonance studies. In Gordon JL (ed): "Platelets in Biology and Pathology." New York: Elsevier/North-Holland Biomedical Press, Vol 2, pp 147–177.

Ugurbil K, Holmsen H, Shulman RG (1979). Adenine nucleotide storage pools and secretion as studied by ^{31}P nuclear magnetic resonance. Proc Natl Acad Sci (USA) 76: 2227–2231.

Ugurbil K, Fukami MH, Holmsen H (1984a). ^{31}P NMR studies of nucleotide storage in the dense granules of pig platelets. Biochemistry 23: 409–415.

Ugurbil K, Fukami MH, Holmsen H (1984b). Proton NMR studies of nucleotide and amine storage in the dense granules of pig platelets. Biochemistry 23: 416–428.

Vargas JR, Radomski M, Moncada S (1982). The use of prostacyclin in the separation from plasma and washing of human platelets. Prostaglandins 23: 929–945.

Verhoeven AJM, Mommersteeg ME, Akkerman JWN (1984a). Metabolic energy is required in human platelets at any stage of aggregation and secretion. Biochim Biophys Acta 800: 242–250.

Verhoeven AJM, Mommersteeg ME, Akkerman JWN (1984b). Quantification of energy consumption during thrombin-induced aggregation and secretion. Tight coupling between platelet responses and the increment in energy consumption. Biochem J 221: 777–787.

Verhoeven AJM, Mommersteeg ME, Akkerman JWN (1985a). The energetics of early platelet responses. Energy consumption during shape change and aggregation with special reference to protein phosphorylation and polyphosphoinositide cycle. Biochem J 228: 451–462.

Verhoeven AJM, Mommersteeg ME, Akkerman JWN (1985b). Balanced contribution of glycolytic and adenylate pool in supply of metabolic energy in platelets. J Biol Chem 260: 2621–2624.

Verhoeven AJM, Mommersteeg ME, Akkerman JWN (1986a). Comparative studies on the energetics of platelet responses induced by different agonists. Biochem J (accepted).

Verhoeven AJM, Tysnes OB, Horvli O, Cook CA, Holmsen H (1986b). Thrombin-induced increase in phosphate-uptake and incorporation into ATP and polyphosphoinositides in human platelets. (To be submitted.)

Walseth TF, Gander JE, Eide SJ, Krick TP, Goldberg, ND (1983). ^{18}O Labeling of adenine nucleotide α- phosphoryls in platelets. Contribution by phosphodiesterase-catalyzed hydrolysis of cAMP. J Biol Chem 258: 1544–1558.

Wegner A (1976). Head to tail polymerization of actin. J Mol Biol 108: 139–150.

Witas H, Duba W, Kotelba-Witkowska B, Leyko B (1974). Changes of adenine nucleotides content and release reaction of human blood platelets following gamma irradiation. Radiat Environ Biophys 14: 317–322.

Yoshino M, Murakami K (1982). AMP deaminase reaction as a control system of glycolysis in yeast. Activation of phosphofructokinase and pyruvate kinase by the AMP deaminase-ammonia system. J Biol Chem 257: 2822–2828.

Modern Methods in Pharmacology, Volume 4
Methods for Studying Platelets and Megakaryocytes, pages 157–183

Methods of Studying Cyclic AMP Metabolism

BARRIE ASHBY and PAUL GRANT

INTRODUCTION

Cyclic AMP is generated from ATP by adenylate cyclase (EC 4.6.1.1) and hydrolyzed by cyclic AMP phosphodiesterases (EC 3.1.4.17). Hence the intracellular level of cyclic AMP represents a steady-state concentration. The second messenger role of cyclic AMP in platelets is clear: a rise in the steady-state level of cyclic AMP due to activation of adenylate cyclase or inhibition of phosphodiesterase leads to an inhibition of platelet responsiveness. Consequently efforts to understand and control the activity of these two enzymes have been coupled to the search for antithrombotic drugs. The concentration of cyclic AMP can be measured in extracts derived from intact platelets, providing a picture of intracellular cyclic AMP fluxes in response to a variety of agents. Adenylate cyclase activity can be determined in membrane preparations of various degrees of purity as well as in detergent solubilized preparations. Platelet cyclic AMP phosphodiesterases have been purified and to date three separate enzymes have been identified.

The purpose of this chapter is to compile the methods for measurement of cyclic AMP in intact platelets and methods for preparing and examining adenylate cyclase and phosphodiesterase activities in cell-free preparations. Agents that act as modifiers or probes of the two enzymes are also discussed, indicating the utility of such agents in elucidating the regulation of cyclic AMP metabolism and perhaps controlling platelet responsiveness.

MEASUREMENT OF CYCLIC AMP

Cyclic AMP is most often determined in extracts of platelets by measuring its production from radiolabeled ATP, derived from nucleotide pool labeling, or by radioimmunoassay. Both methods also can be used effectively with membrane

From the Thrombosis Research Center, Temple University School of Medicine, Philadelphia, Pennsylvania 19140.

preparations of solubilized enzyme in the presence of phosphodiesterase inhibitors to determine the activity of adenylate cyclase. Radioimmunoassay gives a direct measure of the amount of cyclic AMP but is expensive when purchased as a kit from, for example, New England Nuclear.

Measurement of cyclic AMP in cell-free systems is possible by use of [alpha-^{32}P]ATP, as described by Salomon [1979] or by use of [^{3}H]ATP according to modifications of the method of Salomon [1979] due to Van Heyningen et al. [1983]. In intact platelets, use of radiolabeled ATP is restricted to [^{3}H] or [^{14}C] nucleotides generally incorporated into the cell as adenine or adenosine. [^{32}P]PO_4 enters the cell but does not incorporate into the alpha position of ATP and therefore does not label cyclic AMP. The two major methods are discussed below. Other methods of determining cyclic AMP have been employed and also will be described here.

Preparation of Platelets and Platelet Extracts

Platelets are obtained from freshly drawn human blood collected into acid-citrate dextrose anticoagulant. Platelet-rich plasma is prepared as the supernatant following centrifugation at 300 × g for 15 min at room temperature. When radioactive measurement of cyclic AMP is employed, platelet-rich plasma is labeled with 1.0 μCi/ml [^{3}H]- or [^{14}C]adenine for 1 hour at 37°C. Cyclic AMP measurements can be made on platelet-rich plasma. Alternatively, platelet-rich plasma can be gel-filtered according to Lages et al. [1975] or washed to remove plasma and excess label, providing a more controlled system for observing the effects of modifiers on cyclic AMP level.

A suitable washing procedure is described here that results in little activation of the platelets in terms of shape change or secretion. Platelet-rich plasma is centrifuged at 180 × g for 15 min and the platelets resuspended in HEPES buffer, pH 6.6, containing 0.14 M NaCl and 5 μg/ml of apyrase (Sigma, grade I). The suspension is centrifuged (440 × g, 25 min, 4°C) and the platelet pellet resuspended in HEPES buffer, pH 7.4, containing 0.14 M NaCl and 0.05 U/ml hirudin but no apyrase. The resuspended platelets should be warmed to the temperature of the experiment before use.

Platelet-rich plasma, gel-filtered or washed platelets can be challenged with a variety of effectors or inhibitors of adenylate cyclase or phosphodiesterases in appropriate experiments. Following treatment for a measured interval of time, platelets can be sampled into an equal volume of a stopping solution designed to lyse the cells and stop further formation or disappearance of cyclic AMP. Suitable stopping solution agents include an equal volume of ice-cold 15% (w/v) trichlor-acetic acid or 1.2 M perchloric acid. When the metabolism of radiolabeled cyclic AMP is measured, the stopping solution always contains a recovery standard of

1,000–2,000 cpm of radiolabeled cyclic AMP ([^{3}H]cyclic AMP when [^{14}C]adenine is used and [^{14}C]cyclic AMP when [^{3}H]adenine is used).

Samples obtained by these methods can be analyzed for cyclic AMP according to the methods described below.

Analytical Methods

Nucleotide pool labeling. Incubation of platelets with radiolabeled adenine or adenosine results in labeling of all adenine nucleotides in the cytoplasmic pool to the same specific activity [Daniel et al., 1980]. As a result cyclic AMP formation in intact cells is frequently expressed as a percentage of the total radiolabeled ATP. Determination of the mass of cyclic AMP formed can be obtained by measuring the amount of ATP by firefly luminescence [Holmsen et al., 1972] or by high pressure liquid chromatography [Daniel et al., 1980; Brooker, 1971] and hence obtaining the specific radioactivity of the adenine nucleotides. This procedure is complicated by the fact that as much as 40% of the ATP in platelets is sequestered in the secretable dense granules and does not become radiolabeled along with the metabolically active cytosolic pool. Hence the amount of ATP in the cell must be determined on samples obtained before and after secretion.

Radioactive cyclic AMP formed in platelets is determined by separating cyclic AMP from other nucleotides. This is no trivial matter, since the amount of cyclic AMP representing basal levels comprises less than 0.2% of the total nucleotide pool, rising to 6% or higher following stimulation with prostacyclin or forskolin. The most frequently used method for separation of cyclic AMP is the two column method of Salomon [1979]. The method is thoroughly documented by Salomon and only the principle will be discussed here. Samples of nucleotides extracted from platelets, generally in a volume of 1 ml, are passed first through small columns of Dowex 50. Both ATP and ADP elute slightly ahead of cyclic AMP in the first two milliliters of water passed through the columns. The cyclic AMP is still contaminated by significant amounts of other nucleotides and is eluted with water directly into small columns of alumina (aluminum oxide). Cyclic AMP can be readily eluted from the alumina column with 0.1 M imidazole, pH 7.0, while ATP remains tightly bound. The eluted cyclic AMP can be collected directly into scintillation vials and mixed with a suitable aqueous phase scintillant such as Liquiscint (National Diagnostics) or Scinti Verse II (Fisher Scientific Co.). Two channel radioactivity counting is employed to determine the amount of cyclic AMP generated in the sample (generally as [^{3}H]cyclic AMP) and to determine the recovery measured relative to a [^{14}C]cyclic AMP standard included in the stopping solution. Calculation of the amount of cyclic AMP formed requires a cross-over correction.

The method of Salomon [1979] represents an improvement over previous methods of column purification of cyclic AMP. Krishna et al. [1968] originally introduced chromatography on Dowex in combination with selective precipitation of residual ATP with freshly generated $BaSO_4$. This method is still fairly widely used. White and Zenser [1971], and Ramachandran [1971] introduced the method of separation of cyclic AMP from ATP on alumina. The three methods have been carefully compared by Salomon et al. [1974].

Haslam and McClenaghan [1981] have described an alternative method of purification of cyclic AMP. Acidified extracts, obtained by centrifugation of platelet suspensions sampled into trichloroacetic acid, are applied to columns of alumina (15 × 0.7 cm) that have been washed with 10% (w/v) trichloroacetic acid. The columns are then washed with 9 ml of 10% (w/v) trichloroacetic acid, 9 ml of water, and 2 ml of 0.2 M ammonium formate (pH 6.0). Cyclic AMP is eluted with a further 3 ml of 0.2 M formate and applied directly to columns of Dowex 50. These columns are washed with 6 ml of 1 mM potassium phosphate buffer, pH 7.3, and cyclic AMP finally eluted with 9 ml of the same buffer, which is lyophilized and counted.

A further method of isolating radiolabeled cyclic AMP from perchloric acid extracts of platelets has been described by Sinha and Colman [1978] and is called affinity elution chromatography. Radiolabeled adenine nucleotides from the neutralized extract are absorbed to QAE-cellulose. After washing, cyclic AMP is specifically eluted with commercially available cyclic AMP-dependent protein kinase. The method has the advantage of high specificity intrinsic to the method of elution.

Radioimmunoassay for cyclic AMP. A radioimmunoassay for cyclic AMP has been described by Brooker et al. [1979]. The method has the advantage that it gives a direct measure of the amount of cyclic AMP in cell extracts. Antibody to cyclic AMP is prepared by using 2′-O-succinyl cyclic AMP coupled to albumin. The method is based on competition of the tyrosine methyl ester of 2’-O-succinyl cyclic AMP (iodinated with iodine-125) with cyclic AMP in the tissue extract. Cyclic AMP in the extracts is usually acetylated to increase the affinity for the antibody (and hence the sensitivity of the assay) by 10- to 40-fold. The assay is sensitive into the femtomolar range and is highly specific for cyclic AMP. Hence purification of cyclic AMP is not necessary and neutralized platelet extracts can be used directly.

High performance liquid chromatography. Brooker [1971] has demonstrated direct measurement of cyclic AMP by high pressure liquid chromatography in adenylate cyclase assays and tissue extracts, which involves extraction and purification of the nucleotide. However, this method is not feasible for routine assay of cyclic AMP because of the small amounts in platelet samples and the time involved in each determination. Combination of high pressure liquid chromatography with intracellular pool labeling allows the determination of specific radioactivity of cyclic AMP in tissues and hence the mass of the nucleotide.

^{18}O labeling of adenine nucleotide alpha-phosphoryls in platelets. Goldberg and coworkers [Walseth et al., 1983] have used ^{18}O incorporation into the alpha-phosphoryls of adenine nucleotides to follow phosphodiesterase-promoted hydrolysis of cyclic AMP in intact human platelets. The methods employed are complex and involve use of gas chromatography/mass spectrometry to measure the atom percent excess of ^{18}O incorporation, so that this approach is not readily applicable. However, the work has provided a wealth of data on cyclic AMP metabolism, some of which are summarized here. ^{18}O was incorporated into the alpha-phosphoryls at a basal rate of 70 nmol of ^{18}O/min/7.8 $\times$ 10^8 platelets (equivalent to 1 g wet weight). A 10–40-fold increase in platelet cyclic AMP concentration due to prostacyclin increased the total rate of ^{18}O incorporation by 4- to 5-fold during the first 10 min. A decline in rate after 10 min exposure to prostacyclin probably resulted from desensitization. From the rate of ^{18}O labeling of alpha-phosphoryls an apparent Km value of 4 to 5 μM and Vmax of 3 nmol/min/mg of protein can be calculated for the total operational phosphodiesterase activities in intact platelets. Equating ^{18}O labeling of alpha-phosphoryls with hydrolysis of cyclic AMP the half-time for turnover of the entire pool of cyclic AMP can be determined as 200 ms under basal conditions and 1.3 s when the pool size is increased by prostacyclin. These values exceed estimates based on measurements of changes in steady-state levels and prelabeling of adenine nucleotides and indicate that metabolism of cyclic AMP in platelets is a very dynamic process. Inhibition of the ^{18}O labeling rate by the phosphodiesterase inhibitor 1-methyl-3-isobutylxanthine was transient and presumably reflects a readjustment of the level of metabolic intermediates to overcome the influence of this competitive inhibitor.

Perhaps just as interesting as the intracellular kinetic parameters revealed by this method is the idea that cyclic AMP and related nucleotide metabolites must be associated with a discrete compartment or complex of metabolic enzymes. Such compartmentation prevents their dilution by larger pools of adenine nucleotides during metabolic flux but exchange of nucleotide products with other pools can occur, so that, for example, some of the cyclic AMP may fulfill its second messenger function in activation of protein kinases. Goldberg [Walseth et al., 1983] hypothesizes that the rapid flux of cyclic AMP in a small compartment may render the system highly responsive in providing an increased steady-state level of cyclic AMP.

PREPARATION AND ASSAY OF ADENYLATE CYCLASE

All of the components of the adenylate cyclase system are localized and interact in membranes. The most obvious location for interaction with hormones, autocoids, and other endogenous agents acting at the cell-surface receptor is the plasma membrane surrounding the outer surface of the cell. However, histochemical localization studies [Cutler et al., 1985] indicate that the enzyme is located in the dense tubular system. A possible reason for this is that enzyme localized on the cytoplasmic membrane is more labile to fixative than the enzyme localized on internal membranes. Biochemical methods for separation of platelet membrane types are now becoming available (see below) that may resolve this question.

Platelet Membrane Preparation

Membrane preparations are amenable to studies at defined concentrations of ATP, magnesium ions, guanine nucleotides, and other ligands that affect the activity of the enzyme, while still showing responsiveness of receptor-linked activators such as prostacyclin, and inhibitors such as epinephrine and ADP. Membranes are also amenable to treatment with cholera toxin and pertussis toxin that modify the activity of the guanine nucleotide proteins linking the catalytic unit to stimulatory receptors or inhibitory receptors.

Activity is fairly stable at 0–4°C, and remarkable stability can be achieved in the presence of ATP. This is evident from the fact that progress curves are linear for many minutes even at 37°C. Adenylate cyclase activity is quite stable in intact platelets but may be attenuated in platelets stored according to blood banking procedures for more than a week. Hence it is possible to use reasonably outdated platelets for studies of adenylate cyclase, and large quantities of outdated platelets could be used as a starting point for purification of the enzyme.

Platelet membranes that contain active adenylate cyclase responsive to hormonal regulation can be fairly readily prepared with a range of specific activities. A number of methods are described here. It is also possible to solubilize the enzyme from membrane preparations and it has become feasible to purify the enzyme. Steps toward this goal are described.

Freeze and thawing. The simplest method of obtaining a membrane preparation of adenylate cyclase is to freeze and then thaw washed platelets once. The procedure, according to Haslam and Lynham [1972], begins with collection of human blood into acid-citrate-dextrose anticoagulant and centrifugation (300 × g, 15 min, room temperature). The supernatant platelet-rich plasma is centrifuged at 750 × g for 15 min at 4°C in an angle head rotor in plastic, or siliconized glass, tapered tubes. The platelet pellets are washed twice by resuspension and centrifugation in a 13 mM sodium citrate, 5 mM glucose, 135 mM NaCl, adjusted to pH 6.5 with HCl. The washed platelets are finally resuspended in Tris-buffered saline (138.6 mM NaCl, 15.4 mM Tris-HCl, pH 7.4) at 25 mg wet weight/ml. The suspension is rapidly frozen in dry ice/acetone or in liquid nitrogen, and then thawed at 37°C. The lysate is centrifuged at 38,000 × g for 20 min at 4°C and the pellet resuspended in Tris-buffered saline to give 6–12 mg protein/ml. This suspension is stored on ice until used. Freezing and thawing releases 50–60% of the platelet protein into the supernatant. Further cycles of freezing and thawing release no more protein and result in a loss in adenylate cyclase activity. After one cycle of freezing and thawing the specific activity of the membranes is typically 28 pmol/min/mg basal activity and 355 pmol/min/mg in the presence of 10 μM PGE_1.

Glycerol lysis. More highly purified membranes with a high specific activity for adenylate cyclase can be obtained by the method of Barber and Jamieson [1970], as described by Steer and Wood [1979]. Platelet-rich plasma is obtained from 450 ml of freshly donated, aspirin-free blood in acid-citrate dextrose. The platelets are pelleted by centrifugation at 4,300 × g for 10 min at 4°C, and carefully resuspended in a buffer consisting of 1 mM EDTA, 150 mM NaCl, 10 mM Tris-HCl, pH 7.6. This washing procedure is repeated two or three times to remove red cells. The pellet is resuspended in 1 or 2 ml of the same buffer, and layered over 26 ml of a 0 to 40% glycerol gradient prepared in 150 mM NaCl. The intracellular glycerol concentration is raised to 4.3 M by slowly centrifuging the platelets through the glycerol gradient, using a swinging bucket rotor (2,000 × g, 10 min, 4°C). The pelleted platelets are lysed by suspension and rapid mixing in 12 ml of a buffer consisting of 1 mM EGTA, 250 mM sucrose, 10 mM Tris-HCl, pH 7.6. The lysed platelets are pelleted by centrifugation (8,700 × g, 10 min, 4°C). The pelleted membrane preparation is washed four times by resuspension in 1.5 ml of an appropriate buffer and centrifugation (10,000 × g, 3 min, 4°C) in an Eppendorf table-top centrifuge. The membranes are used immediately for adenylate cyclase studies. One unit of blood (450 ml) provides 2–10 mg of platelet membranes. The specific activity of adenylate cyclase obtained by this method was 89 pmol/min/mg basal and 262 pmol/min/mg in the presence of 2 μM PGE_1.

The membranes obtained by glycerol lysis can be further purified by sucrose gradient centrifugation according to Barber and Jamieson [1970]. The lysed platelet suspension in 250 mM sucrose, 10 mM Tris-HCl, pH 7.5, is layered on top of a solution of 27% (w/v) sucrose and centrifuged (63,000 × g, 3 to 5 h, 4°C) in a swing-out rotor (SW 25.1, in a Beckman ultracentrifuge). The membrane fraction remains as a narrow band above the sucrose interface while unbroken platelets, granules, and other debris sediment to the bottom of the tube.

Two subfractions of the membranes can be obtained by centrifugation through a continuous sucrose gradient for 18 hours. However, these subfractions possess negligible adenylate cyclase activity [Krishna et al., 1972], probably because of the extreme lability of the enzyme.

Free-flow electrophoresis. Crawford and coworkers [Lagarde et al., 1981] have described a method for separation of different platelet membrane fractions by free-flow electrophoresis. This method has yet to be exploited for preparation of adenylate cyclase containing fractions and for biochemical localization of the enzyme. The apparatus is also expensive.

Percoll gradient centrifugation. Record and others [Record et al., 1982; Perret et al., 1979; Mauco et al., 1984] have introduced a rapid method for separating cytoplasmic and intracellular membranes by use of Percoll gradients. The method was originally described for use in separating membranes of ascites cells and has since been adapted for use with platelets [Perret et al., 1979; Mauco et al., 1984]. The method has been used to examine the subcellular distribution of diacylglycerol- and monoacylglycerol-lipases in human platelets, and has the potential for localization of other membrane bound enzymes as well.

Washed platelets are suspended in a lysis buffer consisting of 100 mM KCl, 3mM ATP, 3 mM $MgCl_2$, 20 mM Tris-HCl, pH 7.4. The platelets are lysed by nitrogen cavitation in a Parr bomb (1,000 psi, 15 min) and the lysate centrifuged at low speed (1,500 × g, 15 min, 4°C) to remove aggregated contractile proteins and other debris. The membranes suspended in the supernatant are separated from cytosol by high speed centrifugation (100,000 × g, 45 min, 4°C).

Further fractionation of the membranes may be carried out quickly on self-forming Percoll gradients. The membrane pellet is resuspended in 19.2 ml of lysis buffer adjusted to pH 9.6 and mixed with Percoll. The pH is optimal for resolution of membrane subfractions according to the method of Perret et al. [1979]. The mixture is centrifuged at 28,500 rpm for exactly 15 min in a Ti60 rotor. 15× 2 ml fractions are collected and can be assayed for adenylate cyclase assay following adjustment to pH 7.4. Although the requirement for a pH of 9.6 for effective resolution of membrane fractions seems extreme our own experience indicates that active adenylate cyclase, responsive to prostaglandin activation, can be obtained by this method. ATP is added to the buffer mixture to precipitate contactile proteins but also serves to stabilize adenylate cyclase.

Membrane fractions may be characterized by a variety of markers. Treatment of cells with [^{3}H]concanavalin A prior to cell disruption provides a marker for the plasma membrane. Assay of acid hydrolase activity (N-acetyl-beta-D-glucos-aminidase) can be used to identify the lysosomal fraction, and assay of NADH diaphorase provides a marker for the dense tubular system.

Preparation of Solubilized Platelet Adenylate Cyclase

Adenylate cyclase can be solubilized from membrane preparations using methods described for other cell-types [Bitonti et al., 1982; Ross, 1981; Strittmatter and Neer, 1980]. A variety of detergent systems involvi nonionic detergents have been employed. Of various detergent sys determined that solubilization using CHAPS, a zwitterionic deriva acid [Bitonti et al., 1982], in the presence of high salt gives the best yield and specific activity. In addition CHAPS, unlike cholate or nonionic detergents such as Lubrol (26), does not interfere with adenylate cyclase activity and so does not have to be removed or diluted out prior to assay.

Membranes obtained by freeze-thawing are resuspended in a buffer consisting of 50 mM HEPES, pH 7.4, 1 mM ATP, 1 mM EDTA, 1 mM dithiothreitol, and 1 M ammonium sulfate to a protein concentration of 10 mg/ml. The suspension is made 15 mM in CHAPS by addition from a stock solution of 500 mM CHAPS and mixed for 10 min at 4°C before being centrifuged at 100,000 × g for 45 min. The supernatant routinely contains 80% of the adenylate cyclase activity (B. Ashby, unpublished data) of the original membranes and can be stored at −70° for many months with little loss in activity. The solubilized preparation can be activated by forskolin, GTP, and fluoride but is insensitive to receptor-mediated effects such as prostacyclin stimulation or epinephrine inhibition.

Assay of Adenylate Cyclase

Assay components. Adenylate cyclase activity is generally assayed in Tris-HCl or triethanolamine-HCl, at pH 7.4. Tris should be avoided when the effects of manganese ions are investigated, since the buffer catalyzes the oxidation to insoluble manganese hydroxide. Other suitable buffers include HEPES and glycylglycyl-maleate.

Since adenylate cyclase is associated with membranes the enzyme is contaminated with ATPase activity that exceeds the activity of adenylate cyclase. For this reason an ATP regenerating system is used in the assay. Creatine phosphokinase/phosphocreatine or pyruvate kinase/phosphoenol pyruvate are typically employed. It is also possible to use the nonhydrolyzable ATP analog 5′-adenylyl imidodiphosphate (AppNp) as substrate [Krishna et al. 1972]. [alpha-^{32}P]AppNp is available from NEN. This compound is not cleaved by ATPases or adenylate kinase since it lacks the gamma phosphate, but is a substrate for adenylate cyclase. Use of AppNp obviates the need for an ATP regenerating system but its general use is prohibited by its high cost.

Membrane preparations of adenylate cyclase are also contaminated with phosphodiesterase activity so that a phosphodiesterase inhibitor such as 3-isobutyl 1-methylxanthine, papaverine, or theophylline is added to the assay mix.

[alpha-^{32}P]ATP is usually used as substrate, although this can be substituted with [^{3}H]ATP [Van Heyningen et al., 1983]. [alpha-^{32}P]ATP can be purchased or, more conveniently, prepared from carrier-free [^{32}P]phosphoric acid by the method of Johnson and Walseth [1979]. The true substrate for adenylate cyclase is MgATP so that magnesium ions must be added in sufficient concentration to convert all of the ATP to this complex. The Michaelis constant (Km) for MgATP for platelet adenylate cyclase has been estimated to be 21 or 54 μM [Johnson et al., 1979; Awad et al., 1983]. Our own data indicate a Km of 50–100 μM for enzyme stimulated by forskolin or prostacyclin. Care should be taken to ensure that the assay conditions give a linear rate over the time period chosen in terms of substrate concentration and other factors.

Assay procedure. A typical assay for adenylate cyclase, based on that described by Salomon [1979], is presented here. Incubation mixtures contain 50 mM triethanolamine-HCl, pH 7.4, 1 mM 3-isobutyl 1-methylxanthine, 10 mM dithiothreitol, 1 mg/ml bovine serum albumin, 10 mM $MgCl_2$, 0.1 mM EDTA, 20 mM phosphocreatine, 200 μg/ml creatine phosphokinase, 1 mM ATP, [alpha-^{32}P]ATP (2 to 8 $\times$ 10^5 cpm) and adenylate cyclase in a total volume of 100 μl. Reactions are incubated for 10 min at 37°C and terminated by addition of a stopping solution containing 2% sodium dodecyl sulfate, 45 mM ATP, 1.3 mM cyclic AMP, and 2,000 cpm of [^{3}H]cyclic AMP as a recovery standard. [^{32}P]Cyclic AMP is determined by the method of Salomon described above under "Analytical Methods."

Knowing the specific radioactivity of the added [^{32}P]cyclic AMP it is possible to calculate the cyclic AMP formed as pmol/min. Protein concentrations can be determined by the method of Lowry et al. [1951] and results expressed as pmol cyclic AMP/min/mg protein.

The assay can be modified to include effectors of adenylate cyclase activity. In addition membranes can be treated with a variety of modifiers that can be used as probes of the regulation of the enzyme.

EFFECTORS AND PROBES OF ADENYLATE CYCLASE REGULATION

Regulation of Platelet Adenylate Cyclase

An outline of the regulation of platelet adenylate cyclase is provided to clarify discussion of the factors important is assaying and studying this enzyme. A recent and thorough review of the role and regulation of platelet adenylate cyclase has been presented by Mills [1982].

The platelet adenylate system possesses components common to most other hormonally regulated adenylate cyclase systems [for a review, see Gilman, 1984]. Stimulatory ligands, such as prostaglandins and ribose-specific (R-site) analogs of adenosine, bind to stimulatory receptors in the outer membrane. The receptors, in turn, activate the guanine nucleotide-dependent regulatory protein

Ns that activates the catalytic unit (C) of the enzyme. The platelet system is somewhat anomalous in that exogenously added GTP is not required for hormonal stimulation of the enzyme in membrane preparations [Tsai and Lefkowitz, 1979; Olson et al., 1985]. Presumably endogenous GTP tightly bound to Ns is sufficient to transfer hormonal effects on the receptor to the catalytic unit. Inhibitory ligands such as epinephrine and ADP bind to a separate set of receptors that activate the inhibitory protein Ni, leading to inhibition.

Ns and Ni possess GTPase activity so that activation and inhibition are transient in the presence of GTP. However, use of nonhydrolyzable GTP analogs such as 5′-guanylyl imidodiphosphate (GppNp) can cause permanent activation of Ns. Similarly, cholera toxin can bring about permanent activation of Ns through an ADP-ribosylation reaction, whereas Ni inhibition can be abolished by treatment with pertussis toxin. However, unlike other mammalian cell types, platelets apparently lack receptors for toxin binding so that these probes can only be used with permeabilized platelets or membrane preparations. Jakobs and coworkers [Jakobs et al., 1985; Katada et al., 1985] have shown that phosphorylation of Ni by protein kinase C can also abolish Ni mediated inhibition of platelet adenylate cyclase. Hence treatment of intact platelets with tumor-promoting phorbol esters that are potent activators of protein kinase C leads to abolition of epinephrine-induced inhibition in membranes prepared from the treated cells.

The catalytic unit can also be activated directly by several ligands including manganese ions and the plant diterpene forskolin. It can be inhibited directly by adenosine and purine-specific (P-site) analogs of adenosine such as dideoxyadenosine.

Useful Probes for the Study of Adenylate Cyclase Regulation

Forskolin. Forskolin is a diterpene purified from the roots of the Indian medicinal plant *Coleus forskolii*. It is commercially available from Hoechst. Forskolin is a highly specific and potent activator of adenylate cyclase, capable of producing a 10- to 20-fold stimulation above basal activity [Seamon and Daly, 1981; Seamon and Daly, 1983]. The compound is very hydrophobic and only sparingly soluble in water ($< 100\ \mu M$). Forskolin is very soluble in ethanol and is generally added to intact platelets and membranes in ethanolic solution. The amount of ethanol added, however, should be minimized ($<1\%$) because of adverse effects on platelets and reported inhibition of adenylate cyclase [Huang et al., 1982].

Forskolin can diffuse through membranes to activate adenylate cyclase, apparently through direct interaction with the catalytic unit modified by interaction with Ns. In platelets forskolin has been used to inhibit aggregation and secretion

[Siegl et al., 1982] and therefore offers potential as an antithrombotic drug. Binding studies using [12-^{3}H]forskolin [Nelson and Seamon, 1985] reveal 20 to 50 fmol binding sites per mg of platelet protein with a dissociation constant (Kd) of 20 nM. Activation of Ns by GTP or fluoride increases the number of binding sites to 400 fmol/mg of protein.

Apart from the intrinsic interest of forskolin interaction with platelets, the compound can be used to amplify cyclic AMP levels or adenylate cyclase activity to examine phenomena such as epinephrine inhibition of adenylate cyclase, which is difficult to observe at basal levels of cyclic AMP. Forskolin has also been coupled to agarose as 7-succinylforskolin, providing a highly selective ligand for affinity purification of the catalytic unit of myocardial adenylate cyclase [Pfeuffer et al., 1985]. Forskolin affinity chromatography should form a general method for purification of the enzyme from many sources, including platelets.

2′,5′-Dideoxyadenosine. Purine-specific or P-site analogs of adenosine, such as 2′,5′ -dideoxyadenosine and the Squibb compound SQ 22536 (9-(tetrahydro-2-furyl)adenine), are potent noncompetitive inhibitors of adenylate cyclase [Johnson et al., 1979, Harris et al., 1979; Haslam et al., 1978], apparently acting directly on the catalytic unit. Endogenous inhibitors of adenylate cyclase such as ADP or epinephrine also activate platelets, whereas 2′,5′ -dideoxyadenosine has no activating effect on platelets. This fact was used by Haslam [1978] to show that although an increase in cyclic AMP leads to inhibition of platelet responsiveness, the reverse is not true: a decrease in cyclic AMP level is not in itself sufficient to activate platelets. The implication is that ADP and epinephrine act through pathways distinct from their effect on adenylate cyclase to activate platelets, whereas 2′,5′ -dideoxyadenosine is restricted to its effect on adenylate cyclase. SQ 22536 has been used in similar studies, but its use has been complicated by contamination of some preparations with ADP-like substances that cause platelet activation [Haslam et al., 1978].

Cholera toxin and pertussis toxin. Cholera toxin contains an enzyme activity capable of ADP-ribosylating the alpha-subunit of Ns, using NAD as substrate, resulting in abolition of the GTPase activity of this component and permanent activation of adenylate cyclase in the presence of GTP. Pertussis toxin (also called islet activating protein) catalyzes the ADP-ribosylation of the alpha-subunit of Ni, preventing displacement of tightly bound GTP and eliminating the inhibitory influence of Ni on the catalytic unit. Neither toxin can act on intact platelets, since these cells apparently lack the receptors for toxin binding; however, both agents can be used to modify Ns and Ni in platelet membranes. Both toxins are commercially available from List Biological Laboratories Inc., Campbell, CA.

The ability to selectively modify Ns and Ni provides a useful probe for the role of these proteins in various aspects of adenylate cyclase regulation including prostaglandin-induced desensitization. The 45 kilodalton alpha-subunit of Ns and the 41 kilodalton alpha-subunit of Ni can be identified through autoradiography of gels obtained from membranes ADP-ribosylated using the appropriate toxin in the presence of [^{32}P]NAD [Smith and Limbird, 1982; Murayama and Ui, 1983; Bokoch et al., 1983].

Phorbol ester. The phorbol ester phorbol 12-myristate 13-acetate (PMA), also called 12-O-tetradeconylphorbol 13-acetate (TPA), is a potent activator of protein kinase C. Protein kinase C is a ubiquitous enzyme with increasingly apparent pleiotropic effects. In platelets, as in other cell types, the enzyme is activated by calcium and by diacylglycerol generated from phosphoinositol by receptor-activated phospholipase C [Nishizuka, 1984]. Protein kinase C phosphorylates a platelet protein of molecular weight 40–47,000, which has no known function but may play a role in secretion [Imaoka et al., 1983; Kaibuchi et al., 1983]. Phorbol ester mimics the action of endogenously produced diacylglycerol but also persistently activates protein kinase C, resulting in phosphorylation events that may be less obvious under physiological conditions. One of these events is the phosphorylation of Ni observed and examined by Jakobs and coworkers [Jakobs et al., 1985; Katada et al., 1985]. Treatment of intact platelets with phorbol ester followed by lysis resulted in a particulate preparation that was unresponsive to epinephrine inhibition. Study of the phosphorylation pattern revealed that phosphorylation of Ni was responsible for this loss of responsiveness. Hence phosphorylation of Ni provides another selective method of eliminating the action of Ni. This work also suggests a regulatory link between a protein kinase C-mediated pathway of platelet activation and the cyclic AMP-mediated pathway of inhibition of platelet responsiveness.

N-ethylmaleimide. Less selective elimination of epinephrine-induced inhibition can be achieved by use of sulfydryl reagents such as N-ethylmaleimide (NEM) [Jakobs et al., 1982]. Evidence indicates that NEM acts through modification of Ni to bring about this effect and that Ni is somewhat more susceptible to sulfydryl modification than other components of the adenylate cyclase. At concentrations of NEM less than 1 mM, epinephrine inhibition can be abolished in intact platelets but at higher levels nonspecific inactivation of the enzyme takes place. This method has the advantage that it can be used on intact platelets.

Proteases. Mild proteolytic treatment of human platelet membranes with alpha-chymotrypsin increases basal adenylate cyclase activity and abolishes epinephrine-induced inhibition [Ferry et al., 1982]. Evidence indicates that the effects of proteolysis are again on Ni. Johnson and coworkers [Johnson et al., 1985] have purified a protease from bovine sperm that has similar effects on adenylate cyclase activity and epinephrine inhibition, and because the protease seems to be highly specific for Ni, they have named it ninhibin.

PREPARATION AND ASSAY OF cAMP PHOSPHODIESTERASES FROM HUMAN PLATELETS

Subcellular Localization of Phosphodiesterase Activity

Multiple forms of cyclic nucleotide phosphodiesterase activity have been reported in cells from many species and tissue types [Wells and Hardman, 1977; Strada and Thompson, 1978; Vaughn et al., 1981; Appleman et al., 1982; Beavo et al., 1982]. These forms vary in their substrate specificities, kinetic characteristics, physical properties, and their response to pharmacologic effectors. On subcellular fractionation of human platelets most, if not all, of the cyclic nucleotide phosphodiesterase activity was in the soluble or cytoplasmic fraction [Hidaka and Asano, 1976; Grant and Colman, 1984]. Three forms of cyclic nucleotide phosphodiesterase activity have been separated from this cytosolic fraction by DEAE-cellulose chromatography [Hidaka and Asano, 1976; Grant and Colman, 1984]. One form appears to be relatively specific for cGMP, a second form hydrolyzes both cAMP and cGMP at about the same rate with equal K_m's, and the third form appears relatively specific for cAMP. The following discussion focuses on the second and third forms of cyclic nucleotide phosphodiesterase from platelets, as these are the forms that appear to be most important in the intracellular regulation of cyclic AMP levels.

Purification of Cyclic Nucleotide Phosphodiesterases From Platelet Cytosol

Washing platelets. Phosphodiesterases can be prepared using platelets from freshly drawn blood and from outdated platelet concentrates. The platelets in either PRP or outdated platelet concentrates are washed as described by Grant and Colman [1984]. The platelet suspension is made 1 mM in EDTA and centrifuged at 1,500g (3,000 rpm in Sorvall GS3 rotor) for 2.5 min to remove most of the contaminating erythrocytes. The supernatant is carefully decanted and platelets pelleted by centrifugation at 10,000g (8,000 rpm in GS3 rotor) for 20 min at 4°C. The platelet pellet is resuspended in 50 mM tris-acetate, pH 6.0, containing 1 mM EDTA and 0.15 M sodium chloride, taking care to scrape the platelets off the bottom of the tube while disturbing the pelleted erythrocytes as little as possible. The platelets are washed two more times in the same buffer. The washed platelets are then frozen as a pellet in a dry ice bath and stored at −70°C.

Disruption of platelets. We have disrupted platelets using nitrogen bomb decompression [Grant and Colman, 1984]. Others have successfully used homogenization [Pichard et al., 1973], freeze-thaw techniques [Alvarez et al., 1981], and sonication [Hidaka and Asano, 1976] to prepare phosphodiesterases from platelets.

The final platelet pellet is resuspended in 50 mM tris-acetate, pH 6.0, containing 20 mM $MgCl_2$, 2 mM DTT, and a mixture of protease inhibitors [Grant and Colman, 1984]. The suspension is placed in a nitrogen bomb (Paar Instrument Co.) that has been cooled to 0–4°C and pressurized to 1,200–1,300 psi. Pressure is maintained for 30–45 min while stirring the platelet suspension. After release of the pressure, the platelet suspension is centrifuged (15,000g for 10 min) to pellet most of the large cellular debris. The supernatant is decanted and the pellet washed with an aliquot of the suspension buffer and recentrifuged. After centrifugation the supernatants are combined and centrifuged at 150,000g for 1 hr.

DEAE-cellulose chromatography. The supernatant from the 150,000g centrifugation is carefully removed from the pellet and applied directly to a DEAE-cellulose column (Whatman DE-52) equilibrated in the lysis buffer containing protease inhibitors [Grant and Colman, 1984]. The column is then washed and eluted with a linear gradient of sodium acetate with a limiting concentration of 0.6 M. Three peaks of cyclic nucleotide phosphodiesterase activity have been identified from such a column [Hidaka and Asano, 1976; Grant and Colman, 1984]. The first peak eluted from the column appears to be a cGMP-specific phosphodiesterase, which is often not observed if the column fractions are assayed with cAMP as the substrate. The second peak of phosphodiesterase activity hydrolyzes both cAMP and cGMP at similar rates and with similar K_m's [Hidaka and Asano, 1976; Grant et al., 1986]. The third phosphodiesterase has a lower K_m for cAMP than either of the other phosphodiesterases from platelets [Hidaka and Asano, 1976; Grant and Colman, 1984; Umekawa et al., 1984]. The second and third peaks of phosphodiesterase activity can be easily distinguished by assaying the column fractions at cAMP concentrations of 100 μM and 1μM, respectively.

Purification of cyclic GMP-specific phosphodiesterase. The first peak of phosphodiesterase activity eluted from the DEAE-cellulose column has been further purified and characterized by Hidaka and Endo [1984], who purified the enzyme 175-fold by affinity chromatography on a column containing the phosphodiesterase inhibitor MY-5445. This enzyme exhibited negatively cooperative kinetics for cGMP hydrolysis with a K_m of 0.4 μM and Michaelis-Menten kinetics for cAMP hydrolysis with a K_m of 500 μM. At low concentrations (below 10 μM) cGMP stimulated cAMP hydrolysis by this enzyme while inhibiting cAMP hydrolysis at higher concentrations. The molecular weight of this enzyme determined by gel-filtration was 240,000 [Hidaka and Asano, 1976]. The homogeneity of the affinity purified enzyme has not been described.

Purification of cyclic GMP-stimulated cyclic nucleotide phosphodiesterase. The second phosphodiesterase eluted from the DEAE-cellulose column has been further purified by cGMP affinity chromatography using a modification of a method described by Martins et al. [1982]. The DEAE fractions containing the phosphodiesterase activity are pooled, placed in dialysis tubing, and concentrated to about one-quarter volume versus dry sucrose. The sample is then dialyzed against 10 mM MOPS, pH 7.0, containing 1 mM EDTA, 125 mM NaCl, 2 mM DTT, 10 mM benzamidine-HCl, 5 mM ϵ-amino caproic acid, 20 μM N-α-p-tosyl-L-lysine chloromethyl ketone (TLCK), 10 μM leupeptin, and 5 μM pepstatin A. After dialysis the sample is applied at 4°C to a cGMP affinity column prepared by linking cGMP to epoxy activated Sepharose 4B [Martins et al., 1982]. The cGMP affinity column is equilibrated in the same buffer used for dialysis. After washing the column with the same buffer, the column is removed from the cold (4°) and allowed to warm to room temperature (20–25°). The column is then eluted with a linear gradient of cGMP from 0 to 10 mM. Fractions are collected into tubes containing $MgCl_2$ to reconstitute the enzyme activity. The phosphodiesterase activity elutes as a single peak, which is pooled and concentrated versus dry sucrose and stored at 4°C. These steps result in about a 7,400-fold purification of the enzyme with a specific activity of 131 nmol min^{-1} μg^{-1} [Grant et al., 1986].

The enzyme exhibits positively cooperative kinetics for the hydrolysis of both cAMP and cGMP [Grant et al., 1986]. Low levels of cGMP (below 10 μM) stimulate the rate of cAMP hydrolysis by this enzyme at subsaturating levels of cAMP. At cGMP concentrations above 10 μM, cGMP begins to inhibit cAMP hydrolysis [Asano et al., 1977; Grant et al., 1986]. The enzyme hydrolyzes both cAMP and cGMP at similar rates and with $S_{0.5}$ values of about 50 μM for both nucleotides [Hidaka and Asano, 1976; Grant et al., 1986]. On SDS polyacrylamide electrophoresis the purified enzyme gives a single band of M_r 105,000 [Grant et al., 1986].

Purification of cyclic AMP phosphodiesterase. The third peak of cyclic nucleotide phosphodiesterase activity eluting from the DEAE column is further purified by chromatography on blue dextran-Sepharose. Blue dextran-Sepharose is prepared by reacting blue dextran with cyanogen bromide-activated Sepharose 4B [Ryan and Vestling, 1974]. The pooled DEAE fractions are applied directly to a column of blue dextran-Sepharose equilibrated in 50 mM tris-HCl, pH 7.5, containing 20 mM $MgCl_2$ and a mixture of protease inhibitors [Grant and Colman, 1984]. The column is washed and then eluted with a linear gradient of cAMP from 0 to 1 mM. The phosphodiesterase activity elutes as a single peak, which is pooled, concentrated, and stored at 4°C. The enzyme is purified about 2,500-fold by these steps with a specific activity of approximately 2,500 nmol min^{-1} mg^{-1} [Grant and Colman, 1984].

This enzyme exhibits Michaelis-Menten kinetics with a K_m of 0.18 μM for cAMP. The enzyme also hydrolyzes cGMP with a lower K_m (0.02 μM) than for cAMP, but the rate of cGMP hydrolysis is tenfold slower than for cAMP. More detailed characterization of this enzyme has been reported elsewhere [Grant and Colman, 1984].

Assay of Cyclic Nucleotide Phosphodiesterase Activity

The cyclic nucleotide phosphodiesterases catalyze the hydrolysis of a 3′,5′ cyclic nucleotide to the corresponding 5′ nucleotide monophosphate. The assays for cyclic nucleotide phosphodiesterases all measure the production of AMP (or GMP) from cyclic AMP (or cGMP).

Purification of tritiated cyclic nucleotides. Most assays utilize ^{3}H-labeled cAMP and cGMP as a substrate for the enzyme. Purification of the tritiated nucleotide before use in the enzyme assay lowers the backgrounds of the assays and increases the sensitivity of the assays by removing AMP or GMP contamination caused by hydrolysis of the nucleotides and by removing tritiated water produced by proton exchange with the solvent. Such purifications should be performed every 4 to 5 weeks if backgrounds are to be kept as low as possible.

Two procedures for purifying the labeled nucleotides that are effective and simple to use are described below.

Thin layer chromatography. A good system for purifying both cGMP and cAMP by thin layer chromatography on cellulose plates (Baker-flex cellulose) has been described by Thompson et al. [1979]. The tritiated nucleotide is spotted onto the cellulose plate, which is then developed with 2-propanol: NH_4OH: H_2O (7:1:2, v:v). When development is complete the cyclic nucleotide spots are scraped from the plates and eluted with water and stored at −20°C in 50% ethanol. This system works well for both cAMP and cGMP.

Reverse phase chromatography. Van Lookeren Campagne and van Haastert [1983] have described a system for purification of cAMP by reverse phase chromatography on Bondapak C_{18} Porosil B (Waters Associates). A small (0.5 ml) column of Porosil B is poured in a pasteur pipet and equilibrated with 10 mM phosphate, pH 7.0, containing 1% methanol. The tritiated cAMP sample is applied to the column in 10 mM phosphate, pH 7.0, the column washed with at least 1 ml of the equilibration buffer, which removes any tritiated water or AMP. The column is then eluted with 10 mM phosphate, pH 7.0, containing 10% methanol to elute the cAMP. The fractions containing tritiated cAMP are then stored at −20°C in the 10% methanol buffer.

Van Lookeren Campagne and van Haastert [1983] reported that tritiated cGMP can also be purified using this reverse phase system.

Assay procedures for cyclic nucleotide phosphodiesterase. The cyclic nucleotide phosphodiesterases usually have a pH optimum between pH 7.5 and 8.5. Assays are usually run at pH 7.5 to 8.0 in an appropriate buffer such as 50–

100 mM tris-HCl containing 2–10 mM Mg^{+2} and an appropriate concentration of the cyclic nucleotide, often with 2-mercaptoethanol or dithiothreitol (DTT) and 0.1–1.0 mg/ml bovine serum albumin (BSA) present. A typical assay is run in 0.1 ml total volume containing 100 mM tris-HCl, pH 7.5, 2–20 mM $MgCl_2$, 1 mg/ml BSA, 0.5 to 100 μM cAMP or cGMP, and 50–100 nCi of ^{3}H-cAMP or cGMP and is initiated by the addition of the substrate.

Incubations are most often carried out at 30°C for an appropriate time (usually 5–10 min), followed by separation of the product AMP from the nonhydrolyzed cAMP. Multiple systems have been developed to effect this separation including chromatography on anion exhange resins [Thompson et al., 1979], Florisil [Sinha and Colman, 1981], paper [Nakai and Brooker, 1975], thin layer plates [Gulyassy and Farrand, 1976], reverse phase supports [Van Lookeren Campagne and Van Haastert, 1983], polyacrylamide-boronate gel [Davis and Daly, 1979], and immobilized acriflavin [Rochette-Egly and Egly, 1980], as well as barium sulfate precipitation [Poch, 1971; Sinha et al., 1977] and measurement of phosphate release [Butcher and Sutherland, 1962; Forn et al., 1970; Schonhofer et al., 1972]. These techniques have been extensively reviewed as to their advantages and disadvantages [Thompson et al., 1979]. The procedures described below are ones that we have found particularly useful in studying the phosphodiesterase activities in platelets.

Anion exchange chromatography. Anion exchange chromatography is the most widely utilized method for separating the product AMP from the unreacted cAMP. The procedure in general involves the hydrolysis of the cAMP by a cyclic nucleotide phosphodiesterase followed by conversion of AMP to adenosine by a 5′-nucleotidase from a snake venom preparation. The mixture of cAMP and adenosine is then placed on an anion exchange column under conditions in which the cAMP binds but the adenosine does not. The amount of adenosine eluted from the column is then measured to determine the degree of cAMP hydrolysis.

The assay described below is a slight variation of an anion exchange system described in detail by Thompson et al. [1979].

Dowex 1-X8 or BioRad AG1-X8 resin is washed successively with 0.5 N HCl, H_2O, 0.5 N NaOH, H_2O, and 0.5 N HCl. The resin is then washed extensively with H_2O until pH 5 is reached. After washing, a small amount of Tris base is added to adjust and maintain the pH and the resin is stored at 4°C.

Columns are prepared in pasteur pipets or plastic pipet tips. One ml of a 1:4 slurry (resin:methanol) is used to prepare each column. Incubation of the phosphodiesterase is carried out as described above. The reactions are terminated by placing the incubation tubes in a dry ice bath. The samples are then placed in a boiling water bath for 45 sec to inactivate the phosphodiesterase. After heating, the samples are cooled in an ice bath. Twenty-five μl of a 1 mg/ml solution of lyophilized venom from *Ophiophagus hannah* are added to each assay and the tubes incubated 10 min at 30°C. One milliliter of methanol is then added to each assay and the entire contents of the tube are transferred to a column prepared as described above and the eluate collected directly into a scintillation vial. When the column has drained to dryness, the column is washed with an additional milliliter of methanol and allowed to drain to dryness. The radioactivity of the combined eluates is then determined by liquid scintillation counting after the addition of 10 ml of liquid scintillation cocktail.

This method works well for determining the hydrolysis of both cAMP and cGMP.

Barium sulfate precipitation assay. A second method of separating AMP from cAMP that has proven useful involves the binding of AMP to freshly precipitated $BaSO_4$ as described by several investigators [Poch, 1971; Sinha et al., 1977]. The assay is run as described above in 0.1 ml volume in 1.5 ml conical centrifuge tubes. The reaction is stopped by the addition of 0.2 ml of 0.2 N $ZnSO_4$, followed by the addition of 0.2 ml of 0.2 N $Ba(OH)_2$. After mixing the $BaSO_4$ precipitate is collected by centrifugation in a tabletop centrifuge. An aliquot of the supernatant is removed and counted in an aqueous liquid scintillation cocktail. The AMP produced by hydrolysis binds to the $BaSO_4$ and is removed from solution while the cAMP stays in solution. The degree of cAMP hydrolysis is then determined by difference from control assays that contained no phosphodiesterase. Since phosphodiesterase activity is determined by difference this assay is not suitable for measuring low levels of phosphodiesterase activity necessary in studies such as kinetic determinations. However, this assay system has proven very useful for the rapid screening of column fractions for phosphodiesterase activity and for rapid estimates of the level of phosphodiesterase activity in unknown preparations.

Florisil chromatography. Sinha and Colman [1981] have described a separation of cAMP and AMP by chromatography on columns of Florisil, an activated magnesium silicate, eluted with phosphate buffer. The assay is simple, sensitive, and does not require the conversion of AMP to adenosine. The reaction is run as described above in a 0.1 ml volume and the reaction terminated by the addition of one-tenth volume of 50% trichloroacetic acid. The assay mixture is then diluted with 1 ml of 0.5 M phosphate buffer, pH 7.0, and the entire sample applied to a 1 ml column of Florisil prepared in a pasteur pipet and equilibrated in the same 0.5 M phosphate buffer. The column is then eluted with additional aliquots of buffer and fractions collected. AMP elutes from the column first while cAMP is retained. The fractions containing the AMP are then counted by liquid scintillation after acidification of the sample with HCl. This assay is simple, accurate, and sensitive and avoids the problems inherent in coupled enzyme assays such as the anion exchange assay. However, this procedure does not work for cGMP hydrolysis. Also, we have noted that some batches of Florisil have given unsatisfactory results (unpublished results) so that each batch of Florisil needs to be tested before it is used in assays. When the batches of Florisil that proved to be unsatisfactory were washed with water to remove the fines, the supernatant remained milky in appearance regardless of the number of times the Florisil was washed.

REGULATION OF CYCLIC NUCLEOTIDE PHOSPHODIESTERASES IN PLATELETS

Little is known about the role of the different forms of phosphodiesterase in platelets or any regulatory mechanisms that might control the phosphodiesterase activities in platelets. The calcium binding protein calmodulin, which was originally isolated as a phosphodiesterase stimulatory protein [Cheung, 1970; Kakiuchi and Yamazaki, 1970], is found in human platelets [Muszbek et al., 1977] and thus must be considered as a potential regulatory mechanism in platelets. Hidaka and Endo [1984] reported that the calmodulin antagonist W-7 (N-(6-aminohexyl)-5-chloro-1-naphthalenesulfonamide), a potent inhibitor of platelet aggregation, did not increase platelet cyclic nucleotide levels at concentrations up to 0.5 mM, and that added Ca^{2+} produced little stimulation of phosphodiesterase activity in platelet lysates. In addition, TCV-3B, a potent inhibitor of the basal activity of calmodulin-stimulated phosphodiesterase, did not prevent platelet aggregation [Hidaka and Endo, 1984]. We have also found that the cAMP hydrolytic activities of the isolated phosphodiesterases from platelets are neither stimulated by exogenously added Ca^{2+}-calmodulin nor inhibited by EGTA [Grant and Colman, 1984; Grant et al., 1986]. Therefore it appears that a calmodulin-stimulated phosphodiesterase probably does not play an important role in platelet cyclic nucleotide metabolism.

Alvarez and coworkers [1981] reported that treatment of intact platelets with prostacyclin, PGE_1, or PGD_2 produced an increase in cAMP phosphodiesterase activity measured in freeze-thaw lysates of the treated platelets. The level of stimulation showed a dose-dependent increase with increasing prostaglandin concentrations. This increase in phosphodiesterase activity also coincided with the increase in intracellular cAMP levels produced by stimulation of adenylate cyclase. The enhanced phosphodiesterase activity was observed at low cAMP concentrations (0.1–10 μM), suggesting that a low K_m form of the enzyme may have been stimulated by this treatment.

Hamet and coworkers [Hamet et al., 1983; Hamet et al., 1984] reported a similar stimulation of the cAMP phosphodiesterase from rat platelets by PGE_1,

PGE_2, and prostacyclin. They have also reported stimulation of the cGMP-binding phosphodiesterase and the cAMP phosphodiesterase in rat platelets when intact platelets were incubated with forskolin [Tremblay et al., 1985]. The presence of phosphodiesterase inhibitors such as 1-methyl-3-isobutylxanthine (MIX), indomethacin, and dipyridamole potentiated the increase in phosphodiesterase activity produced by PGE_1 and forskolin [Hamet et al., 1983; Tremblay et al., 1985]. Stimulation of both cGMP-binding and cAMP-specific phosphodiesterase activities could also be produced in lysed platelet preparations when cAMP, ATP, and cAMP-dependent protein kinase were added in the presence of the phosphodiesterase inhibitor MIX [Tremblay et al., 1985]. These results suggest that cAMP-dependent phosphorylation may be involved in this stimulation of phosphodiesterase activities, although this has not been directly demonstrated.

A promising approach to the study of the role of the different forms of cyclic nucleotide phosphodiesterase in platelets as well as in other cells is the use of inhibitors that are specific for a single form of phosphodiesterase. In recent years compounds that are more specific for a single form of phosphodiesterase than many of the more "classical" inhibitors such as the methyl xanthines and papaverine have been isolated or synthesized. Some of these compounds, such as amrinone [Endoh et al., 1982; Carpendo et al., 1984], milrinone [Alousi et al., 1983], cilostamide [Hidaka et al., 1979; Lugnier et al., 1983; Yamamoto et al., 1984], RO15-2041 [Muggli et al., 1985], HL 725 [Rupert and Weithman, 1982], Y 590 [Mikashima et al., 1984], and rolipram [Frossard et al., 1981; Lugnier et al., 1983], preferentially inhibit cAMP phosphodiesterase activity, while others such as M & B 22948 [Frossard et al., 1981], MY 5445 [Hidaka and Endo, 1984], and mepacrine [Yamakodo et al., 1984] show a preference for the inhibition of cGMP phosphodiesterase activity. In addition the calmodulin-sensitive forms of phosphodiesterase can be inhibited by compounds such as TCV-3B and HA 558, which appear to inhibit the enzyme directly [Hidaka and Endo, 1984], or the activity of the calmodulin-sensitive enzymes can be inhibited indirectly by calmodulin antagonists such as W-7 [Hidaka and Endo, 1984] and trifluoperazine (or other phenothiazines). The evaluation of these inhibitors with respect to their specificities for the various forms of phosphodiesterase in platelets and their effects on platelet functions should assist in our studies of both the regulation of phosphodiesterase activities in platelets and the role of each form of phosphodiesterase in the regulation of cyclic nucleotide levels and platelet function.

REFERENCES

Alousi AA, Canter JM, Montenaro MJ, Fort DJ, Ferrari RA (1983). Cardiotonic activity of milrinone, a new and potent cardiac bipyridine, on the normal and failing heart of experimental animals. J Cardiovasc Pharmacol 5:792–803.

Alvarez R, Taylor A, Fazzari JJ, Jacobs JR (1981). Regulation of cyclic AMP metabolism in human platelets: Sequential activation of adenylate cyclase and cyclic AMP phosphodiesterase by prostaglandins. Mol Pharmacol 20:302–309.

Appleman MM, Ariano M, Takemoto DJ, Whitson RH (1982). Cyclic nucleotide phosphodiesterases. Handb Exp Pharmacol 58:261–300.

Asano T, Ochiai Y, Hidaka H (1977). Selective inhibition of separated forms of human platelet cyclic nucleotide phosphodiesterase by platelet aggregation inhibitors. Mol Pharmacol 13:400–406.

Awad JA, Johnson RA, Jakobs KH, Schultz G (1983). Interactions of forskolin and adenylate cyclase: Effects on substrate kinetics and protection against inactivation by heat and N-ethylmaleimide. J Biol Chem 258:2960–2965.

Barber AJ, Jamieson GA (1970). Isolation and characterization of plasma membranes from human blood platelets. J Biol Chem 245:6357–6365.

Beavo JA, Hansen RS, Harrison SA, Hurwitz RL, Martins TJ, Mumby MC (1982). Identification and properties of cyclic nucleotide phosphodiesterases. Mol Cell Endocrinol 28:387–410.

Bitonti AJ, Moss J, Hjelmeland L, Vaughn M (1982). Resolution and activity of adenylate cyclase components in a zwitterionic cholate derivative [3-[(3-cholamidopropyl)dimethylammonio]-1-propanesulfonate]. Biochemistry 21:3650–3653.

Bokoch GM, Katada T, Northup JK, Hewlett EL, Gilman AG (1983). Identification of the predominant substrate for ADP-ribosylation by islet activating protein. J Biol Chem 258:2072–2075.

Brooker G (1971). High pressure anion exchange chromatographic measurement of cyclic adenosine 3′,5′-monophosphate and cyclic [^{14}C] adenosine monophosphate specific activity in myocardium prelabeled with [^{14}C] adenosine. J Biol Chem 246:7810–7816.

Brooker G, Harper JF, Terasaki WL, Moylan RD (1979). Radioimmunoassay of cyclic AMP and cyclic GMP. Adv Cyclic Nucleotide Res 10:1–33.

Butcher RW, Sutherland EW (1962). Adenosine 3′,5′-phosphate in biological materials. I. Purification and properties of cyclic 3′,5′-nucleotide phosphodiesterase and use of this enzyme to characterize adenosine 3′,5′-phosphate in human urine. J Biol Chem 237:1244–1250.

Carpenedo F, Floreani M, Cargnelli G (1984). Competitive inhibition of phosphodiesterase activity by amrinone: Its implication in the cardiac effect of the drug. Pharmacol Res Commun 16:969–977.

Cheung WY (1970). Cyclic 3′,5′-nucleotide phosphodiesterase. Biochem Biophys Res Commun 38:533–538.

Cutler LS, Christian CP, Feinstein MB (1985). Cytochemical localization of adenylate cyclase in the dense tubule system of human blood platelets stimulated by forskolin, prostacyclin and prostaglandin D_2. Biochim Biophys Acta 845:403–410.

Daniel JL, Molish IR, Holmsen H (1980). Radiolabeling of the purine nucleotide pool of cells as a method to distinguish among intracellular compartments: Studies on human platelets. Biochim Biophys Acta 632:444–453.

Davis CW, Daly JW (1979). A simple direct assay of 3′,5′-cyclic nucleotide phosphodiesterase activity based on the use of polyacrylamide-boronate affinity gel chromatography. J Cyclic Nucleotide Res 5:65–74.

Endoh M, Yamashita S, Taira N (1982). Positive inotropic effect of amrinone in relation to cyclic nucleotide metabolism in the canine ventricular muscle. J Pharmacol Exp Ther 221:775–783.

Ferry N, Adnot S, Borsodi A, Lacombe M-L, Guellaen G, Hanoune J (1982). Uncoupling by proteolysis of alpha-adrenergic receptor-mediated inhibition of adenylate cyclase in human platelets. Biochem Biophys Res Commun 108:708–714.

Forn J, Schonhofer P, Skidmore I, Krishna G (1970). Effect of aging on adenyl cyclase and phosphodiesterase activity of isolated fat cells of rat. Biochim Biophys Acta 208:304–309.

Frossard N, Landry Y, Pauli G, Ruckstuhl M (1981). Effects of cyclic AMP- and cyclic GMP-phosphodiesterase inhibitors on immunological release of histamine and on lung contraction. Br J Pharmac 73:933–938.

Gilman AG (1984). Guanine nucleotide-binding regulatory proteins and dual control of adenylate cyclase. J Clin Invest 73:1–4.

Grant PG, Colman RW (1984). Purification and characterization of a human platelet cyclic nucleotide phosphodiesterase. Biochemistry 23:1801–1807.

Grant PG, Mannarino AF, Colman RW (1986). Purification of a cGMP-stimulated cyclic nucleotide phosphodiesterase from human platelets (submitted for publication).

Gulyassy PF, Farrand JR (1976). Comparison of batch and chromatographic assays of cyclic nucleotide phosphodiesterases. J Chromatogr 129:107–113.

Hamet P, Coquil JF, Bousseau-Lafortune S, Franks DJ, Tremblay J (1984). Cyclic GMP binding and phosphodiesterase: Implication for platelet function. Adv Cyclic Nucleotide Prot Phosphoryl Res 16:119–136.

Hamet P, Franks DJ, Tremblay J, Coquil JF (1983). Rapid activation of cAMP phosphodiesterase in rat platelets. Can J Biochem Cell Biol 61:1158–1165.

Harris DN, Magdi MA, Phillips MB, Goldenberg HJ, Antonaccio MJ (1979). Inhibition of adenylate cyclase in human blood platelets by 9-substituted adenine derivatives. J Cyclic Nucleotide Res 5:125–134.

Haslam RJ (1978). Cyclic nucleotides in platelet function. In Day HJ, Holmsen H, Zucker MB (eds): "Platelet Function Testing." DHEW Publication (NIH) 78-1087, pp 487–503.

Haslam RJ, Davidson ML, Desjardins JV (1978). Inhibition of adenylate cyclase by adenosine analogues in preparations of broken and intact platelets. Biochem J 176:83–95.

Haslam RJ, Lynham JA (1972). Activation and inhibition of blood platelet adenylate cyclase by adenosine or by 2-chloroadenosine. Life Sci 11(II):1143–1154.

Haslam RJ, McClenaghan MD (1981). Measurement of circulating prostacyclin. Nature 292:364–366.

Hidaka H, Asano T (1976). Human blood platelet 3′:5′-cyclic nucleotide phosphodiesterase. Isolation of low-K_m and high-K_m phosphodiesterase. Biochim Biophys Acta 429:485–497.

Hidaka H, Endo T (1984). Selective inhibitors of three forms of cyclic nucleotide phosphodiesterase. Basic and potential clinical applications. Adv Cyclic Nucleotide Prot Phosphoryl Res 16:245–259.

Hidaka H, Hayashi H, Kohri H, Kimura Y, Hosokawa T, Igawa T, Saitoh Y (1979). Selective inhibitor of platelet cyclic adenosine monophosphate phosphodiesterase, cilostamide, inhibits platelet aggregation. J Pharmacol Exp Ther 211:26–30.

Holmsen H, Storm E, Day JH (1972). Anal Biochem 104:789–801.

Holmsen H, Weiss HJ (1979). Secretable storage pools in platelets. Annu Rev Med 30:119–139.

Huang R-D, Smith MF, Zahler WL (1982). Inhibition of forskolin-activated adenylate cyclase by ethanol and other solvents. J Cyclic Nucleotide Res 8:385–394.

Imaoka T, Lynham JA, Haslam RJ (1983). Purification and characterization of the 47,000-dalton protein phosphorylated during degranulation of human platelets. J Biol Chem 258:11404–11414.

Jakobs KH, Bauer S, Watanabe Y (1985). Modulation of adenylate cyclase of human platelets by phorbol ester. Eur J Biochem 151:425–430.

Jakobs KH, Lasch P, Minuth M, Aktories K, Schultz G (1982). Uncoupling of α-adrenoreceptor-mediated inhibition of human platelet adenylate cyclase by N-ethylmaleimide. J Biol Chem 257:2829–2833.

Johnson RA, Jakobs KH, Schultze G (1985). Extraction of the adenylate cyclase activating factor of bovine sperm and its identification as a trypsin-like protease. J Biol Chem 260:114–121.

Johnson RA, Saur W, Jakobs KH (1979). Effects of prostaglandin E_1 and adenosine on metal and metal-ATP kinetics of platelet adenylate cyclase. J Biol Chem 254:1094–1101.

Johnson RA, Walseth TF (1979). Enzymatic preparation of [α-^{32}P]ATP, [α-^{32}P]GTP, [^{32}P]cAMP and [^{32}P]cGMP, and their use in the assay of adenylate and guanylate cyclases and cyclic nucleotide phosphodiesterases. Adv Cyclic Nucleotide Res 10:135–167.

Kaibuchi K, Takai Y, Sawamura M, Hoshijima M, Fujikura T, Nishizuka Y (1983). Synergistic functions of protein phosphorylation and calcium mobilization in platelet activation. J Biol Chem 258:6701–6704.

Kakiuchi S, Yamazaki R (1970). Calcium dependent phosphodiesterase activity and its activating factor (PAF) from brain. Biochem Biophys Res Commun 41:1104–1110.

Katada T, Gilman AG, Watanabe Y, Bauer S, Jakobs KH (1985). Protein kinase C phosphorylates the inhibitory guanine-nucleotide-binding regulatory component and apparently suppresses its function in hormonal inhibition of adenylate cyclase. Eur J Biochem 151:431–437.

Krishna G, Harwood JP, Barber AJ, Jamieson GA (1972). Requirement for guanosine triphosphate in the prostaglandin activation of adenylate cyclase by platelet membranes. J Biol Chem 247:2253–2254.

Krishna G, Weiss B, Brodie BB (1968). A simple sensitive method for the assay of adenyl cyclase. J Pharmacol Exp Ther 163:379–385.

Lagarde M, Menashi S, Crawford N (1981). Localization of phospholipase A_2 and diglyceride lipase activities in human platelet intracellular membranes. FEBS Lett 124:23–26.

Lages B, Scrutton MC, Holmsen H (1975). Studies on gel-filtered human platelets: Isolation and characterization in a medium containing no added Ca^{2+}, Mg^{2+}, or K^{+}. J Lab Clin Med 85:811–825.

Lowry OH, Roseborough NJ, Farr AL, Randall RJ (1951). Protein measurement with folin phenol reagent. J Biol Chem 193:265–275.

Lugnier C, Stierle A, Beretz A, Schoeffler P, Lebec A, Wermuth CG, Cazenave JP, Stoclet JC (1983). Tissue and substrate specificity of inhibition by alkoxy-aryl-lactams of platelet and arterial smooth muscle cyclic nucleotide phosphodiesterases relationship to pharmacological activity. Biochem Biophys Res Commun 113:954–959.

Martins TJ, Mumby MC, Beavo JA (1982). Purification and characterization of a cyclic GMP-stimulated cyclic nucleotide phosphodiesterase from bovine tissues. J Biol Chem 257:1973–1979.

Mauco G, Fauvel J, Chap H, Douste-Blazy L (1984). Studies on enzymes related to diacylglycerol production in activated platelets: II. Subcellular distribution, enzymatic properties and positional specificity of diacylglycerol- and monoacylglycerol-lipases. Biochim Biophys Acta 796:169–177.

Mikashima H, Nakao T, Goto K, Ochi H. Yasuda H, Tsumagari T (1984). Y-590 (a new pyridazinone derivative), a potent anti-thrombotic agent-II. Inhibition of platelet phosphodiesterase. Thromb Res 35:589–594.

Mills DCB (1982). The role of cyclic nucleotides in platelets. In Kebanian JW, Nathanson JA (eds): "Handbook of Experimental Pharmacology" (Springer-Verlag, Berlin, Heidelberg) 58/II. pp 723–761.

Muggli R, Tschopp TB, Mittleholzer E, Baumgartner HR (1985). 7-bromo-1,5-dihydro-3,6-dimethylimidazo (2,1-b) quinazolin-2(3H)-one (Ro 15-2041), a potent antithrombotic agent that selectively inhibits platelet cyclic AMP phosphodiesterase. J Pharmacol Exp Ther 235:212–219.

Murayama T, Ui M (1983). Loss of the inhibitory function of the guanine nucleotide regulatory component of adenylate cyclase due to its ribosylation by islet-activating protein, pertussis toxin, in adipocyte membranes. J Biol Chem 258:3319–3326.

Muszbek L, Kuznicki J, Szabo T, Drabikowski W (1977). Troponin C like protein of blood platelets. FEBS Lett 80:308–312.

Nakai C, Brooker G (1975). Assay for adenylate cyclase and cyclic nucleotide phosphodiesterases and the preparation of high specific activity ^{32}P-labeled substances. Biochim Biophys Acta 391:222–239.

Nelson CA, Seamon KB (1985). Regulation of [^{3}H]forskolin binding to human platelet membranes by GppNHp, NaF, and prostaglandin E_1. FEBS Lett 183:349–352.

Nishizuka Y (1984). The role of protein kinase C in cell surface signal transduction and tumor promotion. Nature 308:693–698.

Olson CV, Smiley PA, Lad PM (1985). Human platelet adenylate cyclase: Persistent binding of guanine nucleotide is central to the regulation of both hormone-stimulated and basal levels. Biochim Biophys Acta 845:411–420.

Perret B, Chap HJ, Douste-Blazy L (1979). Asymmetric distribution of arachidonic acid in the plasma membrane of human platelets: Determination using purified phospholipases and a rapid method for membrane isolation. Biochim Biophys Acta 556:434–446.

Pfeuffer E, Dreher R-H, Metzger H, Pfeuffer T (1985). Catalytic unit of adenylate cyclase: Purification and identification by cross-linking. Proc Natl Acad Sci USA 82:3086–3090.

Pichard AL, Hanoune J, Kaplan JC (1973). Multiple forms of cyclic adenosine 3′,5′ -monophosphate phosphodiesterase from human blood platelets. I. Kinetic and electrophoretic characterization of two molecular species. Biochim Biophys Acta 315:370–377.

Poch G (1971). Assay of phosphodiesterase with radioactively labeled cyclic 3′, 5′-AMP as substrate. Naunyn Schmiedebergs Arch Pharmacol 268:272–299.

Ramachandran J (1971). A new simple method for separation of adenosine 3′,5′-cyclic monophosphate from other nucleotides and its use in the assay of adenyl cyclase. Anal Biochem 41:227–239.

Record M, Bes J-C, Chap H, Douste-Blazy L (1982). Isolation and characterization of plasma membranes from Krebs II ascite cells using Percoll gradients. Biochim Biophys Acta 668:57–65.

Rochette-Egly C, Egly JM (1980). A rapid direct assay of 3′-5′ cyclic nucleotide phosphodiesterase activity using chromatography on immobilized acriflavin. J Cyclic Nucleotide Res 6:335–345.

Ross EM (1981). Phosphatidylcholine-promoted interaction of the catalytic and regulatory proteins of adenylate cyclase. J Biol Chem 256:1949–1953.

Ruppert D, Weithmann KU (1982). HL 725, an extremely potent inhibitor of platelet phosphodiesterase and induced platelet aggregation in vitro. Life Sci 31:2037–2043.

Ryan LD, Vestling CS (1974). Rapid purification of lactate dehydrogenase from rat liver and hepatoma: A new approach. Arch Biochem Biophys 160:279–284.

Salomon Y (1979). Adenylate cyclase assay. Adv Cyclic Nucleotide Res 10:35–55.

Salomon Y, Londos C, Rodbell M (1974). Highly sensitive adenylate cyclase assay. Anal Biochem 58:541–548.

Schonhofer PS, Skidmore IF, Bourne HR, Krishna G (1972). Cyclic 3′, 5′-AMP phosphodiesterase in isolated fat cells. Simple and sensitive methods for the assay of phosphodiesterase activity in fat cells and studies of the enzyme inhibition by theophylline. Pharmacology 7:65–77.

Seamon KB, Daly JW (1981). Forskolin: A unique diterpene activator of cyclic AMP-generating systems. J Cyclic Nucleotide Res 7:201–224.

Seamon KB, Daly JW (1983). Forskolin, cyclic AMP and cellular physiology. Trends Pharmacol Sci 4:120–123.

Siegl AM, Daly JW, Smith JB (1982). Inhibition of aggregation and stimulation of cyclic AMP generation in intact human platelets by the diterpene forskolin. Molec Pharmac 21:680–687.

Sinha AK, Colman RW (1978). A simple assay for adenylate cyclase in intact cells by affinity elution chromatography. Biochem J 174:699–702.

Sinha AK, Colman RW (1981). A new method for separating cyclic AMP from 5′-AMP with application to the assay for cyclic AMP phosphodiesterase. Anal Biochem 1134:239–245.

Sinha AK, Shattil SJ, Colman RW (1977). Cyclic AMP metabolism in cholesterol-rich platelets. J Biol Chem 252:3310–3314.

Smith SK, Limbird LE (1982). Evidence that human platelet α-adrenergic receptors coupled to inhibition of adenylate cyclase are not associated with the subunit of adenylate cyclase ADP-ribosylated by cholera toxin. J Biol Chem 257:10471–10478.

Steer ML, Wood A (1979). Regulation of human platelet adenylate cyclase by epinephrine, prostaglandin E_1 and guanine nucleotides. J Biol Chem 254:10791–10797.

Strada SJ, Thompson WJ (1978). Multiple forms of cyclic nucleotide phosphodiesterases: anomalies or biologic regulators? Adv Cyclic Nucleotide Res 9:265–283.

Strittmatter S, Neer EJ (1980). Properties of the separated catalytic and regulatory units of brain adenylate cyclase. Proc Natl Acad Sci USA 77:6344–6348.

Thompson WJ, Terasaki WL, Epstein PM, Strada SJ (1979). Assay of cyclic nucleotide phosphodiesterase and resolution of multiple forms of the enzyme. Adv Cyclic Nucleotide Res 10:69–92.

Tremblay J, Lachance B, Hamet P (1985). Hypothesis. Activation of cyclic GMP-binding and cyclic AMP-specific phosphodiesterases of rat platelets by a mechanism involving cyclic AMP-dependent phosphorylation. J Cyclic Nucleotide Prot Phosphoryl Res 10:397–411.

Tsai BS, Lefkowitz RJ (1979). Multiple effects of guanine nucleotides on human platelet adenylate cyclase. Biochim Biophys Acta 587:28–41.

Umekawa H, Tanaka T, Kimura Y, Hidaka H (1984). Purification of cyclic adenosine monophosphate phosphodiesterase from human platelets using new inhibitor Sepharose chromatography. Biochem Pharmacol 33:3339–3344.

Van Heyningen SV, Thom A, Ward W (1983). A modified assay of adenylate cyclase using ^3H and ^{14}C. Anal Biochem 129:457–459.

Van Lookeren Campagne MM, Van Haastert PJM (1983). A sensitive cyclic nucleotide phosphodiesterase assay for transient enzyme kinetics. Anal Biochem 135:146–150.

Vaughn M, Danello MA, Manganiello VC, Strewler GJ (1981). Regulation of cyclic nucleotide phosphodiesterase activity. Adv Cyclic Nucleotide Res 14:263–271.

Walseth TF, Gander JE, Eide SJ, Krick TP, Goldberg ND (1983). ^{18}O labeling of adenine nucleotide α-phosphoryls in platelets. J Biol Chem 258:1544–1558.

Wells JN, Hardman JG (1977). Cyclic nucleotide phosphodiesterases. Adv Cyclic Nucleotide Res 8:119–143.

White AA, Zenser TV (1971). Separation of cyclic 3′,5′-nucleotide monophosphates from other nucleotides on aluminum oxide columns: Application to the assay of adenyl cyclase and guanyl cyclase. Anal Biochem 41:372–396.

Yamakado T, Tanaka F,, Hidaka H (1984). Mepacrine-induced inhibition of human platelet cyclic-GMP phosphodiesterase. Biochim Biophys Acta 801:111–116.

Yamamoto T, Lieberman F, Osborne JC Jr, Manganiello VC, Vaughn M, Hidaka H (1984). Selective inhibition of two soluble adenosine 3′,5′-phosphate phosphodiesterases partially purified from calf liver. Biochemistry 23:670–675.

Modern Methods in Pharmacology, Volume 4
Methods for Studying Platelets and Megakaryocytes, pages 185–215

Methods for the Study of the Role of Calcium in Platelet Function

James L. Daniel, Mary A. Selak, A. David Purdon, and Leon Salganicoff

INTRODUCTION

It was proposed some time ago that calcium is the primary and possibly the only intracellular messenger mediating the secretory and aggregatory responses of platelets to external stimuli. This view was reinforced by the experiments of Feinman and Detwiler [1974], which showed that the Ca^{2+} ionophore A23187 could elicit the same platelet responses as stimulatory agonists. However, it is now known that other mediators also play an important role. For example, diacylglycerol is known to activate protein kinase C, and addition of synthetic diacylglycerols can activate platelets with little or no apparent change in free Ca^{2+}. Thus it no longer appears that calcium alone mediates all the responses of the platelet, but it is still thought to play a central role. The object of this chapter is to present a variety of methods by which to study the importance of calcium in mediating platelet responses. The chapter makes no attempt to present a comprehensive review concerning the importance of calcium to platelet function. For this, the reader is referred to many excellent reviews on the subject, especially by Feinstein et al. [1985] and by Zucker and Nachmias [1985].

For ease of discussion, this chapter is divided into two broad sections, one concerning direct measurement of the internal calcium with fluorescent or luminescent probes and the other concerning indirect methods whereby holes are introduced in the platelet membrane and the internal calcium is manipulated using Ca^{2+} buffers.

METHODS USING INTERNAL PROBES

Three different types of probes have been used to study intracellullar Ca^{2+} in platelets. We have had personal experience with the fluorescent Ca^{2+} chelators,

From the Department of Pharmacology and the Thrombosis Research Center, Temple University School of Medicine, Philadelphia, Pennsylvania 19140.

quin2 and fura-2, and will therefore only give background information on the other two.

Chlortetracycline

Chlortetracycline fluoresces at 520 nm when excited at 400 nm [Mathew and Balaram, 1980]. Chlortetracycline (CTC) binds both Ca^{2+} and Mg^{2+} with relatively low affinity. The dissociation constants are 2.7×10^{-4} M for Mg^{2+} and 4.4×10^{-4} M for Ca^{2+} (assuming a 1:1 stoichiometry of binding) in aqueous solution at pH 7.4 [Caswell and Hutchison, 1971b]. Binding of either divalent ion enhances the fluorescence yield but Ca^{2+} increases fluorescence 65% more than Mg^{2+}. If fluorescence is measured at 530 nm, a rather poor but maximal 1.5-fold selectivity of the fluorescence of the CTC-Ca^{2+} complex over that of the CTC-Mg^{2+} complex is obtained [Blinks et al., 1982; see Figure 15]. CTC can penetrate the plasma and intracellular membranes of cells and, thus, is not specifically located in the cytoplasm but may also enter intracellular organelles. Although CTC can penetrate membranes, it apparently is more hydrophilic than lipophilic and remains mainly in the aqueous compartments of the cell. When CTC binds Ca^{2+}, presumably in the aqueous phase, the complex (for reasons that are not entirely clear) prefers to associate with the membrane; however, this association does not imply that the complex is actually dissolved in the bilayer or that CTC can function as an ionophore [Blinks et al., 1982]. Evidence indicates that CTC does not actually probe membrane-bound Ca^{2+}, since the complex can bind to membranes that contain no previously bound Ca^{2+} [Caswell and Hutchison, 1971a; Millman et al., 1980]. Blinks et al. [1982] point out that five questions need to be answered to interpret signals obtained from chlortetracycline loaded cells; "1) Where is the chlortetracycline? 2) In what compartment or compartments is the Ca^{2+} to which it responds? 3) How quickly does the indicator respond to changes of [Ca^{2+}] in those compartments? 4) To what extent and how quickly does the chlortetracycline redistribute itself in response to changes in the [Ca^{2+}] of the various cell compartments? and 5) How quickly does the chlortetracycline diffuse out of the cell altogether?" Other considerations include 1) the method is difficult to calibrate and the fluorescence is probably not linearly dependent on the free Ca^{2+} concentration; results with CTC may be considered to be qualitative. 2) High levels of the indicator are to be avoided since sufficient Ca^{2+} could be bound to significantly alter cell function. Also, both CTC and its photooxidation products may be cytotoxic.

Le Breton et al. [1976] used CTC-loaded platelets and showed that 10 μM ADP induced a decrease in fluorescence that was temporally correlated with the onset of platelet shape change. It is interesting that this decrease in fluorescence was maintained for up to 4 min after ADP addition (see fura-2 data below). ATP, a competitive antagonist for ADP [MacFarlane and Mills, 1975], blocked the majority of the ADP-induced fluorescence change. These data were interpreted to show that Ca^{2+} -CTC complex moves from a nonpolar to a polar environment during platelet activation. However, in light of the discussion above [Blinks et al., 1982], it is not clear exactly how these data should be interpreted. In another study, the same group [Le Breton and Dinerstein, 1977] showed that the decrease in CTC fluorescence was not blocked by the presumed Ca^{2+} antagonist TMB-8. It is possible that the compound TMB-8 is not a Ca^{2+} antagonist but rather inhibits platelet secretion through inhibition of protein kinase C. Feinstein [1980] compared the thrombin-induced change in CTC fluorescence to secretion of dense granule Ca^{2+} and found that the changes in CTC fluorescence were more rapid than secretion. This result would be consistent with the experiments (above) that correlated CTC fluorescence changes to shape change. Jy and Haynes [1984] used CTC and quin2 (see below) in parallel experiments to correlate changes in cytosolic Ca^{2+} both uptake and release by the dense tubules and mitochondria. They interpreted changes in CTC fluorescence to indicate fluxes in dense tubular and mitochondrial Ca^{2+} pools and changes in quin2 as a measure of cytoplasmic Ca^{2+}. The data were interpreted to indicate that Ca^{2+} sequestration by the dense tubules is rapid but of low capacity, while the mitochondria had high capacity but slow uptake. However, uncertainties in the method including the response time of the CTC for Ca^{2+} and the nonlinearity of the CTC signal, as well as the effects of surface area, charge, composition of the membranes in each compartment, make even these conclusions speculative. At the A23187 concentrations used, the authors state that the ionophore only affected the plasma membrane. However, it is quite clear from experiments with quin2 that intracellular Ca^{2+} is rapidly mobilized under the same conditions, suggesting that the ability of the internal systems to sequester Ca^{2+} would be compromised. Thompson and Scrutton [1985] have performed similar experiments and conclude that while CTC is useful for monitoring Ca^{2+} fluxes under some conditions, CTC does not always present a reasonable picture of the Ca^{2+} metabolism of the platelet.

Aequorin

Aequorin consists of a single polypeptide apoprotein of 20,000 daltons and a tightly bound chromophore, a substituted imidazolopyrazinone [Prendergast and Mann, 1978; Cormier, 1978]. Upon binding Ca^{2+}, the chromophore becomes oxidized, producing a molecule of CO_2 and a photon with a $\lambda_{max} = 469$ nm. The oxidized chromophore has a lower affinity for the protein and dissociates when Ca^{2+} is removed. Addition of reduced chromophore to spent aequorin in the presence of O_2 and absence of Ca^{2+} regenerates fully active aequorin [Shimomura and Johnson, 1975].

The response of aequorin to Ca^{2+} is exponential over the range of 10^{-7}–10^{-4} M [Allen et al., 1977]; there is no response at all below 10^{-8} M. The most important feature of this response is that on a log-log plot the maximum slope is 2.5, suggesting that at least three Ca^{2+} ions interact with aequorin to generate the luminescence. The consequence of this steep slope is that a change in Ca^{2+} produces a greater change in luminescence than if the slope was 1.0. A Ca^{2+} increase in a small localized area would give a greater response than if the same amount of Ca^{2+} were spread uniformly over the cytoplasm. For example, Blinks et al. [1982] have calculated for the case in which Ca^{2+} is localized in 10% of the cytoplasm the intensity of the light signal will be 30 times greater than if the same amount of Ca^{2+} were uniformly distributed. This means that in the case where there are local Ca^{2+} concentration gradients, aequorin does not provide quantitative data about the average value of the cytoplasmic Ca^{2+}. One would expect to see large signals during the initial phases of a Ca^{2+} flux when Ca^{2+} gradients within the cytoplasm are steep. This may explain the "spiky" appearance of some aequorin traces. This behavior contrasts to that of fluorescent probes, quin2 and fura-2, which report the average value of Ca^{2+} in the compartment in which the dye is located.

In the physiologic range, aequorin is relatively insensitive to pH changes; however, temperature must be considered, since the amount of light produced particularly at low Ca^{2+} is strongly temperature dependent [Blinks et al., 1982]. Magnesium probably presents the greatest problem for the use of aequorin in biological systems. While the light reaction is not initiated by Mg^{2+}, the Ca^{2+}-dependence of the aequorin reaction is antagonized by Mg^{2+} [Blinks et al., 1982]. It therefore becomes imperative to know the Mg^{2+} concentration inside a cell before a proper calibration curve can be obtained. In addition, any changes in Mg^{2+} that occur during an experiment may affect the interpretation of the results. Aequorin is especially sensitive to such a change, since, as mentioned, its calibration curve is steep.

Aequorin does not appear to enter intracellular organelles such as mitochondria or sarcoplasmic reticulum since the signals generated in many cells in which it has been used under conditions where the organelles would contain appreciable amounts of Ca^{2+}, indicate that the probe is only in a region of low Ca^{2+} [Blinks et al., 1982]. However, it is possible that this may not be true in all cases. If the cells are large, the time for a uniform steady-state concentration to be achieved must also be considered. A distinct advantage of aequorin is that it can be used at concentrations that are much lower than some fluorescent probes and appears to have very little buffering effect on cytosolic Ca^{2+}.

Because aequorin is a protein, originally the only method that could be used to introduce this probe into cells was microinjection. Platelets could not be studied because of their small size. A procedure has been developed that uses ATP and EGTA to selectively permeabilize the plasma membrane [Morgan and Morgan, 1982]. The membrane is subsequently resealed by addition of Mg^{2+}. The exact mechanism by which this allows such a large protein as aequorin to enter is uncertain, but it appears that no cytoplasmic proteins leak out during the loading procedure. Recently, this method was applied to platelets by Johnson et al. [1985a]. In this study they compared the effects of quin2 and aequorin on platelet function and found that, whereas quin2 severely damped the response of the platelets to A23187, aequorin-loaded cells had the same response as control cells. This methodology has been employed in several subsequent studies by this group [Johnson et al., 1985b; Ware et al., 1985, 1986] to show, for example, that aequorin, in contrast to quin2, could detect changes in Ca^{2+} in response to both epinephrine and 12-O-tetradecanoyl phorbol-13-acetate (TPA). The following criticisms were made of these studies. 1) In experiments in which platelets were loaded with either quin2 or both quin2 and aequorin, the cells were incubated at 22°C rather than the standard 37°C. Temperatures below 37°C are not recommended for loading quin2 by Rink and Pozzan [1985] due to incomplete hydrolysis of quin acetoxymethyl ester (see below). 2) Platelets are subjected to harsh conditions during aequorin loading, i.e., 0°C in the presence of EGTA. These conditions have been shown to alter platelet morphology [White and Krivitt, 1967] and can strip tightly bound membrane Ca^{2+} from the cell [Brass and Shattil, 1982]. 3) The level of Ca^{2+} in the resting cells is 10-fold higher with aequorin than with other techniques (see below). These data have been interpreted to show that there is a localized region of high Ca^{2+} within the resting platelet; however, it could also indicate that a portion of the aequorin has entered an internal organelle that contains higher Ca^{2+} than the cytoplasm. 4) The kinetics of aequorin transients are often not as expected. In some of the published traces, the major component of the increase in the aequorin signal occurs only after a lag of greater than 10 sec and in some cases not until shape change is complete [Johnson et al., 1985b; Ware et al., 1985]. In our experience, there is never a similar lag with either quin2 or fura-2. As discussed above, it would be expected that aequorin signals would rise more rapidly than quin2 or fura-2 signals owing to the potential for local calcium gradients during the early stages of calcium mobilization.

Quin2 and Fura-2

Several polycarboxylic fluorescent Ca^{2+}chelators have been synthesized recently by Roger Tsien and his colleagues [Tsien, 1980; Grynkiewicz et al., 1985]. These indicators change their fluorescent properties upon binding Ca^{2+} and thus can be adapted to measure Ca^{2+} concentrations. The dyes were synthesized with a backbone similar to that of EGTA and thus show a high selectivity for Ca^{2+} over Mg^{2+}. In contrast to EGTA, the compounds do not have significant affinity for protons in the physiological pH range and they more rapidly bind and release Ca^{2+}. Ordinarily such highly charged molecules would not cross the plasma membrane; however, the carboxylic groups can be masked with acetoxymethyl ester groups, thereby rendering the molecule electrically neutral and membrane permeant. Esterases are present in the cytosol of platelets that can cleave the ester groups at a reasonable rate, trapping the free acid in the cytosol. It is the ease with which cells can be loaded that makes these fluorescent indicators both unique and useful.

Quin2

Note: the following discussion incorporates much of the information discussed by Rink and Pozzan [1985]. A careful reading of this excellent discussion is highly recommended.

Quin2 was the first fluorescent probe synthesized that was suitable for use with cells. The advantages of this molecule include: it is commercially available; it can be loaded into platelets in plasma where they could be better maintained (this is in contrast to aequorin); loading is both simple and rapid; it does not appear to enter intracellular organelles; and in larger cells its distribution in the cytoplasm has been shown to be relatively uniform [Rink and Pozzan, 1985].

However, quin2 has several disadvantages as well. Because quin2 has both a low extinction coefficient and fluorescence quantum yield, large cytoplasmic concentrations of the indicator are required for good signal to noise ratios. Quin2 is routinely used in platelets at cytoplasmic concentrations of 1 to 2 mM, concentrations which have significant buffering effects on any mobilized Ca^{2+}. The buffering of free calcium by quin2 is observed as a slowing or in some cases a damping of platelet responses to agonists. When quin2/AM is cleaved by esters, three metabolites are generated: protons, acetate ions, and formaldehyde. However, the cell can probably recover from most of the deleterious effects of the agents. For example, low concentrations of formaldehyde have been shown to deplete metabolic ATP, but the adenylate energy charge is maintained and these cells function as well or perhaps better than untreated platelets. However, Rink and Pozzan [1985] have noted that quin2-loaded platelets are more sensitive to platelet-activating factor. We have found that quin2-loaded platelets are more easily labeled with $[^{32}P]$-PO_4. All of this evidence does suggest that the platelet is in some way altered by loading with quin2.

When quin2 binds Ca^{2+}, the fluorescence intensity increases over sixfold; however, there is no significant change in either the excitation or emission spectrum. If there was a shift in either spectrum, calibration of Ca^{2+} could be performed by measurement of the fluorescence at two different wavelengths (see fura-2). Calibration of quin2 signals requires cell lysis in order to measure the fluorescence at both saturating and zero Ca^{2+}.

Loading quin2 into platelets. Loading of platelets with quin2 is best done before the platelets are separated from plasma. Platelet-rich plasma is incubated at 37°C for 30 min with 20 μM quin2/AM. Loading can be followed by monitoring the changes in the emission spectrum of the suspension as a function of time using an excitation wavelength of 339 nm. The emission spectrum of the ester (λ_{max}=430 nm) is different from that of the free acid (λ_{max}=492 nm). A typical example of the spectral changes that occur during loading of platelets in plasma with quin2 are shown in Figure 1. The fluorescence emission spectrum initially shows the expected peak at 430 nm. The most notable change that occurs during loading is a reduction of the peak at 430 nm (Fig. 1). The increase expected at 492 nm is masked by the strong fluorescence of the plasma. The loading efficiency can be determined by washing and lysing the cells in a Ca^{2+} containing medium. The fluorescence emission spectrum is recorded and corrected for the autofluorescence by determining a similar spectrum for lysed platelets that had not been loaded with quin2. The amount of trapped quin2 free acid is quantitated by comparing the corrected spectrum with spectra of known dilutions in the same medium of a standard solution of quin2 acid. The intracellular concentration of quin2 can then be calculated assuming an average intracellular volume of 0.52 μl/10^8 cells [Wiley et al., 1983]. We routinely observe loading efficiencies of about 35% with intracellular quin2 concentrations of about 2.5 mM. The loading temperature is quite important. Rink and Pozzan [1985] report that if cells are loaded with quin2 below 37°C, unhydrolyzed ester can be trapped in the cell. This unhydrolyzed ester is not converted to free acid by later raising the temperature to 37°C.

Calibration. Calibration must done at the end of the experiment on a sample, since the cells must be lysed. The object of the calibration procedure is to obtain the values of quin2 fluorescence in the absence of Ca^{2+} (Fmin) and in the presence of saturating Ca^{2+} (Fmax). From these two values any measured fluorescence can be converted to a Ca^{2+} concentration. The following two approaches can be used. The first entails cell lysis with digitonin or Triton-X100 in an EGTA containing buffer followed by the addition of a mixture of excess Ca^{2+} and CaDTPA (diethylenetriaminepentaacetic acid) to saturate the quin2 with Ca^{2+}. The DTPA is used to remove contaminating heavy metals that can quench quin2 fluorescence. Care must be taken in this method to maintain the pH above 7, since addition of Ca^{2+} to EGTA will release protons. An alternate method of calibration in which Fmax is determined without lysis is done by adding a saturating concentration of the nonfluorescent Ca^{2+} ionophore, iono-

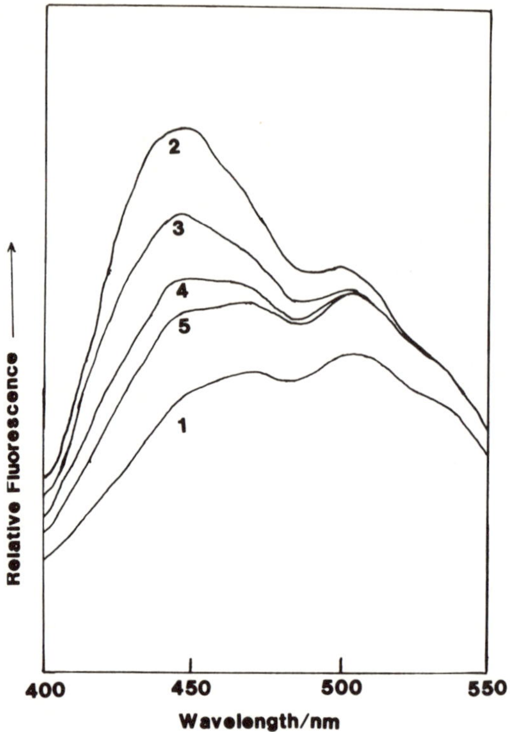

Fig. 1. Changes in fluorescence emission spectra of quin2/AM during uptake and hydrolysis by platelets in plasma. The excitation wavelength was fixed at 339 nm. Twenty μM quin2/AM was added to platelets (5×10^8/ml) in plasma that had been anticoagulated with ACD and were continually stirred at 37°C. Spectra were recorded before quin2/AM addition (#1), immediately after addition (#2), 5.5 min after addition (#3), 15 min after addition (#4), and 30 min after quin2/AM addition (#5).

mycin (now available from Calbiochem), in the presence of a high concentration of extracellular Ca^{2+}. The subsequent addition of excess Mn^{2+} quenches all quin2 fluorescence, leaving only autofluorescence. An example of this type of calibration is illustrated in Figure 2. Since Ca^{2+}-free quin2 fluoresces, Fmin must also be determined in order to calculate the free Ca^{2+}. However, since we know that the fluorescence of quin2 is enhanced sixfold upon binding Ca^{2+}, Fmin can be calculated from the relationship:

$$\text{Fmin} = F_{Mn} + 1/6\,(\text{Fmax} - F_{Mn})$$

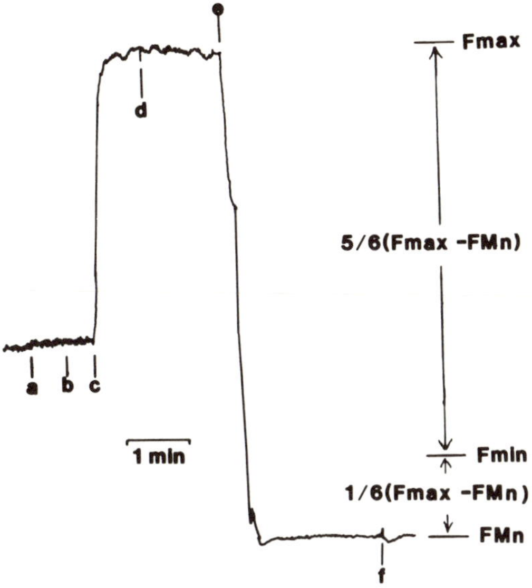

Fig. 2. Calibration of the quin2 response with ionomycin and $MnCl_2$. Washed platelets were loaded with quin2. Additions are: a) 1 mM $CaCl_2$, b) 100 μM CaDTPA, c) 400 nM ionomycin, d) 400 nM ionomycin, e) 5 mM $MnCl_2$, and f) 5 mM $MnCl_2$. Fmin is calculated as described in the text.

The free Ca^{2+} can be calculated form the observed fluorescence (Fobs) by the following equation:

$$Ca^{2+}_{free} \text{ (in nM)} = (\text{Fobs} - \text{Fmin})/(\text{Fmax} - \text{Fobs}) \times 115$$

One should be aware that this calculation is based on an assumed intracellular free Mg^{2+} concentration of 1 mM.

Measurement of quin2 in intact platelets. Measurements of quin2 fluorescence in intact platelets are usually made in a quartz fluorometer cuvette that is continuously stirred at 37°C. The presence of small platelet aggregates does not seem to be a problem, but formation of large clumps may lead to signal loss and make calibration difficult. If light scattering is a problem a 400 nm cutoff filter can be placed in front of the photomultiplier. The autofluorescence of the platelets can represent a large fraction of the signal but under most conditions does not change. However, unloaded cells should be tested using the same experimental protocol to check for any potential problems. A problem can arise if added compounds are themselves fluorescent or quench the quin2 signal. In this regard, ionomycin should be used in preference to A23187, which fluoresces. Photo-bleaching of quin2 can occur if the incident light beam is intense. This has not been a problem in our experience. Correction should also be made for quin2 that has leaked into the suspension medium. Addition of about 100 μM Mn^{2+} will quench the external quin2 fluorescence and give an estimate of the amount of signal that is due to external indicator. The experiment can be continued if excess CaDTPA is added. Another way to assess external quin2 is to gently centrifuge the platelets and measure the fluorescence of the supernatant [Rink and Pozzan, 1985].

Fura-2

Fura-2 and indo-1 can be considered second-generation fluorescent Ca^{2+}-probes [Grynkiewicz et al., 1985]. Since we have used only fura-2 in our own studies, discussion will be restricted to fura-2. While indo-1 and fura-2 have similar properties, indo-1 may be more useful for some applications [Grynkiewicz et al., 1985]. Roger Tsien's goal in synthesizing fura-2 was to overcome two of the major deficiencies of quin2: the low quantum efficiency and the lack of a spectral change upon binding Ca^{2+} [Tsien et al., 1985]. The fura-2-Ca complex has a 30-fold higher fluorescence intensity due to both a greater extinction coefficient and greater fluorescence yield than quin2. Thus at 30-fold lower intracellular concentrations, fura-2 can produce a similar signal to quin2. The benefits of the requirement for lower loading are that the cells are exposed to a lower concentration of the toxic by-products of esterolytic cleavage and the buffering effects of the fluorescent probe are minimized (see below). Another advantage of fura-2 is that calibration does not require cell lysis. The excitation spectrum changes as Ca^{2+} becomes bound to the fluorophore and the excitation maximum gradually shifts from 362 nm to 335 nm. Binding of Ca^{2+} produces a substantial decrease in the excitation spectrum above 365 nm and an increase below this wavelength. By exciting at two different wavelengths (e.g., 340 nm and 380 nm) and measuring the ratio of the emission at a fixed wavelength (i.e., 510 nm), one can determine the free calcium directly. This measurement is independent of dye loading. This property of fura-2 and the fact that reasonable fluorescence measurements can be obtained at excitation wavelengths of 350 nm (the cutoff for glass, the material used for most microscope lenses) and above makes fura-2 suitable for use in microscopic studies of Ca^{2+} mobilization in single cells. In addition to these two primary advantages of fura-2, the newer probe also exhibits a fivefold higher apparent K_d for magnesium (about 5 mM) and a twofold higher apparent K_d for Ca^{2+} than quin2. The former characteristic means that Mg^{2+} has less effect on the fura-2 signal and the latter that slightly higher concentrations of Ca^{2+} can be measured with fura-2 than quin2. In addition, the higher K_d reduces the Ca^{2+} buffering of fura-2 slightly. Fura-2 is also less affected by heavy metals.

Loading of fura-2. Platelets are loaded with fura-2 in plasma in a manner similar to quin2 with one exception. In order to maximize efficiency and lower the cost, we load platelets with fura-2 by concentrating PRP twofold prior to loading. The cells are concentrated by gentle centrifugation of the PRP (800 × g for 20 min). The pellet is resuspended in 1/2 volume of the autologous plasma and the cell suspension is incubated with 5 μM fura-2 for 30 min at 37°C. Loading can be monitored spectrally by recording the time-dependent changes in the fluorescence excitation spectrum between 300 and 400 nm with a fixed emission wavelength of 510 nm (Fig. 3). As the dye is loaded into the cell and converted into the free acid, an increase in the spectrum at about 360 nm is observed. The loading efficiency is determined as discussed for quin2. An intracellular concentration of 100–150 μM fura-2 with about 18% loading efficiency is achieved with this technique.

Calibration. In principle, calibration of the fura-2 signal is quite simple. The concentration of free Ca^{2+} is calculated from the equation given below.

$$[Ca^{2+}] = K_d * ((R - R_{min})/(R_{max} - R) * (S_{f2}/S_{b2}))$$

K_d is the apparent dissociation constant of fura-2 for Ca^{2+} which has been measured to be 224 nM at 37°C in a buffer that approximates the intracellular ionic composition [Grynkiewicz et al., 1985]. R is the ratio at an unknown Ca^{2+} concentration of the fluorescence signal determined at two different excitation wavelengths (in most cases 340 nm/380 nm) after correction for autofluorescence at each wavelength. R_{min} and R_{max} are the 340 nm/380 nm ratios measured at zero and saturating Ca^{2+}, respectively. (S_{f2}/S_{b2}) is the ratio of the fluorescence intensity of the dye again at zero and saturating Ca^{2+} at 380 nm. We have determined that $R_{max} = 22$, $R_{min} = 0.93$, and $(S_{f2}/S_{b2}) = 7.5$ at 37°C in a buffer composed of 110 mM KCl, 20 mM NaCl, 1.2 mM $MgCl_2$, and 25 mM MOPS, pH 7.2. However, it seems that the viscosity of the cytoplasm may be sufficient to significantly alter these values [Tsien et al., 1985]. Tsien et al. [1985] have reported measuring the values of the relevant constants in solutions of fura-2 acid thickened with 20% gelatin. We have not been able to obtain gelatin of sufficient purity to make these measurements ourselves but have estimated the values of Rmin, Rmax, and (S_{f2}/S_{b2}) from the data presented in Figure 3 of the Tsien paper to be 0.44, 18.5, and 7.3, respectively. While these values do not seem very different from those found in nonviscous buffers, the calculated Ca^{2+} can be more than twofold greater using this second set of values.

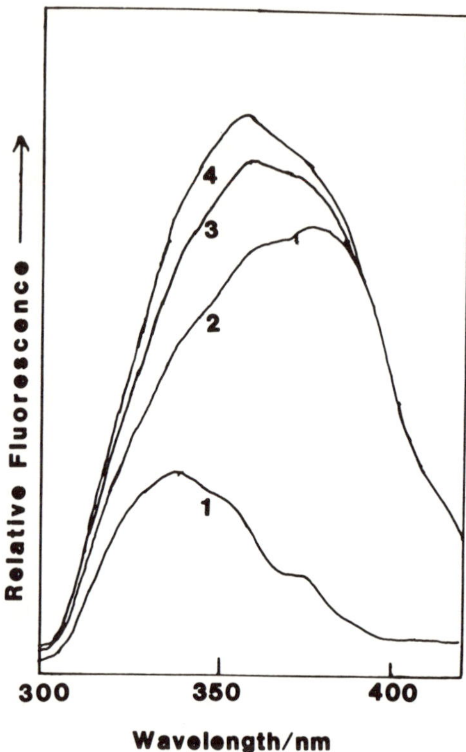

Fig. 3. Changes in fluorescence excitation spectra of fura-2/AM during uptake and hydrolysis by platelets in plasma. The emission wavelength was fixed at 510 nm. Five μM fura-2/AM was added to the platelets (1×10^9/ml) in plasma that were continuously stirred at 37°C. Spectra shown: 1) platelets suspension before fura-2/AM addition, 2) 2 min after fura-2/AM addition, 3) 10 min after fura-2/AM addition, 4) 30 min after fura-2/AM addition.

In addition, measured Ca^{2+} concentrations using the values from the gelatin buffers are in better agreement with measurements made with quin2. As an alternative, fura-2 can be calibrated at 340 nm by a similar technique as used for quin2; however, this method also suffers from the fact that the calibration is made at low viscosity while the viscosity of the cytoplasm is higher.

Measurement of fura-2 fluorescence. Ideally, measurement of fura-2 fluorescence should be made with a fluorometer that can record fluorescence at two excitation wavelengths simultaneously. This can be done if there are two light sources and a chopper that alternates between them. Such fluorometers have recently become commercially available but are very expensive. We have been able to make Ca^{2+} measurements with fura-2 using an ordinary fluorometer

(Perkin Elmer LS-5) by switching the excitation wavelength between 340 and 380. This change requires about 3 sec and, while adequate for most purposes, is not suitable when the signals are changing rapidly. An example of Ca^{2+} transients measured with this technique is shown in Figure 5.

Comparison of the Effects of Fura-2 and Quin2 Loading on Platelet Function

Thrombin-induced platelet aggregation and secretion are compared in Figure 4 for cells loaded either with quin2 or fura-2 by the methods described above. The cells that are loaded with quin2 are distinctly less responsive than those

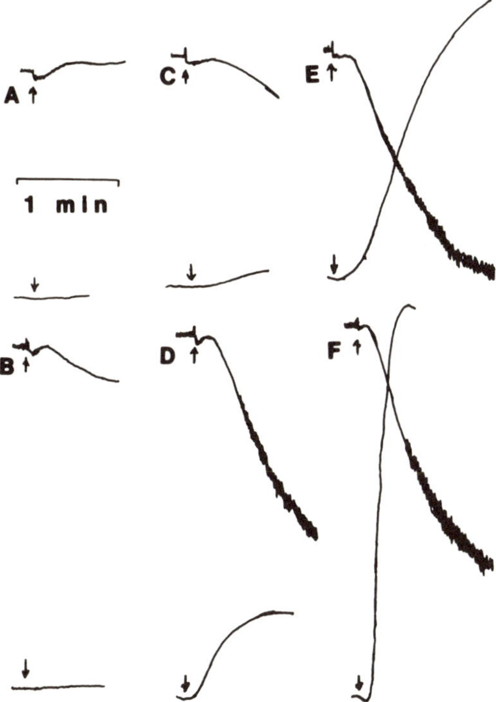

Fig. 4. Comparison of secretion and aggregation of platelets loaded with either quin2 or fura-2. Washed platelets were prepared as described in Hallam et al. [1985]. Aggregation and secretion were measured simultaneously in a Chronolog luminaggregator. Platelets were suspended in a buffer containing nominal Ca^{2+} and were continuously stirred at 37°C. Panels A, C, E show cells loaded with quin2, and B, D, F show cells loaded with fura-2. Platelets were stimulated with 0.05 U/ml thrombin (A and B); 0.1 U/ml thrombin (C and D); 0.5 U/ml thrombin (E and F). Agonist additions are indicated by the arrows.

loaded with fura-2. The greatest differences are observed at the intermediate concentration of thrombin where quin2-loaded cells showed greatly reduced secretion and aggregation. At the lowest concentration of thrombin, quin2-loaded cells showed a diminished rate of shape change. At the highest concentration of thrombin used, the quin2-loaded cells showed decreased rates of aggregation and secretion. These effects are probably largely due to the buffering effect quin2 has on cytosolic Ca^{2+}. The fura-2-loaded cells were not significantly different from unloaded control cells. Similar effects of quin2 loading were also noted when PAF and ADP were used as agonists.

Figure 5 compares the Ca^{2+} transients measured in quin2-loaded cells with those determined in fura-2-loaded platelets. The rise in Ca^{2+} can be seen to occur much more rapidly in the fura-2 record. Maximal Ca^{2+} is reached within

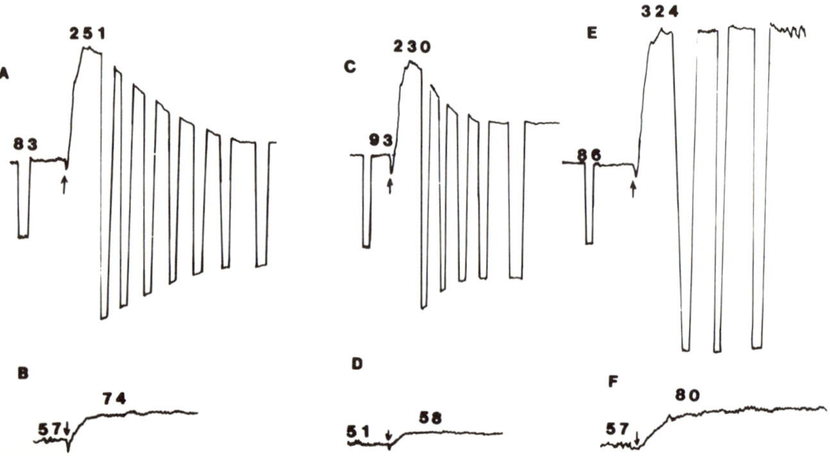

Fig. 5. Comparison of Ca^{2+} mobilization of platelets loaded with either quin2 or fura-2. Washed platelets were suspended in a buffer containing nominal Ca^{2+} and were continuously stirred at 37°C. Panels A, C, E show cells loaded with fura-2, and B, D, F show cells loaded with quin2. Platelets were stimulated with 100 nM platelet-activating factor (A and B); 0.05 U/ml thrombin (C and D); 0.1 U/ml thrombin (E and F). Agonist additions are indicated by the arrows. The rapid changes in the fura-2 spectra represent points where the excitation wavelength was switched. The numbers indicate the basal and maximal calcium attained in nanomolar.

about 8 sec, whereas in quin2-loaded platelets the signal reaches a plateau only after 15 sec. More remarkable, the quin2 signal does not decrease once the maximum has been reached. The fura-2 signal gradually decreases to basal levels, indicating either resequestration of Ca^{2+}, efflux of Ca^{2+}, or both.

METHODS FOR THE STUDY OF Ca^{2+} IN PERMEABILIZED PLATELETS

Calcium Buffer Systems

In the studies discussed below, a good method of maintaining the Ca^{2+} concentration is essential. While any calcium chelator with reasonable affinity is suitable for maintaining the free Ca^{2+} at a fixed concentration, problems arise when one wants to vary the Ca^{2+} concentration by adding Ca^{2+} to samples in small volumes. However, before we discuss buffer systems that overcome these difficulties, we would like to point out the need for a method of calculating the free Ca^{2+} concentrations for a given buffer system. This presents no problem for the simple situation in which only one chelator and one metal ion are present but requires a computer program for more complicated situations. Perrin and Sayce [1967] have published a Fortran computer program called COMICS that can calculate the concentration of all free metals in the presence of multiple ligands if the appropriate stability and proton ionization constants are provided. The values for most common chelators are found in Martell and Smith [1974]. We have adapted this program to a small microcomputer and can calculate free ion concentrations in mixtures of up to five metals and five ligands.

Most simple calcium chelators such as EGTA have one to two protonated carboxyl groups (out of a possible four) in the physiologic pH range; only at high pH (> 11) does EGTA become fully deprotonated. Divalent metals only bind tightly to the unprotonated form of the chelator. Thus when Ca^{2+} is added to solutions containing chelators, up to 2 moles of H^+ are liberated per mole of added Ca^{2+}, and a substantial change in pH can occur even if a pH buffer is present. Because Ca^{2+} binds only to the deprotonated form of the chelator, protons are competitive with Ca^{2+} for the binding site of EGTA and this results in a pH sensitivity for most Ca^{2+} chelators. Figure 6 shows that the level of free Ca^{2+} obtained in an EGTA buffer system will vary greatly with small pH changes. One method usually employed to make EGTA buffers requires two solutions containing equivalent concentrations of EGTA. One solution contains only EGTA, and the other contains equal concentrations of EGTA and Ca^{2+}. The pH of this solution is adjusted to be the same as that of the EGTA-only solution after the Ca^{2+} has been added. The two solutions can then be mixed in different proportions to achieve different free Ca^{2+} concentrations. The EGTA-

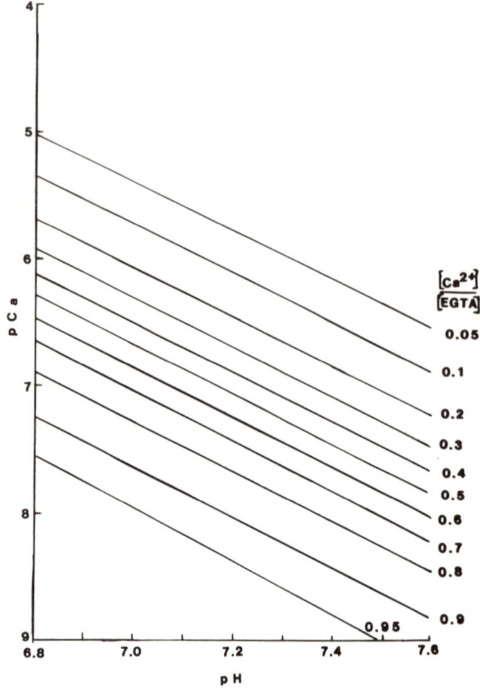

Fig. 6. The pH dependence of an EGTA-Ca^{2+} buffer system.

Ca^{2+} solution should be made in such a way that the chelator and metal are as close to equivalent in concentration as possible. This is usually done by titration of one of the two against the other, either using a Ca^{2+}-sensitive dye such as murexide or a Ca^{2+} electrode to detect the equivalence point. While this method does allow one to be relatively certain of the free Ca^{2+} concentration in most circumstances, it still has two drawbacks. A small change in pH generated during the period of study (e.g., metabolic changes occurring in permeabilized cells) will produce significant and unknown changes in free Ca^{2+}. In addition, the binding constant of EGTA for Ca^{2+} makes it difficult to obtain Ca^{2+} concentrations above 1 μM without decreasing the pH below 7 or operating out of the range in which effective buffering can be assured. (The effective buffering range is from Ca^{2+}/EGTA = 0.05 to 0.95.)

Wolf [1973] proposed a method to make Ca^{2+} buffers that were almost pH insensitive. The buffer system requires that two metals be used, a primary ion whose concentration is to be varied over a given range and a secondary ion that would be added in excess. Typically in most biological experiments, calcium would be the primary ion and magnesium would be the secondary ion. The system will work if the following criteria of Wolf are met: 1) The secondary ion be bound about 100 times weaker than the primary ion. If the binding is much tighter, low concentrations of primary ion cannot be achieved. If the binding is much weaker, the system will become pH sensitive. 2) The concentration of the primary ion should be within the effective buffering range. 3) The sum of the concentrations of the two metals should always be greater than the ligand concentration. In such a system, the secondary ion displaces the protons from the chelator and a change in pH does not change the competition between protons and primary ion. Addition of the primary ion will displace secondary ions rather than protons. Several Ca^{2+} chelators systems including Mg^{2+}-EDTA are able to fulfill the conditions. The pH dependence of a Mg^{2+}-EDTA buffer is shown in Figure 7. It is clear that such a system shows little or no pH dependence. Also Ca^{2+} concentrations greater than 100 μM can be obtained within the effective buffering range. However, two problems remain with this system: calcium

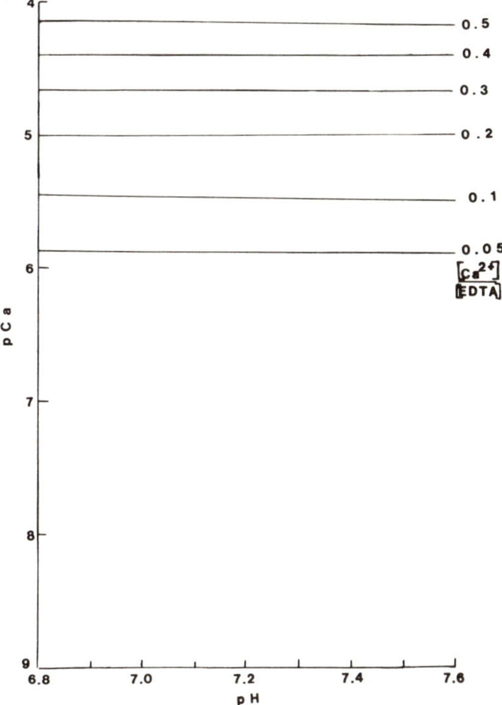

Fig. 7. The pH dependence of an EDTA-Ca^{2+} buffer system in the presence of Mg^{2+}. The Mg^{2+} concentration was 1.2 times the EDTA concentration.

concentrations below 1 μM can only be achieved by using added Ca^{2+} outside the effective buffering range, and the concentration of free Mg^{2+} will vary over a wide range as the free Ca^{2+} is changed. The latter difficulty may be compensated for by varying both the added Mg^{2+} and the added Ca^{2+}, a solution that may not be totally satisfying for all experiments.

Roger Tsien [1980] has synthesized a Ca^{2+}-chelator, BAPTA, that overcomes almost all of these difficulties. BAPTA is similar in structure to EGTA and thus, like EGTA, has 100,000-fold preference for Ca^{2+} over Mg^{2+}. However, it has a much lower affinity for protons than EGTA and at physiologic pH only a small portion of the BAPTA molecules are protonated. The pH sensitivity of a BAPTA buffer system containing 10 mM BAPTA and 1.25 mM Mg^{2+} is shown in Figure 8. Although this system is not quite as pH insensitive as a Wolf system, the pH sensitivity is quite good. The Mg^{2+} concentration is also reasonably constant over the range of Ca^{2+} varying between 0.8 and 1.0 mM. The only difficulty with BAPTA, at the present time, is that it is relatively expensive.

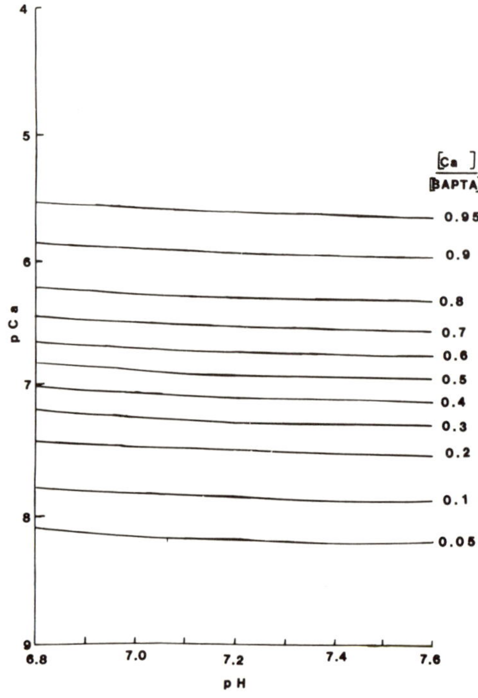

Fig. 8. The pH dependence of a BAPTA-Ca^{2+} buffer system.

Platelet Permeabilization With Digitonin or Saponin

Digitonin treatment of platelets represents a simple technique to permeabilize the plasma membrane to the external milieu. Saponin, a mixture of several related glycosides, is used by some in preference to digitonin owing to its greater water solubility. The basis for the technique lies in the ability of digitonin and related glycosides to form complexes with cholesterol of cell membranes [Haslam and Klyne, 1953; Akiyama et al., 1980]. Other lytic agents such as polyene antibiotics [Kinsky, 1970; DeKruijff, 1974] and lysolecithin [Rand et al., 1975; Purdon et al., 1975] are thought to act in the same manner. Since most of these compounds form micelles, they may also act as detergents, and the possibility that they solubilize membrane components should be considered [Purdon et al., 1980]. The method was first used by Zuurendonck and Tager [1974] in hepatocytes to separate cytosolic from intracellular organelles. The method, if used properly, appears to selectively lyse the plasma membrane leaving internal membranes intact. Two considerations make this possible. The first is kinetic, i.e., because the plasma is the most accessible to external agents it is lysed first. Thus, it is possible that internal membranes may be disrupted if the incubation with detergent is prolonged. The second reason that digitonin acts preferentially on the plasma membrane is that, in general, plasma membranes contain a higher concentration of cholesterol [Monneron and d'Alayer, 1978] than do internal membranes, though it is not certain that this is true for platelets.

This technique was employed with platelets by Akkerman et al. [1980a], who combined the technique with centrifugation through phthalate oils and showed that, under appropriate conditions, cytosolic enzymes and glycolytic intermediates could be separated from internal organelles. They pointed out that the concentrations of digitonin needed were critically dependent on the cell concentration; later [Akkerman et al., 1980b] they showed that increasing concentrations of digitonin would sequentially lyse granules, with dense granule lysis requiring the lowest digitonin concentrations, and lysosomal granule lysis requiring the highest. Alpha granule lysis required an intermediate concentration. Other factors to consider when using this technique are the temperature and whether the cells are stirred. Purdon et al. [1984] showed that lysis is greater in a stirred system at 37°C than when the cells were unstirred and left on ice at 4°C.

It should be clear from this discussion that if one intends to use digitonin permeabilization, the exact lysis conditions should be established under the same conditions in which the experiment will be performed. Since the internal organelle most susceptible to digitonin is the dense granule, this calibration can be performed quite simply using two isotopes. Platelets are incubated with [^{3}H]-adenine, which labels ATP in the metabolic or cytosolic compartment, and with [^{14}C]-serotonin, which is taken up into the dense granules. Platelets at a standardized cell concentration are incubated with varying concentrations of digitonin, and the release of the two radiolabels into the supernatant is determined. An example of such a calibration is shown in Figure 9. A new calibration curve must be made each time a new digitonin stock solution is prepared. We have found that under fixed conditions, the concentration of digitonin needed is reasonably reproducible.

Specific Uses for Digitonin Permeabilization

The null point method for the determination of cytoplasmic free calcium in platelets. Before the advent of calcium-sensitive indicators such as quin2 and fura-2, null point titration [Murphy et al., 1980] was used to determine cytoplasmic free calcium levels in small cells. Such an approach was used by Murphy et al. [1980] to determine the calcium concentration in the cytoplasm of resting and stimulated liver cells. Rink et al. [1982] have also used this method to determine intracellular pH and Mg^{2+} in lymphocytes. The key to the null point method resides in the selective lysis of the plasma membrane without compromising the membrane integrity of intracellular compartments. Stirred (900 rpm) platelets are incubated at 37°C to equilibrate the sample, and a calcium

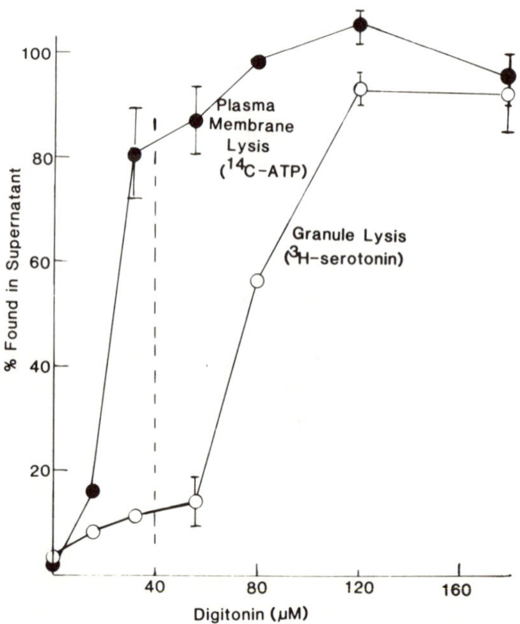

Fig. 9. Assessment of the digitonin concentration required for selective lysis of the platelet plasma membrane. The dotted line indicates the optimal digitonin concentration.

electrode is inserted in the measuring chamber. In the micromolar range and below, the resulting calcium signal is too noisy unless calcium buffers are used. Murphy et al. [1980] have used the metallochromatic indicator arsenazo III in the absence of calcium buffers. Addition of digitonin results in a rapid influx or net decrease in calcium measured in the extracellular space. At a given concentration of digitonin, the null point is achieved when there is no net movement of Ca^{2+} into or out of the cells following permeabilization of the plasma membrane. In liver cells, Becker et al. [1980] have shown that this resting level can be generated in vitro by incubation of mitochondria and endoplasmic reticulum. The influx of calcium seen following digitonin lysis is probably due to uptake by these intracellular organelles as well as buffering by intracellular binding sites for calcium, i.e., the endogenous calcium buffering systems present in the intracellular compartment. The contribution of endoplasmic reticulum or mitochondria can be evaluated by incubating cells with agents known to affect the uptake or sequestration of calcium by these organelles [Murphy et al., 1980; Ronning et al., 1982].

The null point is defined as that concentration of external calcium at which no influx or change in calcium concentration is apparent following lysis. This point of no flow, or the null point, is more precisely defined by a plot of rate of influx versus the external calcium concentration. Such a set of results is shown for resting porcine platelets in Figure 10 [Purdon et al., 1984]. By definition, this is the cytoplasmic free calcium in the cell under conditions in effect at the time of

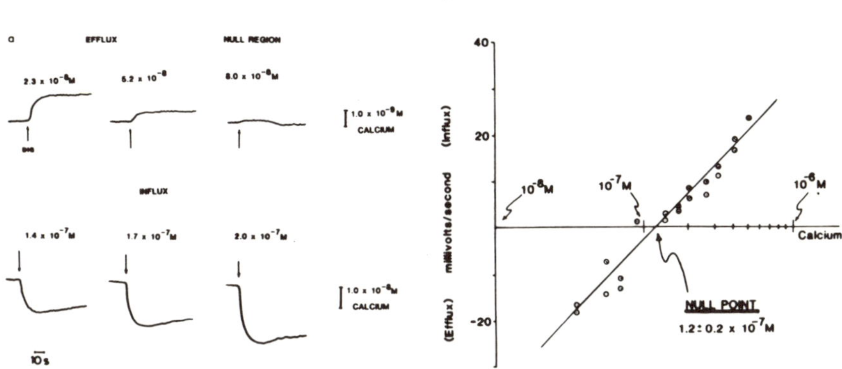

Fig. 10. The null point method for determination of the resting $[Ca^{2+}]$ concentration of platelets. Panel a: Typical recorder outputs from the calcium electrode during digitonin lysis of porcine platelets at different external free calcium concentrations. Addition of digitonin is indicated by the arrow. Panel b: Plot of the rate of calcium flux immediately following digitonin addition vs. the log of the prelytic calcium concentration. The null point is defined as the concentration where the flux is zero. Taken from Purdon et al. [1984] with permission.

lysis. This null point should correspond to the cytosolic free Ca^{2+} concentration even though the calcium is being measured in the bulk phase of the cell incubation medium. If the cell has been stimulated and the cytoplasmic free calcium is higher than in the resting state, then the null point will be reached at a higher level of external calcium [Murphy et al., 1980]. This forms the basis of examining the effect of different agonists. In turn lysis at an external calcium concentration below that of the null point results in an apparent efflux of cytoplasmic calcium. This has been shown to occur in vitro with endoplasmic reticulum and mitochondria and indicates the reversibility of calcium homeostasis by these organelles [Becker et al., 1980]. The agreement between values for free cytoplasmic calcium in resting platelets found using either the null method or quin2 suggests that the toxic substances resulting from the hydrolysis of the quin2 ester have not affected the cell. Again, cytoplasmic free calcium values for platelets are considerably lower than those reported with aequorin [Ware et al., 1985], possibly because different cytoplasmic compartments are being analyzed.

The Calcium Dependence of Myosin Phosphorylation

We have used digitonin-permeabilized platelets to determine the dependence of platelet myosin phosphorylation on Ca^{2+} concentration. Myosin phosphorylation is a Ca^{2+}-dependent event. Ca^{2+} binds to calmodulin, and the complex, in turn, to myosin light chain kinase; the kinase becomes activated and phosphorylates myosin light chain. This event is necessary to activate the contractile activity of this protein. We used digitonin-permeabilized platelets to determine the dependence of myosin phosphorylation in situ on Ca^{2+} [Daniel et al., 1982]. Myosin phosphorylation was seen to be directly dependent on Ca^{2+} between 100 nM and 4 μM (Fig. 11). Myosin phosphorylation was 50% at about 600 nM Ca^{2+}. Since myosin in resting platelets is about 10% phosphorylated [Daniel et al., 1980], this experiment supports measurements of basal Ca^{2+} determined with fluorescent indicators and with the null point method. A comparison of these data with measurements made in intact cells using quin2 as a Ca^{2+} indicator shows that myosin phosphorylation can be as much as 46% at 200 nM Ca^{2+} [Hallam et al., 1985]. These data suggest that factors other than Ca^{2+} may modulate myosin phosphorylation in platelets.

Inositol-Triphosphate-Induced Calcium Mobilization

Inositol 1,4,5-triphosphate (IP_3) is produced by the action of phospholipase C on the membrane phospholipid, phosphatidylinositol 4,5-bisphosphate. Some of the earliest evidence for the possible role of IP_3 as a second messenger in cells came from studies with saponin-treated pancreatic acinar cells and hepatocytes [Berridge and Irvine, 1984]. IP_3 added to these cells was able to release Ca^{2+}

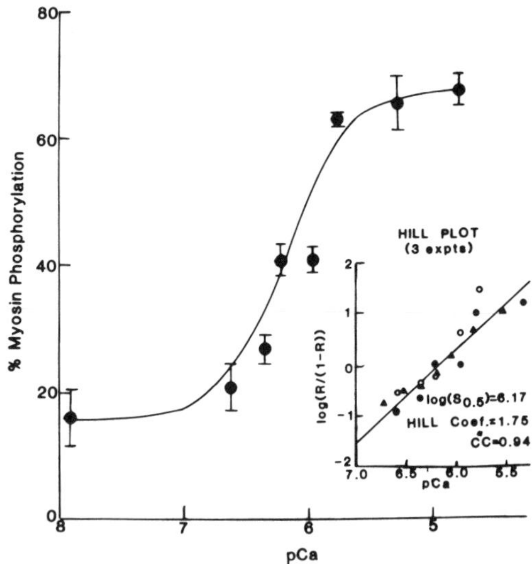

Fig. 11. Calcium dependence of myosin phosphorylation in digitonin permeabilized platelets. Insert to Fig. 11: Hill plot of calcium dependence of myosin phosphorylation. Data shown are from three different experiments. The curve shows the fit to the Hill equation from the insert. The solid points shows the data from one of the three experiments used for the Hill plot with the average values of two determinations.

from an internal organelle as measured either by the release of ^{45}Ca or with a Ca^{2+}-sensitive electrode. Brass and Joseph [1985] have extended these experiments to the platelet and showed that IP_3 was able to release $^{45}Ca^{2+}$ from an internal organelle, which was postulated to be the dense tubular system. Interestingly, an increase in pH was found to potentiate the effects of IP_3.

Electrical Permeabilization of the Platelet Membrane

The technique of electrical permeabilization uses a high voltage electrical field to induce a voltage potential of about 1.5 volts across the plasma membrane of a cell [Knight, 1981]. At this voltage, the lipid bilayer breaks down, leaving a small hole in the membrane. The voltage difference across a membrane at any point will depend on three factors: the applied field strength, the radius of the particle that the membrane surrounds, and the angle made between the membrane and the applied field at that point. The voltage difference across the membrane will be greatest along the direction of the field. For a cell in suspension that is free to tumble, multiple holes of relatively uniform distribution can be achieved by using a series of voltage pulses, since at different times different points on the membrane will be parallel with the field. More important, since the voltage difference is dependent on the particle radius, the voltage difference across the plasma membrane will be greater than across the membranes of internal organelles. By correct choice of voltage, the plasma membrane can be selectively permeabilized without affecting internal organelles. For example, if the voltage across the platelet plasma membrane is 2 V, i.e., above the voltage required for membrane breakdown, the voltage difference across a granule membrane with a radius of less than 10% that of the cell will be below 0.2 V and will not cause membrane perforation. The main advantages of this technique compared to digitonin permeabilization are 1) The method is probably more selective because it depends on the difference in radius between the cell and internal organelles, which may differ by as much as two orders of magnitude. 2) The holes produced are smaller than with digitonin; thus, small molecules such as Ca^{2+} and ATP have access to the cytosolic space but proteins do not diffuse out of the cell. 3) The results obtained depend only on particle size and thus can more easily be predicted. 4) The preparation is stable once made, whereas digitonin over longer times disrupts internal organelles. 5) The preparation appears to be quite homogeneous, i.e., all cells seem to be uniformly permeabilized. The main disadvantages of this method are that a special apparatus is required and preparation of the cells requires more time. For example, this method could not easily be applied to the null point technique described above.

Apparatus

The main elements required in an apparatus are a high voltage power supply capable of at least 4,000 V, a capacitor that is able to take the required voltage, a switch to trigger capacitor discharge, and a chamber in which to place the platelet suspension [Knight, 1981; Knight and Scrutton, 1986]. One simply charges the capacitor with the power supply, the switch is closed, and the stored charge is rapidly discharged through the cell suspension. The voltage pulse required to perforate the plasma membrane need be of about 1–2 μs duration. With cells suspended in physiologic salt solutions, high voltage pulses of this length can be achieved through the discharge of a 4 μf capacitor. Replacement of the majority of the salt with isotonic sucrose will increase the resistance of the solution and allow the use of a smaller capacitor. The platelet with a small radius (about 1 μm) requires a field strength of 20 $kV \cdot cm^{-1}$ to produce lesions in the plasma membrane. In order to reduce the requirements of the power supply and minimize heating, the distance between the electrodes of the chamber in which the cell suspension is placed should be around 1 mm. We use a chamber with a 1.6 mm teflon sheet separating the electrodes and thus need about 3,000 V for permeabilization. While such a narrow chamber may seem to restrict the volume of cells that can be prepared at one time, the volume can be increased by increasing the surface area of the electrodes in contact with the cell suspension. We use two stainless steel plates as electrodes and can fill the chamber with 2.5 ml of platelet suspension. The teflon sheet and two electrodes are sandwiched between two 0.5 inch thick aluminum plates to which leads from the power supply are fastened on terminals that are screwed into the aluminum. Outside each of the aluminum plates is a piece of lucite of similar dimensions and the apparatus is held tightly together with strong clamps. The switch for the apparatus presents a special problem. Since the voltage and current through the switch are quite high, most ordinary switches are not suitable. Knight and Scrutton [1986] recommend a manual switch in which two pieces of metal are pushed together. Not everyone will feel safe with such an approach. We have modified an emergency room defibrillator (Electronics for Medicine, Inc.) to be used as a discharge apparatus by increasing the size of the capacitor found inside the apparatus to 4 μf and suppressing the inductance found in the apparatus, which slows the rise time of the voltage. This apparatus uses a vacuum relay as a switch. The switch operates well for a time and is much safer than using a manual switch. Unfortunately, after a period of time, the relay must be replaced because the surface of its contacts breaks down and the relay remains in the open position. This problem can be overcome by changing this relay to one with a higher current rating. An apparatus of this type can be purchased from Instec Corp., 151 Gilbraltor Rd., Horsham, PA.

Preparation of Permeabilized Platelets

Human platelets are collected using acid citrate dextrose as anticoagulant and platelet-rich plasma prepared by standard procedures. The cells are removed from plasma by centrifugation at 600 $\times$ g for 25 min. In order to minimize the number of samples to be treated in the electrical perforation chamber, the cells are resuspended in a volume 1/2 to 1/4 the original. Concentration of the platelets has no measurable effect on the efficiency of electrical permeabilization. The cells are resuspended in a buffer composed of a modified Ca^{2+}-Tyrode's solution, which also included 5 mM EGTA, 5 mM PIPES, 5 mM HEPES, 0.2% bovine serum albumin, 5 μg/ml apyrase, and 10 μM leupeptin, pH 6.5. The suspension is permeabilized at ambient temperature with a series of 20 discharges at 3–5 sec intervals at 3 kV in the apparatus described above. Each batch of cells is placed on ice immediately after electrical discharge. Originally, we isolated the cells from the suspension medium by gel-filtration as described by Haslam and Davidson [1984b]. However, we often had a problem with the cells aggregating on the column. We now isolate the cells by centrifugation at 900 $\times$ g for 25 min at 4°C. Cells isolated in this way behave the same as cells isolated by gel-filtration. The pellet is resuspended in a buffer containing 140 mM potassium glutamate, 10 mM EDTA, 17 mM $MgCl_2$, 5 mM ATP, and 10 mM HEPES, pH 7.2. The permeabilized platelets are stored on ice.

Measurement of the Quality of the Preparation

The presence of small holes in the plasma membrane of the platelets can be assessed in a manner similar to that used with digitonin. Platelets are preincubated in plasma with [^{3}H]-adenine and [^{14}C]-serotonin. The cell suspension is subjected to electrical discharge and aliquots are centrifuged to separate released materials. Substantial release of the [^{3}H]-label should be detected in the absence of release of the [^{14}C]-label. Leakage of lactate dehydrogenase should be minimal since the holes are not sufficiently large to allow this protein to pass. We have used this method to determine the minimum voltage setting required for platelet permeabilization.

In addition, we also assess the functional integrity of the platelet preparation. We have adopted an experiment first performed by Haslam and Davidson [1984a] to establish that the platelets are responsive and that small molecules can enter. Platelets are preincubated with [^{14}C]-serotonin and the cell suspension is prepared as described above. Samples of permeabilized platelets are preincubated with varying Ca^{2+} concentrations for 15 min on ice. Haslam and Davidson [1984b] have shown that this time is required for the Ca^{2+} to fully equilibrate within the cell. Samples at each Ca^{2+} concentration are warmed to 20°C and treated either with buffer, thrombin, or GTP-γ-S. The amount of [^{14}C]-serotonin released into the supernatant is measured for each sample. An example of such an experiment is shown in Figure 12. The features of this experiment that are important to the assessment of the preparation are: 1) At the lowest concentration of Ca^{2+} addition of thrombin should have a minimal effect on secretion. This indicates very few cells remain unpermeabilized, since intact cells would secrete independently of external Ca^{2+} and the receptor for thrombin remains functional. 2) The cells respond to GTP-γ-S, indicating that the cells are indeed permeabilized, since intact cells do not respond to this agent. 3) The maximal response for all three conditions should be similar. Again this indicates that all cells have been permeabilized, since partial permeabilization would give a larger maximal response for thrombin.

Uses for the Electrically Permeabilized Platelets

This preparation has been extremely useful in demonstrating several aspects of platelet stimulus-response coupling. Only a few relevant findings will be mentioned, since the application of electrical permeabilization to platelets and other cells was the topic of an excellent review [Knight and Scrutton, 1986]. Knight and Scrutton [1980] were the first to use electrical permeabilization with

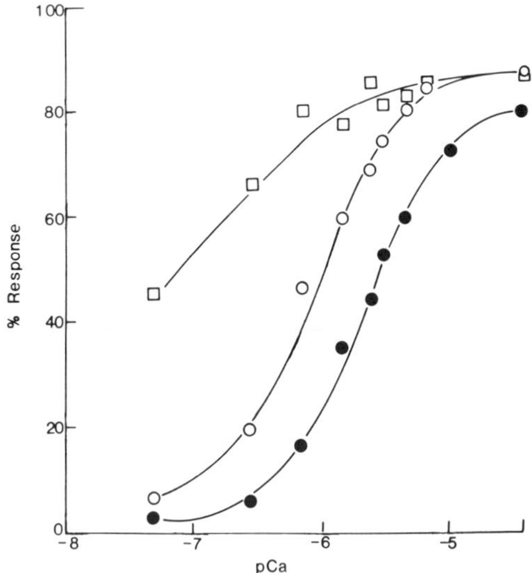

Fig. 12. The effect of thrombin and GTP-γ-S on serotonin secretion in permeabilized platelets. Electrically permeabilized platelets, preloaded with [^{14}C]-serotonin, were prepared in Ca^{2+}-buffers of different free Ca^{2+} concentration. Secretion was monitored after treatment at 2 min at 20°C. Secretion was stopped by addition of 500 μl of platelet suspension to 125 μl of 37 mM EDTA, 75 mM NaCl, and 133 mM formaldehyde. Platelets were either treated with no agonist (control; ●), 2 U/ml of thrombin (○), or 100 μM GTP-γ-S (□).

platelets and provided direct evidence that secretion could be elicited by direct and measurable changes in the Ca^{2+} concentration. The conclusion that the release of granule constituents from permeabilized cells represents a true exocytotic event is based on the observation that large acid hydrolases contained in lysosomes are released to the extracellular space while smaller cytoplasmic proteins are retained within the cell [Knight and Scrutton, 1986]. Knight et al. [1982] made the interesting observation that dense granule secretion has exactly the same Ca^{2+}-dependence as lysosomal secretion. This is in contrast to the situation in the intact cell where higher agonist concentrations are needed to cause lysosomal secretion. The reason for this difference was clarified later by studies that showed thrombin could enhance the Ca^{2+}-sensitivity but not the maximal level of dense granule secretion [Knight et al., 1984]. The effect of thrombin on lysosomal secretion in permeabilized platelets is somewhat different; addition of thrombin does not alter the Ca^{2+}-sensitivity but does increase the amount of secretion obtained at saturating Ca^{2+} concentrations. The effects of thrombin are attributed to agonist-dependent activation of phospholipase C (PLC), since diacylglycerol (DG), a product of PLC, is produced [Knight et al., 1984;

Haslam and Davidson, 1984b]. DG is required for activation of protein kinase C, and protein kinase C-dependent protein phosphorylation is thought to enhance Ca^{2+}-dependent secretion. Substantial DG is produced at 0.1 μM Ca^{2+}, indicating that PLC could be activated at the Ca^{2+} concentration thought to be found in the resting cell. The studies of Haslam and Davidson [1984a] also provided evidence that a guanine-nucleotide binding protein is involved in receptor-dependent stimulation PLC. They showed that DG production is stimulated if GTP or the stable analog GTP-gamma-S is added to permeabilized platelets. At nonsaturating concentrations of GTP, GTP and thrombin act synergistically to produce DG. Finally, electrically permeabilized platelets have been used to study the mechanism by which cyclic AMP inhibits platelet function. Addition of cyclic AMP to a permeabilized platelet preparation has no effect on Ca^{2+}-dependent serotonin secretion in the absence of agonist, but inhibits the enhancement of secretion induced by thrombin [Knight and Scrutton, 1986]. These data suggest that a cyclic AMP-dependent event acts either on phospholipase C or on a step prior to it.

ACKNOWLEDGMENTS

The technical assistance of Marilyn Rigmaiden is appreciated. J.L. Daniel is a recipient of a Research Career Development Award K04 HL00794 from the National Institutes of Health. This work was also supported by N.I.H. grants HL 14127, HL 21128, and BSRG S07 RR05417. This chapter is dedicated to the memory of Mathew J. Daniel, a beloved son.

REFERENCES

Akiyama T, Takayi S, Sankawa U, Inari S, Saito H (1980). Saponin-cholesterol interaction in the multibilayers of egg yolk lecithin as studied by deuterium nuclear magnetic resonance: Digitonin-induced cell damage. Biochemistry 19: 1904–1911.

Akkerman JWN, Ebberink RHM, Lips JPM, Christiaens GML (1980a). Rapid separation of cytosol and particle fraction of human platelets by digitonin-induced cell damage. Br J Haematol 44:291–300.

Akkerman JWN, Niewiarowski S, Holmsen H (1980b). Identification of granular heterogeneity in blood platelets by controlled digitonin-induced cell lysis. Thromb Res 17:249–254.

Allen DG, Blinks JR, Prendergast FG (1977). Aequorin luminescence: Relation of light emission to calcium concentration—a calcium-independent component. Science 196:996–998.

Becker GL, Fiskum G, Lehninger AL (1980). Regulation of free Ca^{2+} by liver mitochondria and endoplasmic reticulum. J Biol Chem 25:9009–9012.

Berridge MJ, Irvine RF (1984). Inositol trisphosphate: A novel second messenger in cellular signal transduction. Nature 312:315–321.

Blinks JR, Wier WG, Hess P, Prendergast FG (1982). Measurement of Ca^{2+} concentration in living cells. Prog Biophys Molec Biol 40:1–114.

Brass LF, Joseph SK (1985). A role for inositol triphosphate in intracellular Ca^{2+} mobilization and granule secretion and platelets. J Biol Chem 260:15172–15179.

Brass LF, Shattil SJ (1982). Changes in surface-bound and exchangeable calcium during platelet activation. J Biol Chem 257:14000–14005.

Caswell AH, Hutchison JD (1971a). Visual of membrane bound by a fluorescent technique. Biochem Biophys Res Commun 42:43–49.

Caswell AH, Hutchison JD (1971b). Selectivity of cation chelation to tetracyclines: Evidence for special conformation of calcium chelate. Biochem Biophys Res Commun 43:625–630.

Cormier MJ (1978). Comparative biochemistry in animal systems. In Herring PJ (ed): "Bioluminescence in Action." London: Academic Press, pp 75–108.

Daniel JL, Purdon AD, Molish IR (1982). Platelet myosin phosphorylation as an indicator of cellular calcium concentration. Fed Proc 41:1118.

Daniel JL, Molish IR, Holmsen H (1980). Myosin phosphorylation in intact platelets. J Biol Chem 256:7510–7514.

DeKruijff B (1974). Polyene-antibiotic sterol interactions in membranes of scholeplasma laidlawwii cells and lecithin liposomes. III. Molecular structure of the polyene antibiotics-cholesterol complexes. Biochim Biophys Acta 339:57–70.

Feinman RD, Detwiler TC (1974). Platelet secretion induced by divalent cation ionophores. Nature 249:172–173.

Feinstein MB (1980). Release of intracellular membrane-bound calcium precedes the onset of stimulus-induced exocytosis in platelets. Biochem Biophys Res Commun 93:593–600.

Feinstein MB, Halenda SP, Zavoico GB (1985). Calcium and platelet function. In Marme D (ed): "Calcium and Cell Physiology." New York: Springer Verlag, pp 345–376.

Grynkiewicz G, Peonie M, Tsien RY (1985). A new generation of Ca^{2+} indicators with greatly improved fluorescence properties. J Biol Chem 260:3440–3450.

Hallam TJ, Daniel JL, Kendrick-Jones J, Rink TJ (1985): Relationship between cytoplasmic free calcium and myosin chain phosphorylation in intact platelets. Biochem J 232:373–377.

Haslam RM, Klyne W (1953). The precipitation of 3- -hydroxysteroids by digitonin. Biochem J 55:340–345.

Haslam RJ, Davidson MML (1984a). Guanine nucleotides decrease the free [Ca^{2+}] required for secretion of serotonin from permeabilized blood platelets. Evidence of a role for a GTP-binding protein in platelet activation. FEBS Lett 174:90–95.

Haslam RJ, Davidson MML (1984b). Potentiation by thrombin of the secretion of serotonin from permeabilized platelets equilibrated with Ca^{2+} buffers. Biochem J 222:351–361.

Johnson PC, Ware JA, Cliveden PB, Smith M, Dvorak AM, Salzman EW (1985a). Measurement of ionized calcium in blood platelets with the photoprotein aequorin. J Biol Chem 260:2069–2076.

Johnson PC, Ware JA, Salzman EW (1985b). Concurrent measurement of platelet ionized calcium and aggregation: Studies with the lumiaggregometer. Thromb Res 40:435–443.

Jy W, Haynes DH (1984). Intracellular calcium storage and release in the human platelet. Chlorotetracycline as a continuous monitor. Circ Res 55:595–608.

Kinsky CL (1970). Antibiotic interaction with model membranes. Annu Rev Pharmacol 10:119–142.

Knight DE (1981). Rendering cells permeable by exposure to electric fields. Tech Cell Physiol P113:1–20.

Knight DE, Niggli V, Scrutton MC (1984). Thrombin and activators of protein kinase C modulate secretory responses of permeabilized human platelets induced by Ca^{2+}. Eur J Biochem 143:437–446.

Knight DE, Hallam TJ, Scrutton MC (1982). Agonist selectivity and second message concentration in Ca^{2+}-mediated secretion. Nature 296:256–257.

Knight DE, Scrutton MC (1980). Direct evidence of a role for Ca^{2+} in amine storage granule secretion by human platelets. Thromb Res 20:437–446.

Knight DE, Scrutton MC (1986). Gaining access to the cytosol: The technique and some applications of electropermeabilization. Biochem J 234:497–506.

LeBreton GC, Dinerstein RJ (1977). Effect of the calcium antagonist TMB-6 on intracellular calcium redistribution associated with platelet shape change. Thromb Res 10:521–523.

LeBreton GC, Dinerstein RJ, Roth LJ, Feinberg H (1976). Direct evidence for intracellular divalent cation redistribution associated with platelet shape change. Biochem Biophys Res Commun 71:362–370.

MacFarlane DE, Mills DCB (1975). The effects of ATP on platelets: Evidence against the central role of released ADP in primary aggregation. Blood 46:309–315.

Martell AE, Smith RM (1974). "Critical Stability Constants," Vol 1. New York: Plenum Press.

Mathew MK, Balaram P (1980). A reinvestigation of chlortetracycline fluorescence: Effect of pH, metal ions and environment. J Inorg Chem 13:339–346.

Millman MS, Caswell AH, Haynes DH (1980). Kinetics of chlortetracycline permeation in fragmented ATPase rich sarcoplasmic reticulum. Membr Biochem 3:291–226.

Monneron A, d'Alayer J (1978). Isolation of plasma membrane and nuclear membranes of thymocytes. J Cell Biol 77:232–245.

Morgan JP, Morgan KG (1982). Vascular smooth muscle: The first recorded transients. Pflugers Archiv 395:75–77.

Murphy E, Coll K, Rich TL, Williamson J (1980). Hormonal effects on calcium homeostasis in isolated hepatocytes. J Biol Chem 255:6600–6608.

Perrin DD, Sayce IG (1967). Computer calculation of equilibrium concentrations in mixtures of metal ions and comlexing species. Talanta 14:833–842.

Prendergast FG, Mann KG (1978). Chemical properties of aequorin and the green fluorescent protein isolated from Aequorea forskalea. Biochemistry 17:3448–3453.

Purdon AD, Hsia JD, Pinteric L, Tinker DO (1975). Lysolecithin-Cholesterol interaction. A spin resonance and electron-micrographic study. Can J Biochem 53:196–206.

Purdon AD, Tinker DO, Neumann AW (1980). The temperature dependence of surface tension and critical micelle concentration of egg lysolecithin. Colloid Sci (Kolloide) 258:1062–1069.

Purdon AD, Daniel JL, Stewart GJ, Holmsen H (1984). Cytoplasmic free calcium in porcine platelets. Biochim Biophys Acta 800:178–187.

Rand RP, Pangborn WA, Purdon AD, Tinker DO (1975). Lysolecithin and cholesterol interact stiochiometrically forming bimolecular lamellar structures in the presence of excess water, or lysolecithin or cholesterol. Can J Biochem 53:189–195.

Rink TJ, Smith SW, Tsien RY (1982). Cytoplasmic free Ca^{2+} in human platelets: Ca^{2+} thresholds and Ca-independent activation for shape change and secretion. FEBS Lett 148:21–26.

Rink TJ, Pozzan T (1985). Using quin2 in cell suspensions. Cell Calcium 6:133–144.

Ronning SA, Heatley GA, Martin TFJ (1982). Thyrotropin-releasing hormone mobilizes Ca^{2+} from endoplasmic reticulum and mitochrondria of GH_3 pituitary cells: Characterization of cellular Ca^{2+} pools by a method based on digitonin permeabilization. Proc Natl Acad Sci 79:6294–6298.

Shimomura O, Johnson FH (1975). Regeneration of the photoprotein aequorin. Nature 256:236–238.

Thompson NT, Scrutton MC (1985) Intracellular calcium fluxes in human platelets. Eur J Biochem 147:421–427.

Tsien RY (1980). New calcium indicators and buffers with high selectivity against magnesium and protons: Design, synthesis, and properties of prototype structures. Biochemistry 19:2396–2404.

Tsien RY, Rink TJ, Poenie M (1985). Measurement of cytosolic free Ca^{2+} in individual cells using fluorescence microscopy with dual excitation wavelengths. Cell Calcium 6:145–157.

Ware JA, Johnson PC, Smith M, Salzman EW (1985). Aequorin detects increased cytoplasmic calcium in platelets stimulated with phorbol ester or diacylglycerol. Biochem Biophys Res Commun 133:98–104.

Ware JA, Johnson PC, Smith M, Salzman EW (1986). Effect of common agonists on cytoplasmic ionized calcium concentration in platelets. J Clin Invest 77:878–886.

White JG, Krivitt W (1967). An ultrastructural basis for the shape changes induced in platelets by chilling. Blood 30:625–635.

Wiley JS, Quinn MA, Connellan JM (1983). Estimation of platelet size by measurement of intracellular water space using an oil technique. Thromb Res 31:261–268.

Wolf HU (1973). Divalent metal ion buffers with low pH-sensitivity. Experientia 29:241–249.

Zucker MB, Nachmias VT (1985): Platelet activation. Arteriosclerosis 5:2–18.

Zuurendonk PF, Tager JM (1974). Rapid separation of particulate components and soluble cytoplasm of isolated rat-liver cells. Biochem Biophys Acta 333:393–399.

Modern Methods in Pharmacology, Volume 4
Methods for Studying Platelets and Megakaryocytes, pages 217–227

Methods of Studying Platelet Arachidonate Metabolism

J. BRYAN SMITH

INTRODUCTION

Arachidonic acid is by far the most commonly occurring precursor of the prostaglandins, leukotrienes, and thromboxanes. In 1974, it was found that PGG_2 and PGH_2, the prostaglandin endoperoxides derived from arachidonic acid, are potent inducers of platelet aggregation [Hamberg et al., 1974]. This discovery, combined with the knowledge that aspirin inhibits prostaglandin synthesis as well as platelet aggregation induced by certain agents, stimulated an enormous interest in studying arachidonic acid metabolism in blood platelets. Further studies on the role of prostaglandin endoperoxides in platelet aggregation indicated that the aggregating factor formed by washed platelets after addition of arachidonic acid was not PGG_2 or PGH_2 because of the extreme lability and greater potency of this factor. This led to the detection of thromboxane A_2 (TxA_2), which is highly unstable in aqueous solution (half life 32 sec at 37°C) and hydrolyses to the stable, but biologically inactive, TxB_2 [Hamberg et al., 1975].

The arachidonic acid used for prostaglandin endoperoxide and thromboxane formation after stimulation of platelets with collagen or thrombin must be made available by release from platelet membranes by the action of one or more phospholipases. Most studies of the mechanisms involved in the release of arachidonic acid have used thrombin as the stimulus, although there have been studies using collagen, trypsin, and the divalent cation ionophore A23187. Bills et al. [1976] presented evidence that most of the arachidonic acid is released by a selective action of phospholipase A_2 on the 2-position of 1-acyl-2-arachidonoyl-phosphatidylcholine. On the other hand, Bell et al. [1979] have presented evidence that arachidonic acid is released by the sequential action of 1) a phospholipase C on phosphatidylinositol producing 1-stearoyl-2-arachidonoyl-diacylglycerol, and 2) a diacylglycerol lipase. The relative importance of the two phospholipases in releasing arachidonic acid is still a matter of some dispute.

From the Department of Pharmacology, Temple University School of Medicine, Philadelphia, Pennsylvania 19140.

Clearly, as evidenced by the differing conclusions in the literature as to the phospholipid source of arachidonate release in thrombin-stimulated platelets, the study of arachidonate metabolism in platelets is not an easy matter. Besides being the source of arachidonic acid, phospholipids that are rich in arachidonic acid may change as a result of stimulation without releasing arachidonic acid but with the formation of other secondary messengers, such as diacylglycerol and inositoltriphosphate. A description of our laboratory's overall methods for the study of arachidonate metabolism in platelets follows.

USE OF PLATELETS PRELABELED WITH [^{3}H]ARACHIDONIC ACID

Prelabeling of platelets with [^{3}H]arachidonic acid, or in some cases [^{14}C]arachidonic acid, prior to performing functional studies has become by far the most popular way of studying platelet arachidonate metabolism. The method allows the investigator to follow which phospholipids release arachidonic acid or otherwise change upon platelet stimulation as well as which transformation products of arachidonic acid are produced. The method works well when platelets are stimulated with strong agonists such as thrombin or collagen but is not suitable for measurement of the release of the small amounts of arachidonic acid induced by weak agonists such as epinephrine or ADP.

Method of Prelabeling the Platelets

Either [^{3}H]arachidonic acid or [^{14}C]arachidonic acid may be used to label the platelets. Most investigators prefer [^{3}H]arachidonic acid as it has a higher specific activity and permits more radioactivity to be incorporated into the cells. Investigators should be aware, however, that tritium is very easily quenched and should ensure that any changes observed are not due to changes in quenching. Another point of caution is that if platelets are incubated with arachidonic acid in the absence of plasma or albumin, they will rapidly oxygenate it rather than incorporate it into phospholipids.

The method we use to prepare prelabeled platelets is as follows: Human blood is obtained from healthy volunteers who have not taken any drug in the previous week. The blood is anticoagulated with citric acid, citrate, dextrose [Aster and Jandl, 1964]. The platelet-rich plasma obtained by centrifugation at 180g for 20 min at room temperature is acidified to pH 6.5 with the anticoagulant mixture and recentrifuged at 1,500g for 15 min at room temperature. The platelet pellet is resuspended in 0.1 volume of autologous plasma and incubated with [^{3}H]arachidonic acid (1 μCi, available from Amersham or New England Nuclear) for 1 hour at 37°C before gel-filtration. Gel-filtration is performed on a column of Sepharose 2B [Lages et al., 1975] using calcium-free Tyrode's buffer (calcium is added after gel-filtration if desired) containing 0.2% fatty acid free bovine serum albumin and 5 mM glucose. The major advantage of this method is that there is a much greater uptake of the radiolabel by the concentrated platelet suspensions as compared to when incubations are performed directly in platelet-rich plasma.

Methods of Lipid Extraction

At the end of the incubations with thrombin or collagen, lipids are extracted by adding sodium EDTA (pH 7.4, 20 mM final concentration) and 3.75 volumes of ice-cold chloroform/methanol: 1/2 by volume plus 1 drop of formic acid (90% w/v). After leaving the samples for 30 min to ensure complete solubilization, they are partitioned into two phases by addition of 1.25 volumes of chloroform and 1.25 volumes of 2 M potassium chloride. The lower phase containing the lipids is removed and the upper phase reextracted with 2.5 volumes of chloroform. The pooled lipid extracts are evaporated to dryness under N_2 at 37°C and stored in chloroform/methanol: 1/2 at −18°C prior to chromatography. All of the organic solvents should contain butylated-hydroxytoluene (50 μg/ml) as an antioxidant. Recovery of label from arachidonic acid prelabeled platelets is better than 90% by this method.

We have found that the most effective method for the extraction of the highly acidic phospholipids, phosphatidylinositol-4-phosphate (PIP), and phosphatidylinositol-4,5-bisphosphate (PIP_2) from platelets is as follows: to 1 volume of platelet suspension is added 3.75 volume of ice-cold chloroform/methanol (1:2 v/v) and EDTA (20 mM final conc.). After thorough mixing, the extract is partitioned into two phases by addition of 1.25 volume of chloroform and 1.25 volume of 2.4 M HCl. The lower phase is removed and the aqueous phase is reextracted with 2.5 volume of chloroform/methanol (2:1 v/v) at −18°C. Again, all solvents contain butylated hydroxytoluene (50 μg/ml) as an antioxidant. Recoveries of PIP and PIP_2 are better than 70% by this method.

Methods of Thin Layer Chromatography

Radioactive phospholipids, phosphatidic acid, and arachidonic acid and its oxygenation products can be resolved by thin layer chromatography on silica gel plates (Merck, Darmstadt, W. Germany; activated for 1 hour at 110°C) using the upper phase of the solvent system: ethyl acetate/ iso-octane/acetic acid/water: 90/50/20/100 by volume [Hong and Levine, 1976], and localized either by means of iodine vapor or by spraying with a solution containing 1% primulin dye in alcohol and exposing to UV light. In order for the primulin dye to stain, it is necessary to first expose the thin layer plates to ammonia vapor for 10 min to neutralize the acid contained in the solvents. Appropriate zones containing (in order of increasing mobility) total phospholipids, phosphatidic acid, thromboxane B_2 (TxB_2), HHT, 12-HETE, and arachidonic acid are scraped from the plates into counting vials and the radioactivity determined.

For the resolution of the phospholipids (phosphatidylcholine, phosphatidylethanolamine, and phosphatidylinositol) that contain arachidonic acid, the solvent system chloroform/methanol/acetic acid/water: 81/10/45/1 by volume is used [Hausser and Eichberg, 1975]. Again the phospholipids can be localized by means of iodine vapor or by using primulin dye. They are scraped from the plates and transferred directly to counting vials containing 1 ml methanol. After allowing 30 min to elute the phospholipid, scintillation cocktail is added and the radioactivity is determined by liquid scintillation counting.

Separation of individual phosphoinositides and other components of the PI cycle can be achieved by thin layer chromatography (TLC) on 0.25 mm silica gel plates (Merck, Darmstadt, W. Germany) using the following solvent systems: 1) chloroform/methanol/4 M ammonia (9:7:2, by volume) for the resolution of PIP and PIP_2 [Lloyd et al., 1973], and 2) chloroform/methanol/conc. HCl (87:13:0.5, by volume) for the resolution of DG. Again all of these compounds can be visualized under ultraviolet (UV) light after exposure to primulin dye and their radioactivity determined as previously described.

The total amount of any of the above phospholipids can be determined by analysis of phosphate content. The silica gel scrapings are digested with boiling perchloric acid, and, after neutralization with potassium hydroxide, inorganic phosphorus is measured by the sensitive malachite green method [Hess and Derr, 1975].

It is advisable to chromatograph known standards on the same plate as is being used to resolve the platelet extracts. Sources for these standards include Sigma Chemical, St. Louis, MO; Serdary, London, Ontario, Canada; Avanti Polar Lipids, Birmingham, AL; Upjohn Diagnostics, Kalamazoo, MI; Cayman Chemical Co., 2280 Peters Road, Ann Arbor, MI; and Biomol Research Labs. Inc., P.O. Box 13247, Philadelphia, PA.

MEASUREMENT OF LIBERATED FREE FATTY ACIDS

Generally in our laboratory quantitative measurements of decreases in phospholipids and increases in arachidonic acid and other free fatty acids are obtained by gas liquid chromatographic (GLC) analysis of fatty acid methyl esters. As far as the phospholipids are concerned, this method is about five times more sensitive than the malachite green method of phosphorus analysis (i.e., we can detect about 40 pmole of fatty acid methyl ester in platelet extracts by this method), and, besides, it gives the fatty acid composition of the phospholipid being analyzed. As far as the free fatty acids are concerned, we prefer to isolate non-radioactive free fatty acids by first developing the thin layer plates for 10 cm in the solvent system isopropyl ether/acetic acid (96:4) and then, after solvent evaporation, redeveloping the plates for 18 cm in petroleum ether/ethyl ether/acetic acid (90:5:0.1, by volume). Care should be taken to minimize the time that the thin layer plates are out of the solvent as oxidation of arachidonic acid (and other polyunsaturated fatty acids) will take place. After development, the acid contained in the solvents is neutralized by exposure to ammonia vapor for 10 min and the resolved free fatty acids are detected by their fluorescence after using a spray containing primulin dye. The phospholipid and free fatty acid zones are scraped from the TLC plate and the scrapings are heated for 10 min at 80°C with boron trifluoride in methanol (a fresh ampoule is used for each experiment, as this reagent is unstable). Heptadecanoic acid (5 μg) is added to the silica gel scrapings to act as an internal standard for the GLC After methylation, the fatty acid methyl esters are extracted into hexane, the hexane is removed under N_2, and the esters are redissolved in 50 μl carbon disulfide.

GLC analysis is presently being performed in our laboratory using a Hewlett-Packard chromatograph model 5730A fitted with two glass columns containing 10% SP-2330 on 100/200 Chromosor W AW (Supelco, Bellafonte, PA). The chromatograph is operated in a differential mode with a temperature gradient as follows: 2 min at 170°C, increasing at 4°C/min to 220°C and holding for 8 min. Injection and flame ionization ports are held at 250°C. The carrier gas is N_2 (20 ml/min). Quantification of the different fatty acid methyl esters is performed with an automatic integrator (Hewlett-Packard model 3390A) with references to the internal standard.

As arachidonic acid is rapidly oxygenated in platelets by the cyclooxygenase and lipoxygenase enzymes (Figs. 1 and 2) little or no free arachidonic acid will normally be detected after stimulation of platelets with agonists such as thrombin or collagen. Indeed any increase that is detected probably reflects released arachidonic acid that has become bound by extracellular albumin. To obtain an estimate of the total arachidonic acid that is released from platelet phospholipids it is necessary to prevent its oxygenation using inhibitors such as propylgallate (200 μM) or BW 755C (100 μM). (Another inhibitor is eicosatetraynoic acid (ETYA). However, the fact that this compound rapidly becomes oxidized complicates its use.) Platelet suspensions are treated with these compounds for 1 min prior to the addition of the agonist, and then incubations are continued for 5 min after agonist addition. The free fatty acids are then extracted, purified by thin layer chromatography, methylated, and quantitated as described above. Using

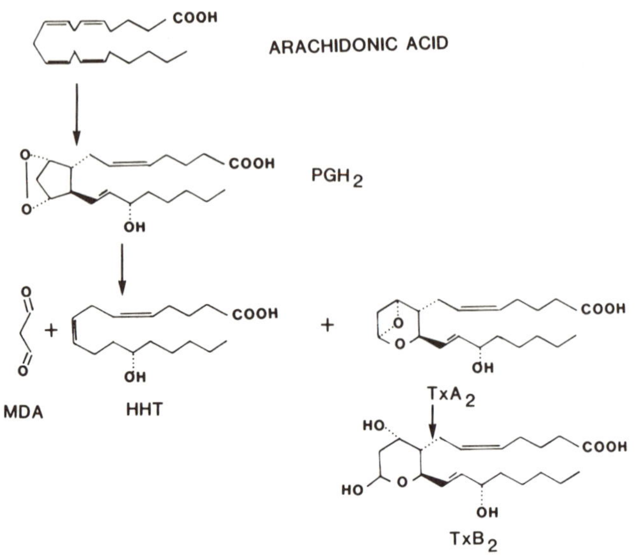

ARACHIDONIC ACID

PGH_2

MDA HHT TxA_2 TxB_2

Fig. 1. Conversion of arachidonic acid via prostaglandin H_2 into malondialdehyde (MDA), 12-hydroxy-5-cis,8-trans,10-trans-heptadecatrienoic acid (HHT), and thromboxane A_2 (TxA_2). The thromboxane A_2 spontaneously hydrolyzes in water into thromboxane B_2 (TxB_2).

this technique we recently demonstrated that human platelets release greater than 20 nmoles/10^9 platelets of arachidonic acid and lesser amounts (2–7 nmole/10^9 platelets) of other fatty acids when stimulated with 5 u/ml thrombin [Smith et al., 1985].

MEASUREMENT OF MALONDIALDEHYDE

As mentioned above, the use of platelets prelabeled with [^{3}H]arachidonic acid is not sensitive or accurate enough to study arachidonate metabolism when platelets are stimulated by weak agonists such as ADP or epinephrine. This is because less than 1% of the arachidonate is liberated from the platelet phospholipids in response to these agonists. Nevertheless, endogenous arachidonic acid is metabolized after addition of these agents and the prostaglandin endoperoxides and thromboxane A_2 so produced are thought to be responsible for the second wave of platelet aggregation observed in stirred, citrated, platelet-rich plasma. A simple and inexpensive method for following arachidonate metabolism after addition of either weak or strong agonists to platelets involves the measurement of malondialdehyde, which is formed in approximately equal amounts with TxB_2

and 12-hydroxy-5,8,10-heptadecatrienoic acid (HHT) by the action of thromboxane synthetase on prostaglandin endoperoxides (Fig. 1).

Malondialdehyde is measured by the thiobarbituric acid reaction. Platelet-rich plasma or platelet suspensions are incubated at 37°C with the agonist under study and then an equal volume of 20% trichloroacetic acid in 1N HCl is added. The precipitate is removed by centrifugation and the supernatant is incubated at 70°C with 0.2 volumes of thiobarbituric acid reagent (0.12 M thiobarbituric acid in 0.26 M Tris-HCl, pH 7.0) for 30 min. The intensity of the pink color that is produced is determined at 532 meters and is directly proportional to the amount of malondialdehyde [Smith et al., 1976].

Three major problems have been encountered in the thiobarbituric acid assay of malondialdehyde. First, while the method readily permits the determination of malondialdehyde formation with agonists such as thrombin, the sensitivity of the assay is at its limits when using agonists such as ADP or epinephrine. Second, while the majority of malondialdehyde that is produced by platelets is derived from prostaglandin endoperoxides, some may be produced from lipoxygenase metabolites of arachidonic acid or from other fatty acids by nonspecific lipid peroxidation. Third, turbidity tends to develop during the incubation with thiobarbituric acid, which interferes with the accuracy of the determinations.

Macfarlane et al. [1977] have developed a method for increasing the sensitivity of the thiobarbituric assay for malondialdehyde. In brief, the pink pigment, produced as described above, is trapped on a small column containing DEAE cellulose. The column is washed with water and 0.2 ml 6 N KOH, and then the pink pigment is eluted with 0.5 ml 6 N KOH. Elution of the color with KOH results in a shift of the peak absorption from 532 to 548 nm, and also makes the color fade on standing, so that readings should be taken with 5 min of elution. Using this method, these authors showed that platelets synthesize malondialdehyde when stimulated by collagen or thrombin and also during the second phase of aggregation induced by ADP or epinephrine.

Nonenzymatic formation of malondialdehyde becomes more of a problem when washed platelet suspensions are being studied, when arachidonic acid is used as the aggregating agent, and when prolonged incubation times (greater than 5 min) are employed. A major factor appears to be the breakdown of peroxidized fatty acids that occurs during the incubation of the acidified platelet extract with thiobarbituric acid at 70°C. Panse et al. [1985] have overcome this problem by including the reducing agent stannous chloride (5% final concentration) instead of HCl in the 20% trichloroacetic acid used to terminate the incubations. This agent reduces peroxides to hydroxides but does not interfere with the assay of preformed malondialdehyde. Turbidity present after incubation of the extracts with thiobarbiturate at 70°C is removed by adding an equal volume of 10% HCl saturated with NaCl followed by centrifugation. Using this assay these authors demonstrated that there was almost a 1:1 correlation between the amounts of thromboxane B_2 and malondialdehyde formed by arachidonic acid-stimulated washed human platelets.

MEASUREMENT OF THROMBOXANE B_2

While the formation of thromboxane B_2 by platelets can be measured by physiochemical methods such as gas chromatography with electron capture detection [Panse et al., 1985], by far the simplest and most rapid method for the measurement of thromboxane B_2 is radioimmunoassay. A detailed discussion of the principles and pitfalls of radioimmunoassay of prostaglandins and thromboxanes is presented elsewhere [Granstrom and Kindahl, 1978] and should be consulted by anyone intending to commence such determinations. Radioimmunoassay is a sensitive technique and sufficient amounts of thromboxane B_2 are made by platelets activated with either strong or weak agonists (second wave) that extraction and concentration of samples prior to radioimmunoassay is not necessary. Furthermore, virtually all of the thromboxane B_2 produced by platelets is released from them. Thus, a sample of the supernatant fluid obtained after activated platelets have been precipitated by centrifugation can simply be added to the radioimmunoassay incubation.

A common mistake made in radioimmunoassay is not to dilute the sample sufficiently to place its competition with tracer on the standard curve. For example, it is impossible to compare a value of >50 pmol/ml (i.e., off the standard curve) with other values of, for example, 1, 3.5, and 7 pmole/ml. The first sample should have been diluted and reassayed.

A useful method for the assay of thromboxane B_2 formed during clotting has been presented by Patrono et al. [1980]. For the investigator interested only in determining the formation of thromboxane B_2 in a few samples, radioimmunoassay kits are available from New England Nuclear or Amersham. However, the investigator interested in performing numerous determinations can save a considerable amount of money by buying commercially available antibodies (e.g., from Seragen), [^{3}H]-thromboxane B_2 (e.g., from New England Nuclear), and standard thromboxane B_2 (e.g., from Upjohn Diagnostics) and developing his own radioimmunoassay.

MEASUREMENT OF LIPOXYGENASE PRODUCTS

Arachidonate released from platelet phospholipids is preferentially utilized by cyclooxygenase [Sautebin et al., 1983] to produce malondialdehyde, HHT, and

TxB_2, as shown in Figure 1. However, platelets also oxygenate arachidonic acid by a lipoxygenase pathway to 12-hydroperoxy-5,8,10,14-eicosatetraenoic acid (12-HPTE), which is reduced to the corresponding 12-hydroxy acid (12-HETE) by a peroxidase (Fig. 2). The simplest way of studying the lipoxygenase pathway in platelets is to use radiolabeled arachidonic acid as discussed above. The radiolabeled 12-HETE generally migrates between HHT and arachidonic acid on thin layer chromatography.

The only satisfactory way presently available to measure the mass of 12-HETE is by gas chromatography-mass spectrometry. Briefly, a total lipid extract is prepared and a crude fractionation is performed using a column of 0.5 g of silicic acid. Free fatty acids are eluted with 15 ml of hexane:diethyl ether (85:15, v/v) and discarded, and 12-HETE together with HHT are recovered using 15 ml chloroform. This fraction is esterified and a sample is injected into a gas chromatograph-mass spectrometer. The 12-HETE has a retention time of 3 min 40 sec on a 1 m × 3 mm glass silanized column packed with 1% SE-30 on Gaschrom Q, with the oven, molecular separator, and ion source at 260°C, 300°C, and 290°C, respectively, and a helium flow rate of 15 ml/min. The mass spectrometer is focused on ion at m/e 295 and 297 for the detection of the unlabeled and ^{14}C-labeled species of 12-HETE, respectively [Sautebin et al., 1983].

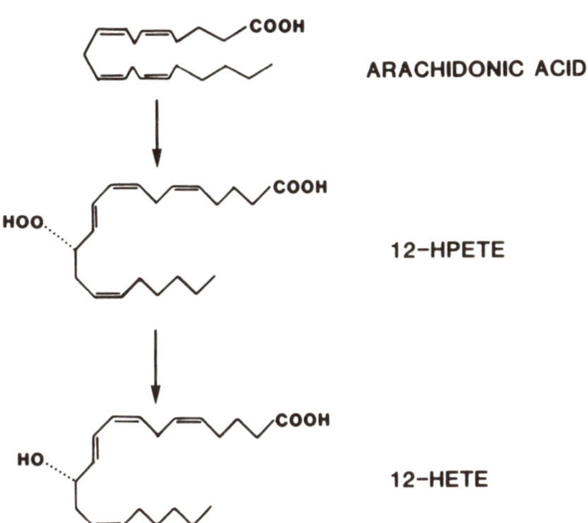

Fig. 2. Conversion of arachidonic acid via intermediary 12L-hydroperoxy-5,8,10,14-eicosatetraenoic acid (12-HPETE) into 12-hydroxy-eicosatetraenoic acid (12-HETE).

CONCLUDING REMARKS

Platelets are rich in arachidonic acid, which is almost entirely present esterified in phospholipids in unstimulated cells. Following stimulation of platelets with an agonist there is metabolism of arachidonate-enriched lipids, particularly phospho- and polyphosphoinositols giving rise to inositoltriphosphate and diacylglycerol, which act as second messengers to bring about platelet aggregation and secretion. It appears that most, if not all, platelet agonists induce phosphatidylinositol turnover, but, on the other hand, only strong agonists such as collagen and thrombin are able to induce substantial arachidonic acid release and thromboxane formation. This, as well as other evidence, indicates that activation of phospholipase A_2 is necessary for the release of considerable amounts of arachidonic acid from phosphatidylcholine and phosphatidylethanolamine in platelets. The mechanism by which agonists activate phospholipase C to cause phosphodiesteric cleavage of phosphatidylinositol-4,5-bisphosphate is unknown, although it has been speculated that it is induced by means of a coupling protein linked to the receptors. Likewise, the mechanism by which strong agonists activate phospholipase A_2 is still unknown. As inositoltriphosphate is known to release intracellular calcium ions and phospholipase A_2 is known to be a calcium-requiring enzyme, it seems plausible that activation of phospholipase A_2 is dependent on activation of phospholipase C. The elucidation of the pathways regulating the metabolism of arachidonate-enriched platelet phospholipids is an important challenge for the future.

REFERENCES

Aster RH, Jandl JH (1964). Platelet sequestration in man. I. Methods. J Clin Invest 43:843–855.

Bell RL, Kennerly DA, Stanford N, Majerus PW (1979). Diglyceride lipase—pathway for arachidonic acid release from human platelets. Proc Natl Acad Sci USA 76:3238–3241.

Bills TK, Smith JB, Silver MJ (1976). Metaboism of [^{14}C]arachidonic acid by human platelets. Biochim Biophys Acta 424:303–314.

Granstrom E, Kindahl H (1978). Radioimmunoassay of prostaglandins and thromboxanes. In Frolich JC (ed). "Advances in Prostaglandin and Thromboxane Research." New York: Raven Press, Vol 5, pp 119–212.

Hamberg M, Svensson J, Wakabayshi T, Samuelsson B (1974). Isolation and structure of two prostaglandin endoperoxides that cause platelet aggregation. Proc Natl Acad Sci USA 71:345–349.

Hamberg M, Svensson J, Samuelsson B (1975). Thromboxanes—a new group of biologically active compounds derived from prostaglandin endoperoxides. Proc Natl Acad Sci USA 72:2994–2998.

Hauser G, Eichberg J (1975). Identification of cytidine diphosphate diglyceride in the pineal gland of the rat and its accumulation in the presence of DL-propranolol. J Biol Chem 250:105–112.

Hess HH, Derr JE (1975). Assay of inorganic and organic phosphorus in the 0.1–5 nanomole range. Anal Biochem 63:607–613.

Hong SL, Levine L (1976). Inhibition of arachidonic acid release from cells as the biochemical action of anti-inflammatory corticosteroids. Proc Natl Acad Sci USA 73:1730–1734.

Lages B, Scrutton MC, Holmsen H (1975). Studies on gel filtered human platelets. Isolation and characterization in a medium containing no added Ca^{2+}, Mg^{2+}, or K^{+}. J Lab Clin Med 85:811–825.

Lloyd JV, Nishizawa EE, Joist JH, Mustard JF (1973). Effect of ADP-induced aggregation on $^{32}PO_4$ incorporation into phosphatidic acid and the phosphoinositides of rabbit platelets. Br J Haematol 24:589–604.

Macfarlane DE, Gardner S, Lipson C, Mills DCB (1977). Malondialdehyde production by platelets during secondary aggregation. Thromb Haemost 38:1002–1009.

Panse H, Block H-U, Forster W, Mest H-J (1985). An improved malondialdehyde assay for estimation of thromboxane synthase activity in washed human blood platelets. Prostaglandins 30:1031–1040.

Patrono C, Ciabattoni G, Pinca E, Pughese F, Castrucci G, de Salvo A, Satte MA, Peskar BA (1980). Low dose aspirin and inhibition of thromboxane B_2 production in healthy subjects. Thromb Res 17:317–327.

Sautebin L, Caruso D, Galli G, Paoletti R (1983). Preferential utilization of endogenous arachidonate by cyclooxygenase in incubations of human platelets. FEBS Lett 157:173–178.

Smith JB, Dangelmaier C, Mauco G (1985). Measurement of arachidonic acid liberation in thrombin-stimulated human platelets. Use of agents that inhibit both cyclooxygenase and lipoxygenase enzymes. Biochim Biophys Acta 835:344–351.

Smith JB, Ingerman CM, Silver MJ (1976). Malondialdehyde formation as an indicator of prostaglandin production by human platelets. J Lab Clin Med 88:167–172.

Modern Methods in Pharmacology, Volume 4
Methods for Studying Platelets and Megakaryocytes, pages 229–265

Phospholipid Metabolism in Platelets

A. DAVID PURDON

INTRODUCTION

Platelets are crucial for hemostasis. The release of arachidonic acid and its conversion to thromboxane A_2 [Hamberg et al., 1975] are important in this regard. Arachidonate is also converted to the lipoxygenase product, 12 HPETE [Aharony et al., 1982]. Platelets are known to contain substantial amounts of both diacyl and ether phospholipid [Mueller et al., 1983] and one subclass, 1-O-alkyl-2-acyl GPC, gains importance as a source of platelet-activating factor. The platelet lacks a nucleus, further simplifying the understanding of its response to agonists, as rapid biosynthesis of enzymes involved in a given response can usually be excluded. Platelets are derived from the much larger megakaryocyte, and the resulting membrane proliferation and demarcation of this larger cell may result in a unique disposition of the phospholipid biosynthetic enzymes/membranes compared to other cells. In addition, to a large degree, the phospholipid and esterified arachidonic acid content of platelet is determined by the biosynthetic capacity of megakaryocytes [Schick et al., 1984].

DE NOVO BIOSYNTHESIS

Preparation of Platelets From Blood

Blood is obtained by venipuncture from healthy human volunteers, free from drug use for at least one week. The blood is collected in ACD (2.5 g of trisodium

Abbreviations: PC, phosphatidylcholine; PE, phosphatidylethanolamine; PI phosphatidylinositol; PS, phosphatidylserine; PIP, phosphatidylinositol-4-phosphate; PIP_2, phosphatidylinositol- 4,5-diphosphate; IP_3, inositol- 1,4,5-triphosphate; TLC, thin layer chromatography; HPLC, high pressure liquid chromatography.

In this review PC, PE, and PI refer to 1-radyl-2-acyl PC, PE, and PI, respectively.

From the Department of Pharmacology and the Thrombosis Research Center, Temple University School of Medicine, Philadelphia, Pennsylvania 19140.

citrate, 1.5 g of citric acid, 2.0 g of glucose/100 ml of H_2O) solution. Following gentle mixing, the blood is centrifuged at 22°C, 180 × g for 15 min and the upper layer of platelet-rich plasma (PRP, which is at pH 6.5) removed. The cells are pelleted by centrifugation of the PRP at 800 × g at 22°C for 15 min. The cells may be resuspended in a number of buffer systems (Tris should be avoided) [Packham et al., 1984] and further "washed" by a number of procedures and finally resuspended in the desired buffer. In general when "washing" platelets, the centrifugation step will result in aggregation in the pellet of cells unless the buffer is pH 6.5 (22°C), 5 mM EDTA (4°C), or contains PGI_2 (22°C). We have found when labeling with carrier-free ^{32}P, [5,6,8,9,11,12,14,15-^3H]-arachidonate, or other radiolabels used to study phospholipid metabolism, that a considerable saving in radiolabel and a more rapid approach to steady state incorporation is achieved by resuspending the pelleted cells in 1/10 volume of the platelet-free plasma with added radiolabel [Purdon and Smith, 1985]. Incorporation can proceed for the required time at 37°C and then the cells are separated from both plasma and radiolabel by gel-filtration [Purdon and Smith, 1985] or washing as mentioned above.

Albumin

Albumin is known to bind a number of amphipathic molecules such as free fatty acids, lysolecithin, and drugs to at least six binding sites [Spector, 1975; Kraigh-Hansen, 1982; Peter, 1970; Ando et al., 1980] with two in particular having a high affinity for fatty acids [Berde et al., 1979]. The normal molar ratio of free fatty acid to albumin in the blood is approximately 0.5 to 2.0 and only the binding of a few weakly bound drugs are thought to be affected at this amount of free fatty acid [Spector and Santos, 1973]. Arachidonate in excess of this ratio becomes effective in stimulating platelets [Dratewka-Kos et al., 1985]. Lipoproteins have also been implicated as carriers of longer-chained fatty acids [Shafrir et al., 1965].

Albumin is a necessary component of buffers used for platelet incubation. It should be noted that the plasma concentration of albumin is approximately 40 g/liter (4%), while in buffers the concentration is in the range of 0.1% to 0.25% (i.e., the order of 1–4 × 10^{-5} M). Absence of albumin is associated with leakage of ADP/ATP presumably because of weakening of the plasma membrane [Tangen et al., 1973]. It aids in the radiolabeling of the cells with fatty acids [Purdon and Smith, 1985], and 1-radyl-2-lyso phosphatidylcholine by facilitating dissolution of these relatively insoluble amphipathic molecules. An equilibrium is set up among albumin, the compound being studied, and the cellular binding site of the molecule. The concentration of free amphipathic ligand is considerably lower than that expected from simple dissolution; for example, the K_a for oleate with albumin is $1.1 \times 10^8\ M^{-1}$ [Goodman, 1958]. The equilibrium set up between the amphipath bound to albumin and its particular cellular binding site(s) is stereospecific. In the absence of albumin or other suitable solubilizing agent, one would expect rapid inclusion of an amphipath in the lipid phase of the cell and stereospecific binding required for enzymic reactions would not have enough time to reach equilibrium.

Given its known binding of amphipaths, albumin can act as a sink for molecules made by the cell. Binding of Paf-acether and arachidonic acid outside the cell, prevents conversion of these molecules to lyso Paf-acether [Ludwig et al., 1985] and TxA_2, respectively, inside the cell. Finally it should be noted that prostaglandin H_2 and thromboxane A_2 react very rapidly with albumin to form covalent derivatives [MacLouf et al., 1980; Fitzpatrick, 1977]. Albumin also catalyzes the isomerization of prostaglandin H_2 to D_2 [Hamberg and Fredholm, 1976].

Fatty Acid Uptake, Incorporation, and Biosynthesis

Fatty acid is rapidly transported across the platelet plasma membrane by an energy-independent mechanism [Spector et al., 1970]. In the resting cell the level of saturates is higher than the unsaturate fatty acid [Spector et al., 1970; Norday et al., 1973; Spector and Santos, 1973; Spector, 1975]. In the cytoplasm of liver cells, fatty acids are bound to a fatty acid binding protein [Glatz and Veerkamp, 1985; Ocker et al., 1982]; however, no such protein has been reported for platelets. Fatty acids are only incorporated into lipid as esters of Coenzyme A (CoA) [Brecher, 1983]. The rate of incorporation of arachidonic acid into phospholipid is much greater than for the other fatty acids, probably due to a specific arachidonoyl-CoA synthetase [Wilson et al., 1982; Neufeld et al., 1983]. A rate of formation of 2.9 nanomole arachidonoyl-CoA/min/10^9 cells was reported. Palmitoyl-CoA synthetase, which also accepts other fatty acids, has also been found in platelets [Vallset and Farstad, 1979, 1980]. In addition, palmitoyl-CoA hydrolase [Vallset and Farstad, 1980; Berge et al., 1980] and carnitine palmitoyl transferase [Vallset and Farstad, 1979] have also been described. Acyl CoA is also oxidized to CO_2 by platelets [Spector et al., 1970; Snyder and Godfrey, 1961].

Human platelets are known to have the acetyl-CoA carboxylase and fatty acid synthetase necessary for the de novo biosynthesis of palmitic acid [Majerus et al., 1969; Abdel-Hakin and Farah, 1985]. Optimum conditions for acetate-1-[^{14}C] incorporation have been described, and free fatty acid, phospholipid, and ceramide were radiolabeled [Deykin and Desson, 1968]. In order to evaluate de novo versus elongation pathways for fatty acids, radioactivity due to acetate incorporation at the C-1 position is determined by its chemical conversion to

CO_2 and comparison with the total fatty acid radioactivity [Brady et al., 1960]. The value for exclusive de novo utilization of acetate in the biosynthesis of palmitate is 12.5% (i.e., 16/2 × 100). However, values higher than this have been obtained for a number of fatty acids, indicating significant chain elongation can occur in platelets [Hennes et al., 1966; Naughton, 1981].

Biosynthesis of Phosphatidic Acid

Platelets are capable of de novo phospholipid biosynthesis [Lewis and Majerus, 1969]. Radioactive glycerol is converted by the enzyme glycerokinase to sn-glycerol-3-phosphate, which is subsequently acylated (2 acyl CoA/sn-glycerol-3-phosphate) to form radiolabeled phosphatidic acid. Phosphatidic acid can be radiolabeled either with acetate (incorporated as fatty acid after de novo biosynthesis or chain elongation), ^{32}P by phosphorylation from donor [^{32}P]-ATP, or [^{3}H]-glycerol by direct incorporation. In platelets most de novo synthesis is studied using [^{3}H]-glycerol as de novo incorporation of ^{32}P in PC, PE, and PS is relatively low.

In other tissues glycerol-3-phosphate is converted to dihydroxyacetone phosphate (DHAP) by glycerol-3-phosphate dehydrogenase. DHAP is also an acyl acceptor [Hajra, 1968; Hajra and Agranoff, 1968] and gains significance as an intermediate in ether lipid biosynthesis [Hajra, 1969; Wykle and Snyder, 1976; Brindley and Stenton, 1982]. In other cell systems the alkyl linkage at sn-1 is formed from fatty alcohol, and subsequently reduction and acylation at sn-2 give the 1-O-alkyl-2-acyl-sn-glycero-3-phosphate which is processed in similar fashion to 1,2 diacyl phosphatidic acid [Wykle and Snyder, 1976; Snyder et al., 1970; Wykle and Snyder, 1969; Wykle and Snyder, 1970; Hajra, 1970].

Ether Phospholipid

Human platelets are reported to have substantial amounts of ether phospholipid; over 60% of their 1,2 diradyl PE and 18% of their 1,2 diradyl PC [Mueller et al, 1983], and 1% of their 1,2 diradyl PI [Natarajan et al, 1983]. Peroxisomes are thought to be involved in β-oxidation of fatty acids and the initial stages of ether lipid biosynthesis. Peroxisomes are capable of conversion of DHAP to 1-O-alkyl-2-lyso glycerolphosphate, but further metabolic steps have not been demonstrated [Hajra et al., 1979; Jones and Hajra, 1980; Hajra and Bishop, 1982; Ballas et al., 1984].

Recently a group of diseases termed "peroxisomopathies" were identified in which peroxisomes are apparently absent in a number of tissues [Goldfischer and Raddy, 1984]. Patients with Zellweger's syndrome lack both peroxisomes and ether lipids and die before 1 year. Wanders et al. [1985] have shown platelets from these patients lack acyl-CoA:dihydroxyacetone phosphate acyltransferase, which nevertheless is present in normal platelets. Presumably, human platelets contain peroxisomes and can synthesize ether phospholipids de novo.

De Novo Biosynthesis of Phospholipid

A significant point for the regulation of phospholipid biosynthesis is the dephosphorylation of phosphatidic acid by phosphotidate hydrolase or phosphotidate phosphatase to give diacylglycerol [Holub and Kuksis, 1978]. In hepatocytes this enzyme is apparently translocated from cytosol to membrane where the hydrolysis of phosphatidic acid occurs [Pittner et al., 1985] and can therefore be considered an ambiquitous enzyme [Wilson, 1978]. A study with human platelets has reported finding the enzyme in the particulate fraction (94% bound) [Call and Williams, 1973]. It is quite active (1–5 nmoles phosphatidic acid hydrolyzed/min/mg protein) and is stimulated by monoglyceride but inhibited by detergent and potassium fluoride. It should be noted that this enzyme's activity can be overestimated [Sturton and Brindley, 1978].

The resulting diglyceride is an acceptor in the biosynthesis of PC, and PE [Holub and Kuksis, 1978]. The biosynthesis of phosphatidylcholine in a number of cells has been reviewed elsewhere [Pelech and Vance, 1984]. Little work has been done on the incorporation of choline into PC in platelets. Choline must be phosphorylated to choline phosphate by a kinase. Subsequently CTP phosphocholine cytidylyltransferase catalyzes the biosynthesis of CDP choline and PPI from phosphocholine and CTP. This enzyme is also ambiquitous and is important in the regulation of PC biosynthesis; its translocation and activation being stimulated by oleate acid and phorbol esters in the bilayer [Pelech et al., 1984a,b; Feldman et al., 1985].

Choline phosphotransferase or CTP choline:1,2-diacylglycerol choline-phosphotransferase is the final step in the Kennedy pathway and CDP choline is transferred to the acceptor diacylaglycerol. Platelets have been shown to possess a membrane bound form of this enzyme [Gorracci et al., 1983]. The assay is problematic as diglyceride must be presented to the enzyme in appropriate fashion. In this study the ratio of the detergent tween-20 to diglyceride (0.5%) was crucial. The incorporation of radioactive CDP choline into PC was monitored. The reaction was stimulated by Mn and Mg and inhibited by Ca. In rat brain microsomes reversal of cholinephosphotransferase has been suggested as a pathway for the degradation of PC [Goracci et al., 1981]. The same enzyme may transfer phosphocholine to 1-O-alkyl-2-acetyl-sn-glycerol to yield platelet-activating factor [Renooij and Snyder, 1981]. The importance of these pathways remains to be assessed.

A similar biosynthetic route exists for PE. Cytidine-5′-diphosphate ethanolamine:1-radyl-2-acyl-sn-glycerol ethanolamine phosphotransferase has also been found in platelets [Call and Rubert, 1975]. This enzyme required Mn and glycodeoxycholate for activity and catalyzed the formation of both 1,2 diacyl and 1-O-alkyl-2-acyl PE with respective 1-radyl-2-acyl-glycerol acceptor. Hydrogen is removed from 1-O-alkyl-2-acyl PE to give the plasmalogen PE with its vinyl ether linkage at sn-1 [Wykle and Snyder, 1976].

Another route for the formation of PC is methylation of PE [Pelech and Vance, 1984]. S-adenosylmethionine is the methyl donor for each of the three methyl groups required. One or more enzymes may be involved. Such enzyme systems have been reported in human platelets. Lysed membrane preparations can methylate phosphatidylethanolamine to the mono-, di-, and trimethyl derivatives with added radioactive S-adenosylmethionine [Hotchkiss et al., 1981; Mori et al., 1981]. In intact platelets [^{3}H]-methionine was used to monitor reaction products, as radioactive S-adenosyl methionine cannot penetrate the plasma membrane [Hotchkiss et al., 1981; Cordasco, 1981].

There has been a considerable amount of interest in correlating the activation of this pathway with stimulus response coupling in a number of cells [Hirata and Axelrod, 1980]. In platelets it was suggested that a substantial amount of 1-acyl-2-arachidonoyl PC made by successive methylations of PE was the source of arachidonic acid released by stimulated cells [Kannagi et al., 1980], or at least a substrate for phospholipase A_2 [Lecompte et al., 1982; Randon et al., 1981]. However, the importance of this pathway has been questioned both in general [Pelech and Vance, 1984; Vance and deKruijff, 1980; Axelrod and Hirada, 1980] and for platelets [Hotchkiss et al., 1981; Cordasco et al., 1981; Shattil et al., 1981; Mori et al., 1983].

The biosynthesis of PI is different from PC and PE in that phosphatidic acid is incorporated into the final reaction product. This has implications for ^{32}P radiolabeling of cells. The enzyme CTP:phosphatidate cytidylyltransferase is found in lysed platelet membranes and incorporates the phosphatidic acid into CDP-diacylglycerol [Call and Williams, 1970]. This molecule is the immediate precursor of PI. CDP-diacylglycerol:inositol phosphatidyltransferase was also found in platelet membrane fractions [Lucas et al., 1970]. Thus enzymes required for the de novo biosynthesis of PI are present in platelets.

Radiolabeling With Radioactive Glycerol

To determine de novo phospholipid biosynthesis [^{3}H]-glycerol is commonly used to radiolabel phospholipid. Radiolabeled glycerol is incorporated into PE, PC, PS, and PI [Lewis and Majerus, 1969; Okuma et al., 1973]. Glycerol cannot be exchanged with endogenous phospholipid but rather is phosphorylated by glycerokinase and acylated to form phosphatidic acid. In general, incorporation of [^{3}H]-glycerol is linear for times of up to 2 hours, with labeling being the order of PC-PI > PE > PS [Lewis and Majerus, 1969; Mahadevappa and Holub, 1984]. Neufeld and Majerus [1983] have calculated that unstimulated platelets synthesize total phospholipid from [^{3}H]-glycerol labeled phosphatidic acid at a rate of 80–300 pmole/min/10^9 cells. In liver, a low amount of the radioactive glycerol is found in the tetraene fraction after incorporation while in platelets, a considerable portion of [^{3}H]-glycerol labeled PC is found in 1-acyl-2-arachidonoyl PC (21%), suggesting the formation of 1-acyl-2-arachidonoyl phosphatidic acid [Mahadevappa and Holub, 1984]. Radioactive glycerol has also been found in highly unsaturated molecular species of phosphatidic acid in retinal microsomes [Gusto and Bazan, 1979; Bazan et al., 1984].

^{32}P Radiolabeling of Platelet Cytoplasmic ATP

^{32}P is transferred into phospholipids by the action of kinases, which transfer the γ-phosphate of ATP to a lipid acceptor. Only one-third of the adenine nucleotides, those residing in the cytoplasm, participate in metabolism, and they can be specifically labeled by incubating platelets with radioactive adenine [Holmsen et al., 1972]. The radiolabeled adenine is distributed evenly among ATP, ADP, AMP, and their metabolic breakdown products [Daniel et al., 1980]. This metabolic compartment can be monitored in contrast to the metabolically inert granule-stored nucleotides, which are secreted when platelets are stimulated.

Platelets can be radiolabeled with carrier-free ^{32}P plasma. Platelet-rich plasma is prepared and ^{32}P added, to give a final concentration of 0.25 mCi/ml. This high concentration is required, owing to the high phosphate content of plasma. ^{32}P concentrations 1/10 of this value can be used if radiolabeling is done in low phosphate buffer. In resting cells the membrane uptake of ^{32}P is rate limiting, while equilibration of cytoplasmic ^{32}P and the γ and β phosphate groups is fairly rapid [Verhoeven et al., 1986; Holmsen et al., 1983]. The α-phosphate group of ATP, ADP, and AMP does not become radiolabeled and ^{32}P is uniformly distributed among the cytoplasmic adenine nucleotides and Pi [Holmsen et al., 1983].

Cells are incubated for 60–90 min at 37°C with the carrier-free ^{32}P, and then cells in plasma can be gel-filtered to separate them from ^{32}P [Holmsen et al., 1981]. Cells labeled in buffer can simply be collected by centrifugation and resuspended in the appropriate buffer. Less than 1% of the ^{32}P added is incorporated into the cells, and the investigator should take precautions when disposing of the considerable amount of unincorporated ^{32}P. In human thrombin-stimulated platelets it is possible to determine the ^{32}P specific activity of cytoplasmic ATP in a number of ways, taking care to make measurements only after nonradioactive ATP of the granule compartment has been removed [Verhoeven et al., 1986]. In thrombin-stimulated cells the specific activity of ^{32}P in phosphatidic acid, Ptd(4,5)P_2, and the γ-phosphate of ATP are the same [Holmsen et al., 1984; Dangelmaier et al., 1986].

THE PHOSPHATIDYLINOSITOL (PI) CYCLE

Introduction

Hokin and Hokin [1953] observed the rapid incorporation of ^{32}P into the phospholipid of slices of pigeon pancreas following stimulation by an agonist. In guinea pig brain (cortex) cells stimulated with acetylcholine, the incorporation of [^{3}H]-inositol and ^{32}P into PI as well as that of ^{32}P into phosphatidic acid was considerably increased, whereas there was no uptake of [^{14}C] glycerol into either phosphatidic acid or PI [Hokin and Hokin, 1958]. This and a considerable amount of other work as reviewed by Michell [1975] led to the concept of a PI cycle, that is, a cycle of reactions excluding de novo biosynthesis, coupled to the increase in cytoplasmic free calcium and stimulation of the cell. At the time of Michell's review the cycle was thought to be initiated by hydrolysis of PI by a PI specific phospholipase C [Mauco et al., 1979] to give 1,2 diacylglycerol and subsequently its phosphorylated derivative phosphatidic acid. However, subsequent work demonstrated that hydrolysis of PIP_2 at low calcium concentration by phospholipase C was the initial event [Berridge et al., 1983; Billah and Lapetina, 1982b; Imai et al., 1983; Mauco et al., 1983; Berridge et al., 1984] and led to the production of both diglyceride, shown to be a second messenger for platelet activation [Kajikawa, 1983; Nishizuka et al., 1984], and IP_3 (inositol-1,4,5-triphosphate), which mobilized and increased intracellular free calcium [Berridge et al., 1984; Brass and Joseph, 1985]. It is now suggested that hydrolysis of PI by phospholipase C is secondary to the action of the same enzyme on PIP_2 and dependent on intracellular calcium [Majerus et al., 1985]. The reader should consider the older and more recent literature from this perspective. Regardless of the source of diglyceride, its phosphorylation by diglyceride kinase is the point at which ^{32}P is transferred into phosphatidic acid from radioactive ATP. Subsequently, as in the de novo synthesis of PI, phosphatidic acid is incorporated intact into CDP-diacylglycerol by CTP:phosphatidate cytidylyltransferase and subsequently with inositol into PI by the action of CDP-diacylglycerol:inositol phosphatidyltransferase, thus completing the PI cycle.

The augmented ^{32}P radiolabeling of phosphatidic acid and phosphatidylinositol reported by the Hokins excluded de novo biosynthesis of phospholipids. However, in platelets there are indications that radiolabeling of "PI cycle" components in stimulated cells may contain a de novo component. Holmsen et al. [1981] have suggested that phosphatidic acid biosynthesis occurring in thrombin-stimulated cells has a de novo component, and Vickers et al. [1984b] have shown [^{3}H]-glycerol turnover in the "PI cycle" components of stimulated cells. Deykin and Snyder [1973] observed an enhanced incorporation of ^{3}H-glycerol into PI in epinephrine-stimulated cells, and Prescott and Majerus [1981] and Imai et al. [1981] provided evidence for de novo synthesis based on the appearance of unsaturated nonarachidonoyl containing molecular species of PI in stimulated cells. Remodeling by deacylation/reacylation reactions increased the arachidonate content within 10 min. It should be noted that [^{3}H]-glycerol-labeled PI has been shown to decrease in thrombin-stimulated platelets [Mahadevappa and Holub, 1983].

In ^{32}P radiolabeled platelets the appearance of PI cycle metabolites occurs within seconds after addition of agonist with the amount of [^{32}P]-phosphatidic acid and subsequently [^{32}P]-PI being in rough proportion to the strength of agonist. Lloyd et al. [1972, 1973, 1974] reported increased ^{32}P labeling of phosphatidic acid, PIP, PIP_2, and subsequently PI in ADP-stimulated platelets. In addition [^{32}P]-phosphatidic acid content was considerably increased for either thrombin or collagen-stimulated cells [Lloyd et al., 1974].

PI Turnover in Stimulated Platelets

There have been some differences on the cause of degradation of PI in stimulated cells. Most investigators implicate a PI-specific phospholipase C in platelets [Mauco et al., 1978, 1979; Rittenhouse-Simmons, 1979; Bell et al., 1979; Chau and Tai, 1981]; however, Billah and Lapetina [1982a] claim that a quinacrine-sensitive phospholipase A_2 is responsible for a significant portion of the PI deacylation, and other workers noted phospholipase A_2 (PLA_2) action on PI was augmented in ionophore (A23187)-stimulated cells, where relatively low amounts of diglyceride and phosphatidic acid were produced [Rittenhouse-Simmons, 1981a].

Mauco et al. [1978, 1979] and Bell et al. [1979] have proposed that diglyceride lipase acting on the diglyceride generated by phospholipase C on PI is responsible for a substantial portion of the total arachidonic acid released in thrombin-stimulated cells. This pathway for arachidonate release was proposed before the importance of phospholipase C action in PIP_2 had been assessed [Berridge, 1983; Berridge and Irving, 1984]; however, only conversion of PI to diglyceride can give the amount of arachidonate release proposed. Out of the 6.4 nmole of arachidonate released per 10^9 cells, Bell et al. [1979] claimed, on the basis of in vitro determinations of diglyceride lipase activity, that this enzyme could account for 5 nmole of arachidonate per 10^9 cells. In maximally thrombin-stimulated human cells the 18.8 nmoles [Mauco et al., 1984] of PI had decreased by 6.6 nmoles per 10^9 cells while phosphatidic acid only increased by 2.2 nmoles per 10^9 cells at 60 sec. The difference of 4.4 nmoles was taken to represent the arachidonic acid released either by diglyceride lipase or phospholipase A_2. Majerus et al. [1985] suggest that the initial release of arachidonic acid is from the diglyceride lipase pathway while later it is released from PC.

Diacylglycerol in Stimulated Platelets

Diacylglycerol stimulates protein kinase C, which phosphorylates a 40-kilodalton protein in platelets [Nishizuka, 1984; Kaibuchi et al., 1983; Kajikawa et al., 1983]. This phosphorylation is correlated with a number of functional responses [Haslam and Lynham, 1977]. In platelets it appears that IP_3 (inositol-1,4,5-triphosphate) and diacylglycerol support two separate pathways which together allow full activation of platelets [Kaibuchi et al., 1983]. Recently an interesting model of protein kinase C/diglyceride/calcium/phosphatidylserine was proposed in which diglyceride is an axial component of a 4 PS/calcium/protein kinase C complex [Ganong et al., 1986].

Phosphorylation of diglyceride by platelet diglyceride kinase [Call and Rubert, 1973] is also thought by some to be an important point of control in the cell's response to agonists. Holmsen et al. [1981, 1984] noted that the appearance of phosphatidic acid and not the disappearance of PI correlated with thrombin receptor occupancy, suggesting the diglyceride kinase was tightly coupled to receptor status with the activation of phospholipase C being an all-or-none event. Billah et al. [1981] have also found evidence for PLA_2 specific for phosphatidic acid, which may also be important for arachidonic acid release.

Hydrolysis of PIP_2 by Phospholipase C in Stimulated Platelets

In resting human platelets the masses of PI, PIP, and PIP_2 are 18.8, 3.1, and 1.1 nmoles/10^9 cells [Mauco et al., 1984]. The work of Lloyd et al. [1972, 1973, 1974] indicated considerable turnover or incorporation of ^{32}P into PIP and PIP_2 in addition to phosphatidic acid and PI. It is now accepted, following results in other cells [Berridge, 1983; Berridge and Irving, 1984], that the initial event in the hydrolysis of inositol-containing phospholipids is the action of phospholipase C on PIP_2 [Billah and Lapetina, 1982b]. This was demonstrated by appearance of 1,4,5-triphosphate (IP_3) preceding that of inositol-1-phosphate and inositol-1,4-diphosphate in stimulated cells [Agranoff et al., 1983]. The PIP_2 is rapidly replenished by kinase(s) acting on PI and PIP, and the decrease and subsequent increase in PIP_2 is more difficult to detect than the release of the water-soluble, charged, head groups of the phospholipids. Thrombin stimulation of ^{32}P radiolabeled platelets showed a transient decrease in PIP_2 at 20 sec, preceding the incorporation of ^{32}P into PIP_2 [Billah and Lapetina, 1982b; Vickers et al., 1982, 1984a; Agranoff et al., 1983; Rendu et al., 1983; Broekman, 1984] and decreases in the other two inositol phospholipids. Weaker agonists such as ADP [Vickers et al., 1982] and Paf-acether [Shukla and Hanahan, 1983] gave similar results.

Phospholipase C can hydrolyze PI, PIP, and PIP_2 in vitro [Wilson et al., 1984, 1985, 1985a; Rittenhouse, 1983], and at low external calcium concentrations PIP_2 breakdown is favored [Majerus et al., 1985; Wilson et al., 1984]. The IP_3 released from PIP_2 has been shown to release nonmitochondrial sequestered calcium from saponin-treated human platelets [Brass and Joseph, 1985] and calcium-sequestering vesicles prepared from platelet sonicates [Adunyah and Dean, 1985; O'Rourke et al., 1985]. [^{32}P]-IP_3 can be isolated, and following removal of 2,3 diglycerolphosphate with phosphoglycerophosphatase, the radioactivity of [^{32}P]-IP_3 can be used to determine mass [Dangelmaier et al., 1986]. Thus the PI cycle in platelets is able to rapidly produce two second-messenger molecules: diglyceride and IP_3. Subsequent to the initial calcium-independent action of phospholipase C on PIP_2, Majerus et al. [1985] favor the calcium-dependent hydrolysis by phospholipase C of PI to release diglyceride following its hydrolysis of PIP_2.

The hydrolysis of PIP_2 is also linked to GTP-binding protein(s). Such proteins are also important for the interaction between adenylate cyclase and its receptors [Gilman, 1984]. Haslam and Davidson [1984] showed the calcium sensitivity of secretion in permeabilized platelets was considerably increased by guanine nucleotides. Thus coupling of phospholipase C hydrolysis of PIP_2 is probably modulated by a guanidine nucleotide-binding protein(s) following receptor occupancy. This regulatory unit is probably different from the N_s and N_i associated with adenylate cyclase. Platelet activating factor and U44069 stimulate a GTPase activity in human platelets, which is distinct from guanine nucleotide regulatory proteins, N_s and N_i [Houslay et al., 1986].

Lipolytic Enzymes Involved in the PI Cycle

Phospholipase C. The action of phospholipase C, at least that responsible for the hydrolysis of PIP_2, is probably modulated by a guanine nucleotide-binding protein(s) [Haslam and Davidson, 1984]. This enzyme has been isolated from platelet cytosol and assayed on ^{32}P labeled phosphoinositides of platelets [Rittenhouse, 1983], exogenous phosphatidyl[U-^{14}C]inositol [Seiss and Lapetina, 1983; Lenstra et al., 1984] or 1-acyl-2-[^{3}H]-arachidonoyl PI [Mauco et al., 1979]. Usually deoxycholate is required for substrate solubilization and 1 mM calcium and pH 7.0 is necessary for optimum activity of the enzyme [Lenstra et al., 1984]. Use of [^{3}H]-inositol radiolabeled PI allows one to monitor enzyme activity by measuring the release of [^{3}H]-inositol in the aqueous supernatant of a Bligh and Dyer [1959] extract [Lenstra et al., 1984]. It should be noted that phospholipase C has also been shown to reside in lysosomes; however, this enzyme will have a lower (acid) pH optimum, no calcium requirement, and probably also degrades other phospholipids [Irving et al., 1977; Matsuzawa and

Hostetler, 1980]. Finally the action of phospholipase C has been demonstrated in platelet membranes following addition of calcium and deoxycholate [Plantavid et al., 1986].

Diglyceride kinase. In addition to converting diglyceride to phosphatidic acid, the appearance of which some workers claim is tightly coupled to lysosomal enzyme secretion [Holmsen et al., 1984], another function of diglyceride kinase may be to attenuate the action of diglyceride as a second messenger [Bishop et al., 1986]. Structural characteristics of a number of activator and inhibitor diglycerides for diglyceride kinase have been deduced [Bishop et al., 1986]. Further demonstration of diglyceride kinase receptor coupling is the dose dependence of epidermal growth factor stimulation of [^{32}P]-phosphatidic acid production in plasma membrane vesicles of A431 cells [Kato et al., 1985]. The importance of this enzyme is shown by its absence in the photoreceptor cells of Drosophila vision mutants [Yoshioka, 1984]. A portion of diglyceride kinase activity has been found associated with microtubule protein in chick embryonic muscle [Daleo et al., 1974; Daleo et al., 1976], and coupled with the known association of phospholipase C with other intracellular proteins [Quinn, 1973; Creutz et al., 1985] suggests some interaction of these structures with receptor-linked events of the PI cycle.

The problems of the diglyceride kinase assay are presentation of the sn-3 hydroxyl function of a virtually nonwettable molecule at the lipid/water interface [Kanoh and Ono, 1984]. The reaction has been done using diglyceride bound in molar excess to albumin [Mauco et al., 1984a], solubilized by detergents [Bishop et al., 1986; Holub and Piekarski, 1978], or in combination with detergents and phospholipids [Lin et al, 1986; Preiss et al., 1986; Call and Rubert, 1973]. An excellent method for preparing [^{32}P]-ATP for the assay is the approach of Walseth and Johnson [1979].

Diacylglycerol lipase. Similar problems are involved in the assay of diacylglycerol and monoacylglycerol lipase. Assay methodology for these enzymes has been deduced for platelets [Mauco et al., 1984a; Bell et al., 1979; Prescott and Majerus, 1983]. Diglyceride lipase is inhibited by indomethacin [Rittenhouse-Simmons, 1980] and RHC 80267 [Oglesby and Gorman, 1984]. Chau and Tai [1983] have used RHC 80267 to argue against the involvement of the diglycerol lipase in arachidonate release.

Modulation of the PI Cycle

The PI cycle is open to modulation by a number of approaches. Pretreatment of platelets with either 1,2 diacylglycerol or phorbol ester inhibits the release of IP_3 [Watson and Lapetina, 1985] or phosphatidic acid formation [MacIntyre et al., 1985] in response to thrombin; however, it has also been claimed that prostacyclin can decrease the phosphatidic acid formed in thrombin-stimulated cells in the presence of activated protein kinase C [Lapetina, 1984]. In resting cells a number of workers have noted that incubation of platelets with either phorbol esters or 1,2 diacylglycerols results in an increase in [^{32}P]-polyphosphoinositides [de Chaffoy et al., 1984a,b; Halenda and Feinstein, 1984]. In ionophore (A23187)-stimulated cells phospholipase C activation is reported to be dependent on both ADP and cyclooxygenase products [Rittenhouse, 1984] and a thromboxane A_2 analog 9,11-epoxymethanoprostaglandin H_2 was shown to elevate phosphatidic acid and cytoplasmic-free calcium in direct proportion to its concentration [Pollock et al., 1984]. Short-chain diacylglycerols [Lapetina et al., 1985] as well as 1-oleoyl-2-acetyl glycerol [Nishizuka, 1984] are known to have similar effects as well as the stimulation of protein kinase C; 1-oleoyl-2-acetyl glycerol is phosphorylated to form phosphatidic acid [Nishizuka, 1984] and short-chained diglycerides are incorporated into PI as well as phosphatidic acid [Lapetina, 1986]. It remains to be seen to what degree these diglycerides can monitor or in turn modulate the PI cycle.

Lithium is known to inhibit the enzyme myo-inositol-1-phosphatase, which is the final step in the generation of free inositol from the various polyphosphoinositides generated in the stimulated cell [Hallcher and Sherman, 1980; Berridge et al., 1982] and lithium has been reported to augment IP_3 formation in certain cells [Berridge et al., 1982]. Some changes have been reported for platelets suitably preincubated with lithium, especially at lower concentrations of agonist, but the effect is not marked [Vickers et al., 1984b]. It is our experience that the equilibration time and concentration of lithium used are crucial in the application of this methodology to platelets.

Extraction and Radiolabeling of Inositol-Containing Phospholipids

In order to get maximum extraction of all the inositol-containing phospholipids and particularly the polyphosphoinositides, acid conditions are required during the extraction [Downes and Michell, 1982]. Thus the Bligh and Dyer extraction procedure [1959] must be done in the presence of 1.2 N HCl. It should be recognized that the vinyl ether linkage of plasmalogens is labile in acid [Mueller et al., 1983] and thus 1-O-lyso-2-acyl forms of GPC and GPE will be generated and can confuse subsequent thin layer chromatography or high pressure liquid chromatography. In addition, acid conditions hydrolyze the cyclic phosphate ester bond of inositol cyclic phosphates [Dawson et al., 1971; Wilson et al., 1985]. Cyclic polyphosphoinositides have shown to be produced by phospholipase C hydrolysis of PI, and 1:2-cyclic 4,5-triphosphate can also release calcium from intracellular pools [Wilson et al., 1985a]. The status of such cyclic inositol phosphates and the plethora of additional inositol polyphosphoinositols, such as

Inositol (1,3,4,5)P_4 reported in other cells [Michell, 1986], is at present unknown for platelets.

In radiolabeling platelets for study of the PI cycle, [^{3}H]-arachidonate, ^{32}P, and [^{3}H]-inositol have been used. The inositol-containing phospholipids all contain substantial amounts of 1-stearoyl-2-arachidonoyl glycerol [Mauco et al., 1984] and a substantial incorporation of [^{3}H]-arachidonate can be achieved. Incorporation of [^{3}H]-arachidonate into the inositol-containing phospholipids is roughly in proportion to mass, which is 18.8, 3.1, and 1.1 nmoles/10^9 cells for PI, PIP, and PIP_2, respectively [Mauco et al., 1984]. Platelets contain an active 1-acyl-glycerophosphorylinositol acyltransferase [Kameyama et al., 1983], which is probably mainly responsible for the incorporation of [^{3}H]-arachidonate into PI. Diglyceride and phosphatidic acid produced by stimulated cells can also be measured by their content of [^{3}H]-arachidonate. ^{32}P incorporation can be utilized in different ways. Following incorporation of ^{32}P into platelets in platelet-rich plasma, we find that the ratio of ^{32}P radioactivity is roughly 1:2:4 for PI, PIP, PIP_2 in resting cells. Cells can be equilibrated to steady-state, for example radiolabeling for 1 hour at 37°C, or a pulse labeling approach can be used with incubation being done for a much shorter time [Wilson et al., 1985b]. It is claimed that in non-steady-state conditions the flux of components through the PI cycle can be determined in the stimulated cell. However, it should be noted that if such studies are done in the presence of external ^{32}P, that influx of the radiolabel has been reported to occur for thrombin-stimulated cells [Verhoeven et al., 1986]. This can also explain the increased radioactivity in the polyphosphoinositides under the same conditions. Finally, another approach with ^{32}P labeled cells is to apply metabolic poisons known to inhibit the production of ATP and note their effect on PI cycle intermediates and different platelet responses [Holmsen et al., 1982, 1984]. In all experiments using ^{32}P labeled cells to study the turnover of the PI cycle metabolites, the cells should be equilibrated for 3 min at 37°C before addition of agonists. [^{3}H]-inositol has also been used to radiolabel the inositol-containing phospholipids (for example, Shukla and Hanahan, 1983; Watson et al., 1984), but under normal conditions only very small amounts of the radiolabel are taken up by platelets, making the use of [^{3}H]-inositol very expensive. [^{3}H]-inositol is used for experiments in which the release of inositol-phosphates is monitored, while ^{32}P is the radiolabel of choice when analyzing the inositol-containing phospholipids.

Mass Determination of PI Cycle Components

Mass determinations of PI cycle intermediates have also been reported. Diglyceride can be measured using *E. coli* diglyceridekinase [Preiss et al., 1986] or by GLC of methylesters of the TLC-purified material [Mauco et al., 1984.

GLC of fatty acid methyl esters has shown that the inositol-containing phospholipids contain a stearoyl-arachidonoyl backbone as does the phosphatidic acid and diglyceride generated in the stimulated cell [Mauco et al., 1984; Broekman et al., 1981]. The solvent systems used in the work of Mauco et al. [1984] are recommended because they are one-dimensional and thus save time; also, the phospholipids are completely resolved and can be used to determine mass and composition. Generally 2×10^8 cells were used for PI determination and 2×10^9 cells were used for determination of PIP, PIP_2, and phosphatidic acid. The location of the polyphosphoinositides was determined by autoradiography for 2 hours or if enough mass were present by use of primulin spray after the TLC plates were neutralized by NH_3 fumes. The following TLC systems are recommended: PI, chloroform/methanol/acetic acid/water (81:10:45:1 by volume) [Hauser and Eichberg, 1975]; PIP and PIP_2, chloroform/methanol/4M-NH_3 (9:7:2 by volume) [Lloyd et al., 1972, 1973] or [Jolles et al., 1981]; phosphatidic acid, upper layer of ethylacetate/iso-octane/acetic acid/water (9:5:2:10 by volume) [Hong and Levine, 1976]; diacylglycerols, the double development method of Skipski [1968].

In order to monitor the ^{32}P incorporation in PI and phosphatidic acid at the molecular species level, these phospholipids must be resolved intact. Analyses of molecular species of PI [Holub and Kuksis, 1971] and phosphatidic acid [Suguira and Waku, 1984; Kato et al., 1984] have been reported using argentation thin layer chromatography. Molecular species of PI can be resolved by the high pressure liquid chromatography (HPLC) reverse phase method of Patton et al. [1982]. Probably the same HPLC system could be used with dimethyl ester of phosphatidic acid made by reacting the sodium salt form of phosphatidic acid [Renkonen, 1968] with diazomethane [Cohen, 1984; Schwartz and Bright, 1974; Hsieh et al., 1981]. In closing, it should be noted that PI cycle components have been shown to reside in both receptor-linked and de novo pools in other cells [Koreh and Monaco, 1986; Monaco, 1986], and such pools should be considered when interpreting results from experiments using platelets.

ARACHIDONIC ACID METABOLISM

Resolution and Mass of Phospholipids

In human platelets we have determined the following phospholipid composition [Mueller et al., 1983]: sphingomyelin (17.7%), choline-containing phospholipids (38.0%), inositol-containing phospholipids (4.4%), phosphatidylserine (10.8%), and ethanolamine-containing phosphoglycerides (25.3%). Human platelets have 380 nmoles of phospholipid phosphate/10^9 cells and the mass of individual phospholipids is 67.3, 144.4, 18.8, 41.0, and 96.1 nmoles/10^9 cells, for sphingomyelin, PC, PI, PS, and PE, respectively. This agrees with results of others [Cohen and Derksen, 1969; Broekman et al., 1980; Mahadevappa and Holub, 1982]. These results were obtained by extraction of platelet phospholipid by the method of Bligh and Dyer [1959], followed by resolution of the phospholipids by TLC [Skipski et al., 1964; Mahadevappa and Holub, 1982; Purdon and Smith, 1985] on silica gel H plates (no binder). No acid is included during the extraction in order not to hydrolyze plasmalogen; however, as mentioned previously, the polyphosphoinositides will not be extracted quantitatively. Mass is determined by phosphate determination and standard procedures are recommended [Rouser et al., 1966; Hess and Derr, 1975]. Other TLC system have been suggested for resolution of phospholipids, especially to resolve PS and PI, which can sometimes be a problem [Fine and Sprecher, 1982; Allan and Cockcroft, 1982].

Ether Phospholipid

It has been known for some time that a major component of phosphatidylethanolamine in platelets is 1-O-alk-1′enyl-2-acyl GPE, or the plasmalogen form [Cohen and Derksen, 1969]. The function of plasmalogen is presently unknown; however, Rittenhouse-Simmons et al. [1977] demonstrated that there was an increased [^{3}H]-arachidonate content in 1-O-alk-1′-enyl-2-acyl GPE following thrombin stimulation.

Considerable interest was generated in ether lipids when the lipid nature of structure of PAF-acether was determined [Benveniste et al., 1977], and an ether linkage was found at position sn-1 [Demopoulos et al., 1979]. Evidence for the formation of PAF-acether (1-O-alkyl-2-acetyl GPC) by a deacylation/reacylation pathway was found for several tissues [Wykle et al., 1980; Ninio et al., 1982; Lee et al., 1982]. Platelets were found to synthesize PAF-acether [Chignard et al., 1979; Chap et al., 1981; Benveniste et al., 1982; Alam and Smith, 1983] and thus a search for 1-O-alkyl-2-acyl GPC was initiated and found by a number of groups [Mueller et al., 1983; Natarajan et al., 1983; Tence et al., 1985] using different procedures. Natarajan et al. [1983] reported the lowest value (4.5% of total PC fraction as 1-O-alkyl-2-acyl GPC) using reductive alkylation with $LiAlH_4$. The approach of Tence et al. [1985] utilizes guinea pig pancrease PLA_1 [Fauvel et al., 1981] specific for the ester linkage at position sn-1. Hydrolysis of the PC fraction leaves the ether lipid unhydrolyzed and it is separated from 1-lyso-2-acyl PC, by TLC. The plate is then exposed to HCl fumes for 10 min, and rerun in a second dimension to separate the intact 1-O-alkyl-2-acyl PC from hydrolyzed plasmalogen [Tamer et al., 1984; Diagne et al., 1984; Colard et al., 1984, 1986]. It is important that the enzyme preparation used be absolutely free of PLA_2 and also that hydrolysis of 1,2 diacyl PC go to completion. It should be noted that the hydrolyzed 1,2 diacyl PC and plasmalogen GPC cannot be subsequently analyzed as intact molecular species in contrast with other methodologies. We have used yet another approach for the analysis of 1-O-alkyl-2-acyl GPC [Mueller et al., 1983; Purdon and Smith, 1985] in which an ether solution of the total PC fraction is incubated with B. Cereus phospholipase C in 0.01 N Tris buffer, pH 7.4, 5 mM $CaCl_2$. Routinely the PC fraction from 10^9 cells is processed. It is important that the PLC hydrolysis go to completion in order to avoid any preferential hydrolysis of a particular molecular species or subclass that might occur if hydrolysis was not complete [Kuksis, 1984]. To ensure that this is so, the incubation must be extended to 12 hours, particularly when hydrolyzing the PE fraction. The resulting diglyceride is extracted with diethyl ether and acetylated with acetic anhydride/pyridine [Mueller et al., 1982]. The subclasses of diglyceride acetates are then resolved by double development TLC, first, hexane/ethyl ether (70:30: v/v) and, second, toluene [Purdon and Smith, 1985; Renkonen, 1966; Suguira et al., 1984; Mueller et al., 1982]. Alternatively, plasmalogen can also be separated before hydrolysis with phospholipase C by exposing the total phospholipid to HCl gas and separating out the lysoplasmalogen by TLC. This will leave only 1,2 diacyl and 1-O-alkyl-2-acyl subclasses to be separated as diglyceride acetates [Mueller et al., 1983]. Our choice has been to use this latter approach, that is, separating the lysoplasmalogen after formation by HCl treatment, when initially examining a given cell type for the presence of ether lipid. When performing metabolic studies involving [^{3}H]-arachidonate the HCl gas treatment is avoided and the three subclasses are resolved by TLC of diglyceride acetates [Purdon and Smith, 1985]. HPLC methodology for the resolution of alkenylacyl, alkylacyl, and diacyl acetylglycerols has been reported by Nakagawa and Horrocks [1983]. This same methodology can be applied to other phospholipids such as the PE fraction.

Results from analysis of platelet phospholipid are shown in Table I. 1,2 diacyl PC represents 80% of total PC, while 1,2 diacyl PE is only 36% of the ethanolamine-containing phospholipids. 1-O-alkyl-2-acyl GPC is 10% of the total phosphatidylcholine fraction. Of interest is the enrichment of arachidonate in ether lipids compared to their respective 1,2 diacyl subclasses. Relatively high amounts of palmitate are also found at position sn-2 of 1-O-alkyl-2-acyl GPC. The fatty acid composition of (sn-1 + sn-2) for 1,2 diacyl diglyceride acetates and sn-2 of 1-O-alkyl-2-acyl diglyceride acetates and lysoplasmalogen is determined by GLC of fatty acid methyl esters generated by treatment of the lipid with 6% H_2SO_4 in methanol for 12 hours at 80°C [Mueller et al., 1982] or BF_3 in methanol [Mauco et al., 1984]. Heptadecanoate is added during esterification in order to allow quantification of the fatty acids and hence the 1,2 diacyl and ether subclasses, keeping in mind that each mole of methyl ester represents 1

TABLE I. 1,2 Diacyl and Ether Phospholipid Subclasses of Human Platelets and Their Arachidonate Content

	Arachidonate content			
	CCPL⁺ M%	%AA*	ECPL⁺⁺ M%	%AA*
Subclass				
1,2 Diacyl	81.8	23.2	36.1	60.0
1-O-alkyl-2acyl	9.7	43.7	3.5	20.4
1-O-alk-1′-enyl 2-acyl	8.8	25.1	60.4	68.4

*%AA at position sn-2 (AA-arachidonic acid).
⁺Choline-containing phospholipids, excluding sphingomyelin.
⁺⁺Ethanolamine-containing phospholipids.

mole of 1-O-alkyl-2-acyl, 1 mole of 1-O-alk-1′-enyl-2-acyl, and 0.5 mole of 1,2 diacyl PC or PE. To determine 1-O-alkyl chain distribution the intact phospholipid separated from lysoplasmalogen following acid treatment is reduced with vitride [Snyder et al., 1971] and 1-O-alkylglycerol purified by TLC (ethyl ether/hexane, 60:40, v/v). The isopropylidene derivatives are prepared [Mueller et al., 1982] and analyzed by GLC-MS analysis. In the case of sn-1 for plasmalogen, aldehydes released by acid treatment are reduced by vitride to the corresponding alcohols, which are acetylated [Waku et al., 1974] and analyzed by GLC-MS [Mueller et al., 1982].

In order to study arachidonate metabolism in platelets the cells are radiolabeled with [^{3}H]-arachidonic acid. Blood is collected in ACD as previously discussed and the platelets from 50 ml of platelet-rich plasma are resuspended in one-tenth volume of platelet-poor plasma and added to 50 μCi of [^{3}H]-arachidonate (solvent evaporated) and incubated for 1 hour at 37°C. We find that the incorporation in this time reaches a so-called steady state, that is, there is no further increase in the radiolabeling of PC, PE, and PI. The cells are then separated from unincorporated radiolabel by gel-filtration [Purdon and Smith, 1985].

Suguira et al. [1984] found that in resting macrophages there was a slow decrease in [^{3}H]-radioactivity of 1-acyl-2-[^{3}H]-arachidonoyl PC and PE and a corresponding increase in 1-O-alk-1′-enyl-2-[^{3}H]-arachidonoyl GPE and 1-O-alkyl-2-[^{3}H]-arachidonoyl GPC; similar results were shown for human platelets [Purdon and Smith, 1985]. To study this transfer of [^{3}H]-arachidonate, the cells are simply incubated at 22°C following removal of exogenous [^{3}H]-arachidonate for the time intervals desired, usually 1 to 5 hours, at which point cellular phospholipids are extracted and purified by TLC, converted to diglyceride acetates, and resolved into subclasses by TLC. Most of such transfer is assumed to be done by CoA-independent transacylation [Purdon and Smith, 1985]. Colard et al. [1986, 1984] have more thoroughly studied this transfer in rat platelets and claim the process reaches equilibrium in 5 hours.

Remodeling Reactions

In a number of other cells, it is known that the fatty acid composition of phospholipid has a higher content of the higher unsaturated fatty acids, including arachidonic acid, than would be expected based on the composition of phosphatidic acid and its incorporation into phospholipid by the de novo pathway [Holub and Kuksis, 1978; Infante, 1984]. Tetraenoic fatty acids are thought to be introduced by remodeling reactions or deacylation-reacylation cycles [Hill and Lands, 1968; Van Golde et al., 1969]. Infante [1984] has proposed alternative biosynthetic routes for the production of tetraenoic phospholipid.

In platelets both acyltransferases and transacylases have been defined. The reactions involve the acylation of a lysolipid acceptor. Acyltransferases utilize acyl-CoA, while transacylases transfer a sn-2 fatty acid esterified in phospholipid. Acyl transferases have a requirement for either acyl CoA or fatty acid and Mg, ATP, and CoA plus the necessary enzyme to generate the acyl-CoA. In the case of acyl-CoA:1-acyl-sn-glycero-3-phosphocholine acyltransferase [McKean et al., 1982] fatty acyl esters of CoASH were synthesized according to Bishop and Hajra [1980], and enzymic activity was determined at 22°C by the spectrophotometric fatty acyl-CoA transferase assay of Lands and Hart [1965]. Following transfer of the fatty acid, CoASH is liberated and reduces dithionitrobenzene to 2-nitro-thiobenzoic acid, which has an absorption maximum at 414 nm. The assay is followed in a dual beam spectrophotometer [Baker and Thompson, 1973]. Kinetic analysis demonstrated a much higher Vmax with unsaturated fatty acyl-CoAs than saturated ones.

Transacylation involves the transfer of fatty acid, usually arachidonate from intact phospholipid to a lyso phospholipid acceptor. Transacylation can be CoA dependent [Kramer et al., 1984a] or CoA independent [Kramer et al., 1983, 1984]. Platelets are radiolabeled with [^{32}H]-arachidonate and then disrupted by freeze-thawing and sonication. Platelet membranes free of cytosol are isolated by centrifugation and resuspended in buffer with lyso phospholipid acceptor. In the absence of CoA, lysoplasmenylethanolamine was the preferred acceptor, while in the presence of CoA, lysophosphatidylserine was the preferred acceptor. The donor phospholipid was mainly 1-acyl-2-[^{3}H]-arachidonoyl PC and to a lesser degree 1-acyl-2-[^{3}H]-arachidonoyl PE, while inositol lysophosphatides were not acylated contrary to the proposal of Irvine and Dawson [1979]. CoA-independent transacylation also results in acylation of 1-O-alkyl-2-lyso GPC, which is produced by a DFP-sensitive cytosolic hydrolase from PAF-acether

[Alam et al., 1983]. The transacylation of 1-O-alkyl-2-lyso GPC results exclusively in 1-O-alkyl-2-arachidonoyl GPC [Kramer et al., 1984], while acylation of 1-acyl-2-lyso PC yields predominantly 1-acyl-2-arachidonoyl PC [Mahadevappa and Holub, 1984]. The transacylation reactions discussed above are defined by the acylation of a lyso phospholipid acceptor at sn-2. Presumably in the intact cell such a lyso-acceptor is generated by PLA_2.

Following incubation of platelets with [^{3}H]-arachidonate for 1 hour at 37°C in PRP and separation of the cells from the external radiolabel by gel-filtration, the total counts are distributed approximately as follows: PC (50%), PE (25%), PI (15%), and PS (10%). In 1-radyl-2-acyl PC, 91% of the radioactivity is found in 1,2 diacyl PC; 7.5% in 1-O-alkyl-2-acyl GPC, and 1.5% in 1-O-alk-1′-enyl-2-acyl GPC. In 1-radyl-2-acyl PE, 84% of the radioactivity was found in the 1,2 diacyl PE, with 14% and 2.0% being in 1-O-alk-1′-enyl and 1-O-alkyl-2-acyl PE, respectively [Purdon and Smith, 1985]. Addition of thrombin (5 U/ml, 37°C, no stirring), results in almost a 50% deacylation of 1-acyl-2-[^{3}H]-arachidonoyl PC and PE and slight and marked transacylation of [^{3}H]-arachidonate into 1-O-alkyl-2-acyl GPC and 1-O-alk-1′-enyl-2-acyl GPE, respectively [Purdon and Smith, 1985]. The deacylation is rapid and at high levels of thrombin it is about 75% complete in 1 min; however, transacylation is slower and increases throughout a 10-min time course.

Deacylation of 1-O-alkyl-2-arachidonoyl GPC by PLA_2 can lead to the production of two agonists, PAF-acether and thromboxane A_2, as well as possible synergism between the two. The work of Purdon and Smith [1985] indicated that 1-acyl-2-arachidonoyl PC was the major source of [^{3}H]-arachidonate in human platelets. However, Benveniste et al. [1982] and Chignard et al. [1984] have measured PAF-acether and 1-O-alkyl-2-lyso GPC (after acetylation) produced in thrombin-stimulated rabbit platelets by rabbit platelet bioassay, and found that approximately a nanomole of 1-O-alkyl-2-acyl GPC/10^9 cells was deacylated. The ratio of lyso PAF-acether/PAF-acether in rabbit platelets was approximately 100.

Sources of Arachidonic Acid in Stimulated Cells

The source of arachidonic acid in thrombin-stimulated platelets has been a question in platelet biochemistry for some time. Bills et al. [1976] demonstrated deacylation of PC and PI following thrombin stimulation. Subsequently, Bell et al. [1979] proposed that PI was a major source of arachidonate due to the sequential action of PLC and diglyceride lipase on PI and the resulting diglyceride, respectively. However, the amount of arachidonate released by thrombin-stimulated platelets has been underestimated until recently. In order to quantify the arachidonate release, its interactions with cyclooxygenase and lipoxygenase must be completely inhibited. This is only accomplished with the dual inhibitor BW 775C [Smith et al., 1985]. In the presence of 100 μM BW 775C, thrombin stimulation of platelets (5 U/ml) releases well over 20 nmoles of arachidonate/10^9 cells. The cells are extracted by the method of Bligh and Dyer [1959], with heptadecanoate added as internal standard. One drop of formic acid is added to ensure recovery of the fatty acids. Subsequently arachidonate is isolated by TLC and the mass determined by GLC after methylation using BF_3 in methanol [Smith et al., 1985]. In other work, Mauco et al. [1984] have demonstrated that 4–5 nmoles of arachidonate could be released from PI. However, the release from PI cannot be a major pathway for the arachidonate release; the amount is too small. We have proposed that 1-acyl-2-arachidonoyl PC is the major source of arachidonate with 1-acyl-2-arachidonoyl PE and 1-acyl-2-arachidonoyl PI being minor sources. Mahadevappa and Holub [1986], using a similar approach, have concurred with this finding. Work already completed in our lab, using HPLC methodology to quantify deacylation in phospholipids, demonstrated that individual molecular species of 1-acyl-2-arachidonoyl PC contributed almost 15 nmoles while 1-acyl-2-arachidonoyl PE yielded only 5 nmoles of arachidonate/10^9 cells.

Phospholipase A_2

Lipomodulin has been proposed as a protein inhibitor of PLA_2 in other cells [Hirata, 1981]. In platelets A23187 mobilizes calcium [Purdon et al., 1984] and activates PLA_2 [Rittenhouse, 1982], even in the absence of activation of phospholipase C [Rittenhouse and Horne, 1984]. Phorbol esters and oleoyl acetoyl glycerol are known to synergistically increase platelet responses when added with ionophore A23187 [Sano et al., 1983; Kaibuchi et al., 1983; Kajikawa et al., 1983; Nishizuka, 1984]. Halenda et al. [1985] have observed similar synergism in the deacylation of 1-radyl-2-[^{3}H]-arachidonoyl PC in human platelets. Ten to 100 ng/ml PMA (phorbol 12-myristate 13-acetate) by itself did not deacylate 1-radyl-2-[^{3}H]-arachidonoyl PC, while 1 μM ionophore A23187 did cause some deacylation of PC, which was considerably increased by 100 ng/ml PMA. This work suggested an effect of PMA on the PLA_2 inhibitor, lipomodulin. Touqui et al. [1986] have suggested that phosphorylation of lipomodulin by protein kinase C inhibits the action of lipomodulin, thereby allowing the PLA_2 activity to increase up to a level determined by cytoplasmic free calcium.

PLA_2 is assumed to be a membrane-bound enzyme, and the initial problem in purification is solubilization of the protein. Activity (which may or may not be the same enzyme) can be solubilized by 0.18 N H_2HSO_4 [Jesse and Franson, 1979; Apitz-Castro et al., 1979], 1 M KCl and sonication [Kannagi and Koizumi, 1979; Aarsman et al., 1986], and octylglucoside [Ballou et al., 1986]. Aarsman et al. [1985] and Kannagi and Koizumi [1979] found a molecular weight of

12,000 daltons using gel chromatography in 1 M KCl. This suggested that higher molecular weights found by other workers were due to aggregation. Affinity supports have been used to purify the platelet enzyme [Aarsman, 1984; Rock and Snyder, 1975] and are mandatory for purification, as the enzyme represents less than 0.1% of the total protein.

PLA_2 can be assayed on sonicated dispersions of phospholipid or the aqueous enzyme (pH 8.0, 5 mM $CaCl_2$) can be added to the lipid dissolved in ether. Radiolabeled E. coli (that is, PE) has been used as a substrate [Jesse and Franson, 1979] and also 1-acyl-2-[^{3}H]-arachidonoyl PC. The work of Kannagi and Kaizumi [1979] in which the enzyme was shown to be most active at the transition temperature of phosphatidylcholine suggests that the mechanism of hydrolysis is comparable to pancreatic phospholipase A_2 [Verheij et al., 1981]. Thus perturbation of the bilayer by detergents such as cholate and deoxycholate, and lipids such as phosphatidic acid (perhaps also a charge effect) [Apitz-Castro et al., 1981] and diglyceride [Dawson et al., 1983] augment the activity. Perturbation of an arachidonate-rich PC bilayer phase [Kannagi et al., 1981] by PI cycle intermediates, such as phosphatidic acid and diglyceride, may facilitate PLA_2 action in stimulated platelets. The work of Smith et al. [1985] demonstrated that arachidonate was by far the major fatty acid released from thrombin-stimulated platelets, suggesting strongly that phospholipase action is selective for arachidonate-containing phospholipids.

There is probably more than one phospholipase acting in stimulated cells. The enzyme of Jesse and Franson [1979] is assayed on phosphatidylethanolamine, while that of Kannagi and Koizumi [1979] was assayed on 1-acyl-2-arachidonoyl PC. Ballou et al. [1986] claim the presence of phospholipase A_2 specific for PC and PE in human platelets; however, the PE-specific enzyme did not require calcium and may have been lysosomal in origin. Most investigators have only assayed phospholipase on 1,2 diacyl phospholipids; however, in heart tissue there are indications that phospholipases are present that are specific for both 1,2 diacyl and plasmalogen phospholipids [Wolf and Gross, 1985], and given the known incorporation of [^{3}H]-arachidonate into 1-O-alk-1′-enyl-2-acyl GPE in thrombin-stimulated platelets [Purdon and Smith, 1985] the action of phospholipase on ether lipid is indicated.

A thorough molecular species analysis of platelet 1,2 diacyl phospholipid has been reported by Mahadevappa and Holub [1982]. Recently HPLC has been applied to resolve molecular species of phospholipid. Patton et al. [1982] reported an isocratic reverse phase HPLC system that resolves molecular species of PC, PE, PS, and PI. However, this system is not amenable to quantitation due to the fact that elution of phospholipid is monitored at 206 nm, which monitors unsaturation; in addition, all subclasses are analyzed together, which can be confusing.

The approach of Blank et al. [1984] allows quantification and resolution of subclasses before the HPLC step. Following PLC hydrolysis the diglycerides are converted into benzoate derivatives and these can be monitored at 230 nm with O.D. being proportional to mass. Before HPLC these benzoates are resolved into subclasses by TLC. In order to allow on-line quantification an internal standard must be included for each subclass at the time of extraction. It is important that the hydrolysis by PLC go to completion and thus give a representative diglyceride sample. Using such an approach, the action of PLA_2 on a given molecular species in a given subclass can be assessed.

We have found that in human platelets [^{3}H]-arachidonate is incorporated into five different molecular species of 1-acyl-2-arachidonoyl PC, namely 20:4–20:4, 10:2–20:4, 18:1–20:4, 16:0–20:4, and 18:0–20:4 PC. Thrombin stimulation (5 U/ml, 5 min, 37°C) results in almost 50% deacylation of each arachidonoyl-containing molecular species and gives a total deacylation of 15 nmol for 1-acyl-2-arachidonoyl PC. The two major molecular species are 16:0–20:4 and 18:0–20:4 PC and they contributed the most arachidonate. In the case of 1-acyl-2-arachidonoyl PE the major molecular species contributing arachidonate following thrombin stimulation was 18:0–20:4 PE. Non-arachdionoyl-containing molecular species were not deacylated, indicating that phospholipase A_2 action was selective for arachidonoyl-containing molecular species of 1,2 diacyl PC and PE. Thus the application of HPLC methodology to deacylation of individual molecular species of phospholipid gives new insight into the action of phospholipase A_2.

ACKNOWLEDGMENTS

This work has been supported by N.I.H. grants HL 14217 and HL 30783 and the American Heart Association, Southeastern Pennsylvania Chapter.

REFERENCES

Aarsman AJ, Neys F, van den Bosch H (1984). A simple and versatile affinity column for phospholipase A_2. Biochim Biophys Acta 792:363–366.

Aarsman AJ, Roosenboom CFP, van Geffen GEW, van den Bosch H (1985). Some aspects of rat platelet and serum phospholipase A_2. Biochim Biophys Acta 837:288–295.

Abdel-Halim MN, Farah SI (1985). Short-term regulation of acetyl-CoA carboxylase is the key enzyme in long-chain fatty-acid synthesis regulated by an existing physiological mechanism. Comp Biochem Physiol 81B:9–19.

Adunyah SE, Dean WL (1985). Inositol triphosphate-induced Ca^{2+} release from human platelet membranes. Biochim Biophys Acta 128:1274–1280.

Agranoff BW, Murthy EB, Seguin EB (1983). Thrombin induced phosphodiesteratic cleavage of phosphatidylinositol bisphosphate in human platelets. J Biol Chem 258:2076–2078.

Aharony D, Smith JB, Silver MJ (1982). Regulation of arachidonate-induced platelet aggregation by the lipoxygenase product, 12 hydroperoxyeicosatetranoic acid. Biochim Biophys Acta 718:193–200.

Alam I, Smith JB, Silver MJ (1983). Metabolism of platelet activating factor by blood platelets and plasma. Lipids 18:534–538.

Alam I, Smith JB, Silver MJ (1983). Human and rabbit platelets form platelet-activating factor in response to calcium ionophore. Thromb Res 30:71–79.

Allan D, Cockcroft S (1982). A modified procedure for thin-layer chromatography of phospholipids. J Lipid Res 23:1373–1374.

Ando S, Kon K, Tanaka Y, Nagase S, Nagai Y (1980). Characterization of hyperlipidemia in Nagase analbuminemia rat (NAR). J Biochem 87:1859–62.

Apitz-Castro RJ, Mas MA, Cruz MR, Jain MK (1979). Isolation of homogeneous phospholipase A_2 from human platelets. Biochem Biophys Res Commun 91:63–71.

Apitz-Castro RJ, Cruz M, Mas M, Jain MK (1981). Further studies on a phospholipase A_2 isolated from human platelet plasma membranes. Thromb Res 23:347-354.

Axelrod J, Hirata F (1980). Reply. Nature 288:278–279.

Baker RR, Thompson W (1973). Selective acylation of 1-acylglycerophosphorylinositol by rat brain microsomes. J Biol Chem 248:7060–7065.

Ballas LM, Lazarow PB, Bell RM (1984). Glycerolipid synthetic capacity of rat liver peroxisomes. Biochim Biophys Acta 795:297–300.

Ballou LR, DeWitt LM, Cheung WY (1986). Substrate-specific forms of human platelet phospholipase A_2. J Biol Chem 261:3107–3111.

Bazan HEP, Sprecher H, Bazan NG (1984). De novo biosynthesis of docosahexaenoyl-phosphatidic acid in bovine retinal microsomes. Biochim Biophys Acta 796:11–19.

Bell RL, Kennerly DA, Stanford N, Majerus PW (1979). Diglyceride lipase: A pathway for arachidonate release from human platelets. Proc Natl Acad Sci USA 76:3238–3241.

Benveniste J, Chignard M, Le Couedic JP, Vargaftig BB (1982). Biosynthesis of platelet activating factor (Paf-acether). Thromb Res 25:375–385.

Benveniste J, Le Couedic JP, Polonsky J, Tence M (1977). Structural analysis of purified platelet-activating factor by lipases. Nature 269:170–173.

Berde CB, Hudson BS, Simoni RD, Sklar LA (1979). Human serum albumin. Spectroscopic studies of binding and proximity relationships for fatty acids and bilirubin. J Biol Chem 254:391–400.

Berge RK, Vollset SE, Farstad M (1980). Intracellular localization of palmitoyl-CoA hydrolase and palmitoyl CoA synthetase in human blood platelets and liver. Scand J Clin Lab Invest 40:471–278.

Berridge MJ (1983). Rapid accumulation of inositol trisphosphate reveals that agonists hydrolyze polyphosphoinositides instead of phosphatidylinositol. Biochem J 212:849–858.

Berridge MJ, Downes CP, Hanley MR (1982). Lithium amplifies agonist dependent phosphatidylinositol responses in brain and salivary glands. Biochem J 206:587–595.

Berridge MJ, Heslop JP, Irvine RF, Brown KD (1984). Inositol trisphosphate formation and calcium mobilization in Swiss 3T3 cells in response to platelet-derived growth factor. Biochem J 222:195–201.

Berridge MJ, Irving RF (1984). Inositol trisphosphate: A novel second messenger in cellular signal transduction. Nature 312:315–321.

Billah MM, Lapetina EG, Cuatrecasas P (1981). Phospholipase A_2 activity specific for phosphatidic acid. A possible mechanism for the production of arachidonic acid in platelets. J Biol Chem 256:5399–5403.

Billah MM, Lapetina EG, Cuatrecasas P (1981a). Lysophosphatidic acid potentiates the thrombin induced production of arachidonic acid metabolites in platelets. J Biol Chem 256:11984–11987.

Billah MM, Lapetina EG (1982a). Formation of lysophosphatidylinositol in platelets stimulated with thrombin or ionophore. J Biol Chem 257:5196–5200.

Billah MM, Lapetina EG (1982b). Rapid decrease of phosphatidylinositol 4,5-bisphosphate in thrombin-stimulated platelets. J Biol Chem 257:12705–12708.

Bills TK, Smith JB, Silver MJ (1976). Metabolism of [^{14}C]-arachidonate by human platelets. Biochim Biophys Acta 424:303–314.

Bishop WR, Ganong BR, Bell RM (1986). Attenuation of sn-1,2-diacylglycerol second messengers by diacylglycerol kinase. J Biol Chem 261:6993–7000.

Bishop JE, Hajra AK (1980). A method for the chemical synthesis of ^{14}C-labelled fatty acyl coenzyme A's of high specific activity. Anal Biochem 106:344–350.

Blank ML, Robinson M, Fitzgerald V, Snyder F (1984). Novel quantitative method for determination of molecular species of phospholipids and diglycerides. J Chromatogr 298:473–482.

Bligh EG, Dyer WJ (1959). A rapid method for total lipid extraction and purification. Can J Biochem Physiol 37:911–918.

Brady RO, Bradley RM, Trams EG (1960). Biosynthesis of fatty acids. Studies with enzymes derived from liver. J Biol Chem 235:3093–3098.

Brass LF, Joseph SK (1985). A role for inositol triphosphate in intracellular Ca^{2+} mobilization and granule secretion in platelets. J Biol Chem 260:15172–15179.

Brindley DN, Stenton RG (1982). Phosphatidic acid biosynthesis. In Hawthorne JN, Ansell GB (eds). "Phospholipids, New Comprehensive Biochemistry." Vol. 4. Amsterdam, NY: Elsevier Sci Pub Co, pp 179–207.

Brecher P (1983). The interaction of long-chain acyl CoA with membranes. Mol Cell Biochem 57:3–15.

Broekman J (1984). Phosphatidylinositol 4,5-biphosphate may represent the site of plasma membrane bound calcium upon stimulation of human platelets. Biochem Biophys Res Commun 120:226–331.

Broekman MJ, Ward JW, Marcus AJ (1980). Phospholipid metabolism in stimulated human platelets. J Clin Invest 66:275–283.

Broekman MJ, Ward JW, Marcus AJ (1981). Fatty acid composition of phosphatidylinositol and phosphatidic acid in stimulated platelets. J Biol Chem 256:8271–8274.

Call FL, Rubert M (1973). Diglyceride kinase in human platelets. J Lipid Res 14:466–474.

Call FL, Rubert M (1975). Synthesis of ethanoamine phosphoglycerides by human platelets. J Lipid Res 16:352–359.

Call FL, Williams WJ (1970). Biosynthesis of cytidine diphosphate diglyceride by human platelets. J Clin Invest 49:392–399.

Call FL, Williams WJ (1973). Phosphatidate phosphatase in human platelets. J Lab Clin Invest 82:663–673.

Chap H, Mauco G, Simon M, Benveniste J, Douste-Blazy L (1981). Biosynthetic labelling of platelet activating factor from radioactive acetate by stimulated platelets. Nature 289:312–314.

Chau LY, Tai HH (1981). Release of arachidonate from diglyceride in human platelets requires the sequential action of a diglyceride lipase and a monoglyceride lipase. Biochem Biophys Res Commun 100:1688–1695.

Chau LY, Tai HH (1983). Diglyceride/monoglyceride lipase pathway is not essential for arachidonate release in thrombin-activated platelets. Biochem Biophys Res Commun 113:241–247.

Chignard M, Le Couedic J, Coeffier E, Benveniste J (1984). Paf-acether formation and arachidonic acid freeing from platelet ether-linked glyceryl-phosphorylcholine. Biochem Biophys Res Commun 124:637–643.

Chignard M, Le Couedic JP, Tence M, Vargaftig BB, Benveniste J (1979). The role of platelet activating factor in platelet aggregation. Nature 279:799–800.

Cohen JD (1984). Convenient apparatus for the generation of small amounts of diazomethane. J Chromatogr 30:193–196.

Cohen P, Derksen A (1969). Comparison of phospholipid and fatty acid composition of human erythrocytes and platelets. Br J Haematol 17:359–371.

Cohen P, Derksen A, van Den Bosch (1970). Pathways of fatty metabolism in human platelets. J Clin Invest 49:128–139.

Colard O, Breton M, Bereziat G (1984). Arachidonoyl transfer from diacyl phosphatidylcholine to ether phospholipids in rat platelets. Biochem J 222:657–662.

Colard O, Breton M, Bereziat G (1986). Arachidonate mobilization in diacyl, alkylacyl and alkenylacyl phospholipids on stimulation of rat platelets by thrombin and the Ca^{2+} ionophore A23187. Biochem J 233:691–695.

Cordasco DM, Segarnick DJ, Rotrosen J (1981). Human platelet phospholipid methylation. Life Sci 29:2299–2309.

Creutz CD, Dowling LG, Kyger EM, Franson RC (1985). Phosphatidyl-specific phospholipase C activity of chromaffin granule-binding protein. J Biol Chem 260:7171–7173.

Daleo GR, Piras MM, Piras R (1974). The presence of phospholipids and diglyceride kinase activity in microtubules from different tissues. Biochem Biophys Res Commun 61:1043–1050.

Daleo GR, Piras MM, Piras R (1976). Diglyceride kinase activity of microtubules. Characterization and comparison with protein kinase and ATPase activities associated with vinblastine-isolated tubulin of chick embryonic muscles. Eur J Biochem 68:339–346.

Dangelmaier CA, Daniel JL, Smith JB (1986). Determination of basal and stimulated levels of inositol triphosphate in [^{32}P]orthophosphate-labelled platelets. Anal Biochem 154:414–419.

Daniel JL, Molish IR, Holmsen H (1980). Radioactive labelling of the adenine nucleotide pool of cells as a method to distinguish among intracellular compartments. Studies of human platelets. Biochim Biophys Acta 632:444–453.

Dawson RMC, Freinkel N, Jungawala FB, Clarke N (1971). The enzymic formation of myoinositol 1:2-cyclic phosphate from phosphatidylinositol. Biochem J 122:605–607.

Dawson RMC, Hemington NL, Irvine RF (1983). Diacylglycerol potentiates phospholipase attack upon phospholipid bilayers. Biochem Biophys Res Commun 117:196–201.

de Chaffoy de Courcelles D, Roevens P, van Belle H (1984a). 1-oleoyl-2-acetyl-glycerol (OAG) stimulates the formation of phosphatidyl 4-phosphate in intact human platelets. Biochim Biophys Res Commun 123:589–595.

de Chaffoy de Courcelles D, Roevens P, van Belle H (1984b). 12-O-tetradecanoylphorbol 13-acetate stimulates inositol lipid phosphorylation in intact human platelets. FEBS Lett 173:389–393.

Demopoulos CA, Pinckard RN, Hanahan DJ (1979). Platelet-activating factor. Evidence for 1-O-alkyl-2-acetyl-sn-glyceryl-3-phosphorylcholine as the active component. J Biol Chem 254:9355–9358.

Deykin D, Desser RK (1968). The incorporation of acetate and palmitate into lipids by human platelets. J Clin Invest 47:1590–1602.

Deykin D, Snyder D (1973). Effect of epinephrine on platelet lipid metabolism. J Lab Clin Med 82:554–559.

Diagne A, Fauvel J, Record M, Chap H, Douste-Blazy L (1984). Studies on ether phospholipid. Comparative composition of various tissues from human, rat and guinea-pig. Biochim Biophys Acta 793:221–231.

Downes P, Michell RH (1982). Phosphatidylinositol 4-phosphate and phosphatidylinositol 4,5-bisphosphate: Lipids in search of a function. Cell Calcium 3:467–502.

Dratewka-Kos E, Kindl B, Tinker DO, Hsia JC (1985). The modulation by serum albumin of rabbit platelet aggregation in response to exogenous sodium arachidonate. Can J Biochem Cell Biol 63:792–800.

Fauvel J, Bonnefis MJ, Sarda L, Chap H, Thouvenot JP, Douste-Blazy L (1981). Purification of two lipases with high phospholipase A_1 from guinea pig pancreas. Biochim Biophys Acta 663:446–456.

Feldman DA, Rounsifer ME, Weinhold PA (1985). The stimulation and binding of CTP:phosphorylcholine cytidylyltransferase by phosphatidylcholine and oleic acid vesicles. Biochim Biophys Acta 429:437–443.

Fine JB, Sprecher H (1982). Unidimensional thin layer chromatography of phospholipids on boric acid impregnated plates. J Lipid Res 23:660–663.

Fitzpatrick FA, Gorman RR (1977). Platelet rich plasma transforms exogenous prostaglandin and endoperoxide H_2 into thromboxane A_2. Prostaglandins 14:881–889.

Ganong BR, Loomis CR, Hannin YA, Bell RM (1986). Specificity and mechanism of protein C activation by sn-1,2-diacylglycerols. Proc Natl Acad Sci USA 83:1184–1188.

Gilman AG (1984). Guanidine nucleotide-binding regulatory proteins and dual control of adenylate cyclase. J Clin Invest 73:1–4.

Glatz JFC, Veerkamp JH (1985). Intracellular fatty acid-binding proteins. Int J Biochem 17:13–22.

Goldfischer S, Reddy JK (1984). Peroxisomes (microbodies) in cell pathology. Int Rev Exp Pathol 26:45–84.

Goodman DS (1958). The interaction of human serum albumin with long chain fatty acid anions. J Am Chem Soc 80:3892–3898.

Gorracci G, Francescangeli E, Horrocks LA, Poicellati G (1981). The reverse reaction of cholinephosphotransferase in rat brain microsomes. A new pathway for degradation of phosphatidylcholine. Biochim Biophys Acta 664:373–379.

Goracci G, Gresele P, Arienti G, Porrovecchio P, Nenci GG, Porcellati G (1983). Choline phosphotransferase activity in human platelets. Lipids 18:179–185.

Gusto NM, Bazan NG (1979). Phosphatidic acid of retinal microsomes contains a high proportion of docosahexaenoate. Biochem Biophys Res Commun 91:791–794.

Hajra AK (1968). Biosynthesis of acyl dihydroxyacetone phosphate in guinea pig liver mitochondria. J Biol Chem 243:3458–3465.

Hajra AK (1969). Biosynthesis of alkyl-ether containing lipid from dihydroxyacetone phosphate. Biochem Biophys Res Commun 37:486–492.

Hajra AK (1970). Acyldihydroxyacetone phosphate. Precursor of alkyl ethers. Biochem Biophys Res Commun 39:1037–1044.

Hajra AK, Bishop JE (1982). Glycerolipid biosynthesis in peroxisomes via the acyl dihydroxyacetone phosphate pathway. Ann NY Acad Sci 386:170–181.

Hajra AK, Agranoff BW (1968). Acyl dihydroxyacetone phosphate. Characterization of a ^{32}P-labelled lipid from guinea pig liver mitochondria. J Biol Chem 243:1617–1622.

Hajra AK, Burke CL, Jones CL (1979). Subcellular localization of acyl coenzyme A: Dihydroxyacetone phosphate acyltransferase in rat liver peroxisomes. J Biol Chem 254:10896–10900.

Halenda SP, Feinstein MB (1984). Phorbol myristate acetate stimulates formation of phosphatidylinositol 4-phosphate and phosphatidylinositol 4,5-bisphosphate in human platelets. Biochem Biophys Res Commun 124:507–513.

Halenda SP, Zavoico GB, Feinstein MB (1985). Phorbol esters and oleoyl acetoyl glycerol enhance release of arachidonic acid in platelets stimulated by Ca^{2+} ionophore A23187. J Biol Chem 260:12484–12491.

Hallcher LM, Sherman WR (1980). The effects of lithium ion and other agents on the activity of myo-inositol-1-phosphatase from bovine brain. J Biol Chem 255:10896–10901.

Hamberg M, Fredholm G. (1976). Isomerization of prostaglandin H_2 into prostaglandin D_2 in the presence of serum albumin. Biochim Biophys Acta 431:189–193.

Hamberg M, Svensson J, Samuelsson B (1975). Thromboxanes: A new group of biologically active compounds derived from prostaglandin endoperoxides. Proc Natl Acad Sci USA 72:2994–2998.

Haslam RJ, Davidson MML (1984). Guanine nucleotides decrease the free calcium required for secretion of serotonin from permeabilized blood platelets. Evidence of a role for a GTP-binding protein in platelet activation. FEBS Lett 174:90–95.

Haslam RJ, Lynham JA (1977). Relationship between phosphorylation of blood platelet proteins and secretion of platelet granule constituents. Biochem Biophys Res Commun 72:714–721.

Hauser G, Eichberg J (1975). Identification of cytidinediphosphate-diglyceride in the pineal gland of the rat and its accumulation in the presence of DL-propranolol. J Biol Chem 250:105–112.

Hennes AR, Awai K, Hammerstrand K, Duboff GS (1966). Carbon-14 in carboxyl carbon of fatty acids formed by platelets from normal and diabetic subjects. Nature 210:839–841.

Hess HH, Derr JE (1975). Assay of inorganic and organic phosphorus in the 0.1-0.5 nanomole range. Anal Biochem 63:607–613.

Hill EE, Lands WEM (1968). Incorporation of long-chain and polymer saturated acids into phosphatidate and phosphatidylcholine. Biochim Biophys Acta 152:645–648.

Hirata F (1981). Lipomodulin and endogenous inhibitor of phospholipase A_2. J Biol Chem 256:7730–7733.

Hirata F, Axelrod J (1980). Phospholipid methylation and biological signal transmission. Science 209:1082–1090.

Hokin LE, Hokin MR (1958). Acetylcholine and the exchange of inositol and phosphate in brain phosphoinositide. J Biol Chem 233:818–821.

Hokin MR, Hokin LE (1953). Enzyme secretion and the incorporation of ^{32}P into phospholipids of pancreas slices. J Biol Chem 203:967–977.

Holmsen H, Dangelmaier CA, Akkerman JWN (1983). Determination of levels of glycolytic intermediates and nucleotides in platelets by pulse-labelling with [^{32}P] orthophosphate. Anal Biochem 131:266–272.

Homsen H, Dangelmaier CA, Holmsen H (1981). Thrombin-induced platelet responses differ in requirement for receptor occupancy. J Biol Chem 256:9393–9396.

Holmsen H, Dangelmaier CD, Rongved S (1984). Tight-coupling of thrombin-induced acid hydrolase secretion and phosphatidate synthesis to receptor occupancy in human platelets. Biochem J 222:157–167.

Holmsen H, Day HJ, Setkowsky CA (1972). Behavior of adenine nucleotides during the platelet release reaction induced by adenosine diphosphate and adrenaline. Biochem J 129:67–82.

Holmsen H, Kaplen KL, Dangelmaier CA (1982). Differential energy requirements for platelet responses. Biochem J 208:9–18.

Holub BJ, Kuksis A (1971). Resolution of intact phosphatidylinositols by argentation thin layer chromatography. J Lipid Res 12:510–512.

Holub BJ, Kuksis A (1978). Metabolism of molecular species of diacylglycerophospholipids. Adv Lipid Res 16:1–125.

Holub BJ, Piekarski J (1978). Suitability of different molecular species of 1,2 diacylglycerol as substrates for diacylglycerol kinase in rat brain microsomes. J Neurochem 31:903–908.

Hong SL, Levine L (1976). Inhibition of arachidonic acid release from cells as the biochemical action of anti-inflammatory corticosteroids. Proc Natl Acad Sci USA 73:1730–1734.

Hotchkiss A, Jordan JV, Hirate F, Shulman NR, Axelrod J (1981). Phospholipid methylation and human platelet function. Biochem Pharm 300:2089–2095.

Houslay MD, Bojanic D, Wilson A (1986). Platelet activating factor and U44069 stimulate a GTPase activity in human platelets which is distinct from guanine nucleotide regulatory proteins, Ns and Ni. Biochem J 234:737–740.

Hsieh JYK, Welch DK, Turcotte JG (1981). High pressure liquid chromatographic separation of molecular species of phosphatidic acid methyl esters derived from phosphatidylcholine. Lipids 16:761–763.

Imai A, Yana K, Kemeyama Y, Nozawa Y (1981). Reversible thrombin-induced modification of positional distribution of fatty acids in platelet phospholipids. Biochem Biophys Res Commun 103:1092–1099.

Imai A, Nakashima S, Nozawa Y (1983). The rapid polyphosphoinositide metabolism may be a triggering event for the thrombin-mediated stimulation of human platelets. Biochem Biophys Res Commun 110:108–115.

Infante JP (1984). Biosynthesis of acyl-specific glycerophospholipids in mammalian tissues. Postulation of new pathways. FEBS Lett 170:1–14.

Irving RF, Dawson RMC (1979). Transfer of arachidonic acid between phospholipids in rat liver microsomes. Biochem Biophys Res Commun 91:1399–1405.

Irving RF, Hemington N, Dawson RMC (1977). Phosphatidylinositol-degrading enzymes in liver lysosomes. Biochem J 164:277–280.

Jesse RL, Franson RC (1979). Modulation of purified phospholipase A_2 activity from human platelets by calcium and indomethacin. Biochim Biophys Acta 575:467–470.

Jolles J, Zwiers H, Dekku A, Wirtz KWA, Gispan WH (1981). Corticotropic-(1-24)-tetracosapeptide affects protein phosphorylation and polyphosphoinositide metabolism in rat brain. Biochem J 194:283–291.

Jones CL, Hajra AK (1980). Properties of guinea pig liver peroxisomal dihydroxyacetone phosphate acyltransferase. J Biol Chem 255:8289–8295.

Kaibuchi K, Takai Y, Sawamura M, Hoshijima M, Fujikura T, Nishizuka Y (1983). Synergistic functions of protein phosphorylation and calcium mobilization in platelet activation. J Biol Chem 258:6701–6704.

Kajikawa N, Kaibuchi K, Matsubara T, Kikkawa U, Takai Y, Nishizuka Y (1983). A possible role of protein kinase C in signal-induced lysosomal enzyme release. Biochem Biophys Res Commun 116:743–750.

Kameyama Y, Yoshioka S, Imai A, Nozawa Y (1983). Possible involvement of 1-acylglycerophosphorylinositol acyltransferase in arachidonate enrichment of phosphatidylinositol in human platelets. Biochim Biophys Acta 752:244–250.

Kannagi R, Koizumi K (1979). Effect of different physical states of phospholipid substrates on partially purified platelet phospholipase A_2 activity. Biochim Biophys Acta 556:423–433.

Kannagi R, Koizumi K, Masuda T (1981). Limited hydrolysis of platelet membrane phospholipids. J Biol Chem 256:1177–1184.

Kannagi R, Koizumi K, Hata-Tanoue S, Masuda T (1980). Mobilization of arachidonic acid from phosphatidylethanolamine fraction to phosphatidylcholine fraction in platelets. Biochem Biophys Res Commun 96:711–718.

Kanoh H, Ono T (1984): Utilization of diacylglycerol in phospholipid bilayer by pig brain diacylglycerolkinase and Rhizopus arrhizus lipae. J Biol Chem 259:11197–11202.

Kato M, Homma Y, Nagai Y, Takenawa T (1985). Epidermal growth factor stimulates diacylglycerol kinase in isolated plasma membrane vesicles from A431 cells. Biochem Biophys Res Commun 129:375–380.

Kato H, Ishidate K, Nakazawa Y (1984). Developmental changes in molecular species of phosphatidic acid in rat lung and liver during the perinatal stage. Biochim Biophys Acta 796:262–268.

Koreh K, Monaco ME (1986). The relationship of hormone-sensitive and hormone-insensitive phosphatidylinositol to phosphatidylinositol 4,5-bisphosphate in the WRK-1 cell. J Biol Chem 261:88–91.

Kraigh-Hansen U (1981). Molecular aspects of ligand binding to albumin. Pharmacol Rev 33:17–53.

Kramer R, Deykin D (1983). Arachidonoyl transacylase in human platelets. Coenzyme A-independent transfer of arachidonate from phosphatidylcholine to lysoplasmenylethanolamine. J Biol Chem 258:13806–13811.

Kramer RM, Patton GM, Pritzker CR, Deykin D (1984). Metabolism of platelet activating factor in human platelets. Transacylase-mediated synthesis of 1-O-alkyl-2-arachidonoyl-sn-glycero-3-phosphocholine. J Biol Chem 259:13316–13320.

Kramer RM, Pritzher CR, Deykin D (1984a). Coenzyme A-mediated arachidonic acid transacylation in human platelets. J Biol Chem 259:2403–2406.

Kuksis A (1984). Quantitative and positional analysis of fatty acids. Lab Res Methods Biol Med 10:77–131.

Lands WEM, Hart P (1965). Metabolism of glycerolipids. Specificities of acyl coenzyme A:phospholipid acyltransferase. J Biol Chem 240:1905–1911.

Lapetina EG (1984). Prostacyclin inhibition of phosphatidic acid synthesis in human platelets is not mediated by protein kinase C. Biochem Biophys Res Commun 120:37–44.

Lapetina EG (1986). Incorporation of synthetic 1,2 diacyl-glycerol into platelet phosphatidylinositol is increased by cyclic AMP. FEBS Lett 195:111–114.

Lapetina EG, Reep B, Ganong BR, Bell RM (1985). Exogenous sn-1,2-diacylglycerols containing saturated fatty acids function as bioregulators of protein kinase C in human platelets. J Biol Chem 260:1358–1361.

Lecompte T, Randon J, Chignard M, Vargaftig BB, Dray F (1982). Interference of transmethylation inhibitors with thromboxane synthesis in rat platelets. Biochem Biophys Res Commun 106:566–573.

Lee TC, Malone B, Wasserman SI, Fitzgerald V, Snyder F (1982). Activities of enzymes that metabolize platelet activating factor in neutrophils and eosinophils from humans and the effect of calcium ionophore. Biochem Biophys Res Commun 105:1303–1308.

Lenstra R, Mauco G, Chap H, Douste-Blazy L (1984). Studies on enzymes related to diacylglycerol production in activated platelets. Biochim Biophys Acta 792:199–206.

Lewis N, Majerus PW (1969). Lipis metabolism into human platelets. De novo phospholipid synthesis and the effect of thrombin on the pattern of synthesis. J Clin Invest 48:2114–2123.

Lloyd JV, Mustard JF (1974). Changes in ^{32}P-content of phosphatidic acid and the phosphoinositides of rabbit platelets during aggregation induced by collagen or thrombin. Br J Haem 26:243–253.

Lloyd JV, Nishizawa EE, Haldon I, Mustard JF (1972). Changes in ^{32}P-labelling of platelet phospholipids in response to ADP. Br J Haem 23:571–585.

Lloyd JV, Nishizawa EE, Joist JH, Mustard JF (1973). Effect of ADP-induced aggregation on ^{32}P incorporation into phosphatidic acid and the phosphoinositides of rabbit platelets. Br J Haem 24:589–604.

Lin CH, Bishop H, Strickland KP (1986). Properties of diacylglycerol kinase purified from bovine brain. Lipids 21:206–211.

Lucas CT, Call FL, Williams WJ (1970). The biosynthesis of phosphatidylinositol in human platelets. J Clin Invest 49:1949–1955.

Ludwig JC, Hoppens CL, McManus LM, Mott GE, Pinckard RN (1985). Modulation of platelet-activating factor synthesis and release from human polymorphonuclear leukocytes (PMN): Role of extracellular albumin. Arch Biochem Biophys 241:337–347.

MacIntyre DE, McNicol A, Drummond AH (1985). Tumor-promoting phorbol esters inhibit agonist induced phosphatidate formation and Ca^{2+} flux in human platelets. FEBS Lett 180:160–164.

MacLouf J, Kindahl H, Granstrom E, Samuelson B (1980). Interactions of prostaglandin H_2 and thromboxane A_2 with human serum albumin. Eur J Biochem 109:561–566.

Mahadevappa VG, Holub BJ (1982). The molecular species composition of individual diacyl phospholipids in human platelets. Biochim Biophys Acta 713:73–79.

Mahadevappa VG, Holub BJ (1983). Degradation of different molecular species of phosphatidylinositol in thrombin-stimulated human platelets. J Biol Chem 258:5337–5339.

Mahadevappa VG, Holub BJ (1984). The incorporation of [^{3}H]-glycerol and [1-^{14}C]-acyl-sn-glycero-3-phosphocholine into different molecular species of phosphatidylcholine in human platelets. Can J Biochem Cell Biol 62:827–830.

Mahadevappa VG, Holub BJ (1986). Diacylglycerol lipase pathway is a minor source of released arachidonic acid in thrombin-stimulated human platelets. Biochem Biophys Res Commun 134:1327–1333.

Majerus PW, Smith MB, Clamon GH (1969). Lipid metabolism in human platelets. Evidence for a complete fatty acid synthesizing system. J Clin Invest 48:156–163.

Majerus PW, Wilson DB, Connolly TM, Bross TE, Neufield EJ (1985). Phosphoinositide turnover provides a link in stimulus-response coupling. TIBS: April, 168–171.

Matsuzawa Y, Hostetler KY (1980). Properties of phospholipase C isolated from rat liver lysosomes. J Biol Chem 255:646–652.

Mauco G, Chap H, Douste-Blazy L (1978). Phosphatidic and lysophosphatidic acid production in phospholipase C- and thrombin-treated platelets. Possible involvement of a platelet lipase. Biochimie 60:653–661.

Mauco G, Chap H, Douste-Blazy L (1979). Characterization and properties of a phosphatidylinositol phosphodiesterase (Phospholipase C) from platelets. FEBS Lett 149:367–370.

Mauco G, Chap H, Douste-Blazy L (1983). Platelet activating factor promotes an early degradation of phosphatidylinositol-4,5-bisphosphate in rabbit platelets. FEBS Lett 153:361–365.

Mauco G, Dangelmaier CA, Smith JB (1984). Inositol lipids, phosphatidate, diacylglycerol share stearoylarachidonoyl as a common backbone in thrombin-stimulated human platelets. Biochem J 224:933–940.

Mauco G, Fauvel J, Chap H, Douste-Blazy L (1984a). Studies on enzymes related to diacylglycerol production in activated platelets. Biochim Biophys Acta 196:169–177.

McKean ML, Smith JB, Silver MJ (1982). Phospholipid biosynthesis in human platelets. Formation of phosphatidylcholine from 1-acyl lysophosphatidylcholine by acyl-CoA 1-acylophosphatidylcholine by acyl-CoA 1-acyl-sn-glycerol-3-phosphocholine acyltransferase. J Biol Chem 256:1522–1524.

Michell RH (1975). Inositol phospholipids and cell surface receptor function. Biochim Biophys Acta 415:81–147.

Michell R (1986). Inositol phosphates. Profusion and confusion. Nature 319:176–177.

Monaco ME (1982). The phosphatidylinositol cycle in WRK-1 cells. J Biol Chem 257:2137–2139.

Mori K, Taniguichi S, Kurnada K, Nakazawa K, Fujiwara M, Fujiwara M (1983). Enzymic properties of phospholipid methylation in rabbit platelets. Thromb Res 29:215–224.

Mueller HW, O'Flaherty J, Wykle RL (1982). Ether lipid content and fatty acid distribution in rabbit polymorphonuclear neutrophil phospholipids. Lipids 17:72–77.

Mueller HW, Purdon AD, Smith JB, Wykle RL (1983). 1-O-alkyl-linked phosphoglycerides of human platelets: Distribution of arachidonate and other acyl residues in the ether-linked and diacyl species. Lipids 18:814–819.

Nakagawa Y, Horrocks LA (1983). Separation of alkenylacyl, alkylacyl and diacyl analogues and their molecular species by high performance liquid chromatography. J Lipid Res 24:1268–1275.

Natarajan V, Zuzarte-Augustin M, Schmid HHO, Graff G (1983). The alkylacyl and alkenylacyl glycerophospholipids of human platelets. Thromb Res 30:119–126.

Naughton JM (1981). Supply of polyenoic fatty acids to the mammalian brain. Int J Biochem 13:21–32.

Neufeld EJ, Majerus PW (1983). Arachidonate release and phosphatidic acid turnover in stimulated human platelets. J Biol Chem 258:2461–2467.

Neufeld EJ, Sprecher H, Evans RW, Majerus PW (1984). Fatty acid structural requirements for activity of arachidonyl CoA synthetase. J Lipid Res 25:288–293.

Ninio E, Menscia-Huerta JM, Heymans F, Benveniste J (1982). Biosynthesis of platelet activating factor. Evidence for an acetyl-transferase activity in murine macrophages. Biochim Biophys Acta 710:23–31.

Nishizuka Y (1984). The role of protein kinase C in cell surface signal transduction and tumor promotion. Nature 308:693–697.

Nordoy A, Bjorge J, Strom E (1973). Comparison of the main lipids in platelets and plasma in man. Acta Med Scand 193:59–64.

Ockner RK, Manning JA, Kane JP (1982). Fatty acid binding protein. Isolation from liver; characterization and immunochemical quantification. J Biol Chem 257:7872–7878.

Oglesby TD, Gorman RR (1984). The inhibition of arachidonic acid metabolism in human platelets by RHC 80267, a diacylglycerol lipase inhibitor. Biochim Biophys Acta 793:269–277.

Okuma M, Yamashita S, Numa S (1973). Enzymic studies on phosphatidic acid synthesis in human platelets. Blood 41:379–389.

O'Rourke FA, Halenda SP, Zavoico GB, Feinstein MB (1985). Inositol 1,2,5-triphosphate releases calcium from calcium-transporting membrane vesicle fraction derived from human platelets. J Biol Chem 260:956–962.

Packham MA, Guccione MA, Nina M, Kinlough-Rathbone RL, Mustard JF (1984). Effect of Tris on responses of human and rabbit platelets to aggregating agents. Thromb Haemost 51:140–144.

Patton G, Fasulo JM, Robbins SJ (1982). Separation of phospholipids and individual molecular species by high performance liquid chromatography. J Lipid Res 23:190–196.

Pelech SL, Cook HW, Paddon HB, Vance DE (1984a). Membrane-bound CTP: Phosphocholine cytidylyltransferase regulates the rate of phosphatidylcholine synthesis in HeLA cells treated with unsaturated fatty acids. Biochim Biophys Acta 795:433–440.

Pelech SL, Paddon HB, Vance DE (1984b). Phorbol esters stimulate phosphatidylcholine biosynthesis by translocation of CTP:phosphocholine cytidylyltransferase from cytosol to microsomes. Biochim Biophys Acta 795:447–451.

Pelech SL, Vance DE (1984). Regulation of phosphatidylcholine biosynthesis. Biochim Biophys Acta 779:217–251.

Peter T (1970). Serum albumin. Adv Clin Chem 13:37–111.

Pittner RA, Fears R, Brindly DN (1985). Interactions of insulin, glucagon, and dexamethasone in controlling the activity of glycerol acyltransferase and the activity and subcellular lular distribution of phosphatidate phosphohydrolase in cultured rat hepatocytes. Biochem J 230:525–534.

Plantavid M, Rossignol L, Chap H, Douste-Blazy L (1986). Studies of endogenous polyphosphoinositide hydrolyis in human platelet membranes. Biochim Biophys Acta 875:147–156.

Pollock K, Armstron RA, Brydon LJ, Jones RL, MacIntyre DE (1984). Thromboxane-induced phosphatidate formation in human platelets. Relationship to receptor occupancy and to changes in cytosolic free calcium. Biochem J 219:833–842.

Preiss J, Loomis CR, Bishop WR, Stein R, Niedel JE, Bell RM (1986). Quantitative measurement of sn-1,2 diacylglycerols present in platelets, hepatocytes, and vas- and cis-transformed normal rat kidney cells. J Biol Chem (In Press).

Prescott SM, Majerus PW (1981). The fatty acid composition of phosphatidylinositol thrombin-stimulated human platelets. J Biol Chem 256:579–582.

Prescott SM, Majerus PW (1983). Characterization of 1,2 diacylglycerol hydrolysis in human platelets. J Biol Chem 258:764–769.

Purdon AD, Daniel JL, Stewart GJ, Holmsen H (1984). Cytoplasmic free calcium concentration in porcine platelets. Regulation by an intracellular non-mitochondrial calcium pump and increase after thrombin stimulation. Biochim Biophys Acta 800:178–187.

Purdon AD, Smith JB (1985). Turnover of arachidonic acid in the major diacyl and ether phospholipids of human platelets. J Biol Chem 260:12700–12704.

Quinn PJ (1973). The association between phosphatidylinositol phosphodiesterase activity and a special subunit of microtubular protein in rat brain. Biochem J 133:273–281.

Randon J, Lecompte T, Chignard M, Seiss W, Marfas G, Dray F, Vargaftig BB (1981). Dissociation of platelet activation from transmethylation of their membrane phospholipids. Nature 293:660–662.

Rendu F, Marche P, Maclou J, Girard A, Levy-Toledano S (1983). Triphosphoinositide breakdown and dense body release as the earliest events in thrombin induced activation of human platelets. Biochem Biophys Res Commun 116:513–519.

Renkonen O (1966). Individual molecular species of phospholipids. Molecular species of ox-brain lecithins. Biochim Biophys Acta 125:288–309.

Renkonen O (1968). Mono and dimethyl phosphatidates from different subtypes of choline and ethanolamine glycerophosphatides. Biochim Biophys Acta 152:114–135.

Renooij W, Snyder F (1981). Biosynthesis of 1-O-alkyl-2-acetyl-sn-Glycero-3-phosphocholine (platelet activating factor and a hypotensive lipid) by cholinephosphotransferase in various rat tissues. Biochim Biophys Acta 663:545–556.

Rittenhouse SE (1982). Inositol lipid metabolism in the response of stimulated platelets. Cell Calcium 3:311–322.

Rittenhouse SE (1983). Human platelets contain phospholipase C that hydrolyzes phosphoinositides. Proc Natl Acad Sci USA 80:5417–5420.

Rittenhouse SE (1984). Activation of human platelet phospholipase C by ionophore A23187 is totally dependent upon cyclo-oxygenase products and ADP. Biochem J 222:103–110.

Rittenhouse SE, Horne WC (1984). Ionomycin can elevate intraplatelet CA^{2+} and activate phospholipase A_2 without activating phospholipase C. Biochem Biophys Res Commun 123:393–397.

Rittenhouse-Simmons SE (1979). Production of diglyceride from phosphatidylinositol in activated human platelets. J Clin Invest 63:580–587.

Rittenhouse-Simmons SE (1980). Indomethacin induced accumulation of diglyceride in activated human platelets. The role of diglyceride lipase. J Biol Chem 255:2259–2262.

Rittenhouse-Simmons SE (1981a). Differential activation of platelet phospholipases by thrombin and ionophore A23187. J Biol Chem 256:4153–4155.

Rittenhouse-Simmons W, Deykin D (1981b). Release and metabolism of arachidonic acid in human platelets. In Gordon JL (ed) "Platelets in Biology and Pathology, II." Amsterdam, NY: Elsevier/North-Holland, Biomedical Press, pp 349–372.

Rittenhouse-Simmons S, Russel FA, Deykin D (1977). Mobilization of arachidonate acid in human platelets, kinetics and Ca dependency. Biochim Biophys Acta 488:370–380.

Rock CO, Snyder F (1975). Rapid purification of phospholipase A_2 from croatalus adamanteus venum by affinity chromatography. J Biol Chem 250:6564–6566.

Rouser G, Siabotos AN, Fleisher S (1966). Quantitative analysis of phospholipids by thin layer chromatography and phosphorus analysis of spots. Lipids 1:85–86.

Sano K, Takai Y, Yamanishi J, Nishizuka Y (1983). A role of calcium-activated phospholipid dependent kinase in human platelet activation. J Biol Chem 258:2010–2013.

Schick PK, Shick BP, Foster K, Block A (1984). Arachidonate synthesis and uptake in isolated guinea-pig megakaroycytes and platelets. Biochim Biophys Acta 795:341–347.

Schukla SD, Hanahan DJ (1983). An early transient decrease in phosphatidylinositol 4,5 bisphophate upon stimulation of rabbit platelets with acetylglyceryletherphosphorylcholine. Arch Biochem Biophys 227:626–629.

Schwartz DP, Bright RS (1974). A column procedure for esterification of organic acid with diazomethane at the microgram level. Anal Biochem 61:271–274.

Seiss W, Lapetina EG (1983). Properties of distribution of phosphatidylinositol-specific phospholipase C in human and horse platelets. Biochim Biophys Acta 752:329–338.

Shafrir E, Gatt S, Khasis S (1965). Partition of fatty acids of 20-24 carbon atoms between serum albumin and lipoproteins. Biochim Biophys Acta 98:365–373.

Shattil SJ, McDonough M, Burch JW (1981). Inhibition of platelet phospholipid methylation during platelet secretion. Blood 57:537–544.

Skipski VP, Good JJ, Barclay M, Reggio RB (1968). Quantitative analysis of simple lipid classes by thin layer chromatography. Biochim Biophys Acta 152:10–19.

Skipski VP, Peterson RF, Barclay M (1964). Resolution of phospholipids by thin layer chromatography. Biochem J 90:374–378.

Smith JB, Dangelmaier C, Mauco G (1985). Measurement of arachidonic acid liberation in thrombin-stimulated human platelets. Use of agents that inhibit both the cyclooxygenase and lipoxygenase enzymes. Biochim Biophys Acta 835:344–351.

Snyder F, Blank M, Wykle RL (1971). The enzymic synthesis of ethanolamine plasmalogens. J Biol Chem 246:3539–3645.

Snyder F, Godfrey P (1961). Collecting $^{14}CO_2$ in a Warburg flask for subsequent scintillation counting. J Lipid Res 2:195.

Snyder F, Malone B, Blank ML (1970). Enzymic synthesis of O-alkyl bonds in glycerolipids. J Biol Chem 245:1790–1799.

Spector AA (1968). The transport and utilization of free fatty acids. Ann NY Acad Sci 149:768–683.

Spector AA (1975). Fatty acid binding to plasma albumin. J Lipid Res 16:165–179.

Spector AA, Hoak JC, Warner ED, Fry GL (1970). Utilization of long chain free fatty acids by human platelets. J Clin Invest 49:1489–1496.

Spector AA, Santos EC (1973). Influence of free fatty acid concentration on drug binding to plasma albumin. Ann NY Acad Sci 226:247–258.

Sturton RG, Brindley DN (1978). Problems encountered in measuring the activity of phosphatidate phosphohydrolase. Biochem J 171:263–266.

Suguira T, Katayama O, Fukui J, Nakagawa Y, Waku K (1984). Mobilization of arachidonic acid between diacyl and ether phospholipids in rabbit alveolar macrophages. FEBS Lett 165:273–276.

Suguira T, Waku K (1984). Enhanced turnover of arachidonic acid-containing species of phosphatidylinositol and phosphatidic acid of concanavalin A-stimulated lymphocytes. Biochim Biophys Acta 796:190–198.

Tamer AE, Record M, Fauvel J, Chap H, Douste-Blazy L (1984). Studies on ether lipids. A new method of determination using PLA_1 from guinea pig pancreas. Biochim Biophys Acta 793:213–220.

Tangen O, McKinnon EL, Berman HJ (1973). On the fine structure and aggregation requirements of gel filtered platelets. Scand J Haemat 10:96–105.

Tence M, Jouvin-March E, Besson G, Record M, Benveniste J (1985). Ether phospholipid composition in neutrophils and platelets. Thromb Res 38:207–214.

Touqui L, Rothhut B, Shaw AM, Fradin A, Vargaftig BB, Russo-Marie F (1986). Platelet activation—a role for a 40K anti-phospholipase A_2 protein indistinguishable from lipocortin. Nature 321:177–180.

Vance DE, de Kruijff B (1980). The possible functional significance of phosphatidylethanolamine methylation. Nature 288:277–278.

Vallset SE, Forstad M (1979). A study of assay conditions for palmitoyl-CoA synthetase and carnitine palmitoyltransferase in homogenates of human blood platelets. J Clin Lab Invest 39:15–21.

Vallset SE, Forstad M (1980). Intracellular localization of palmitoyl-CoA hydrolase and palmitoyl-CoA synthetase in human blood platelets and liver. Scand J Clin Lab Invest 40:271–278.

Van Golde LMG, Scherphof GL, van Deenen LLLM (1969). Biosynthetic pathways in the formation of individual molecular species of rat liver phospholipids. Biochim Biophys Acta 176:635–637.

Verheij HM, Slotboom AJ, deHaas GH (1981). Structure and function of phospholipase A_2. Rev Physiol Biochem Pharmacol 91:92–203.

Verhoeven A, Horvli O, Holmsen H (1986). Is polyphosphatidylinositol turnover increased upon platelet activation. TIBS 11:67–68.

Vickers JD, Kinlough-Rathbone RL, Mustard JF (1982). Changes in phosphatidylinositol 4,5-bisphosphate 10 seconds after stimulation of washed rabbit platelets with ADP. Blood 60:1247–1250.

Vickers JD, Kinlough-Rathbone RL, Mustard JF (1984a). Changes in the platelet phosphoinositides during the first minute after stimulation of washed rabbit platelets with thrombin. Biochem J 219:25–31.

Vickers JD, Kinlough-Rathbone RL, Mustard JF (1984b). Accumulation of the inositol phosphates in thrombin-stimulated, washed rabbit platelets in the presence of lithium. Biochem J 224:399–405.

Waku K, Ito H, Bito T, Nakazawa Y (1974). Fatty chains of acyl, alkenyl, and alkyl phosphoglycerides of rabbit sarcoplasmic reticulum. J Biochem 75:1307–1312.

Walseth TF, Johnson RA (1979). The enzymic preparation of [α^{32}P] nucleoside triphosphates, cyclic [^{32}P]AMP, and cyclic [^{32}P]GMP. Biochim Biophys Acta 562:11–31.

Wanders RJA, van Weringh G, Schrakamp G, Tager JM, van den Bosch H, Schutgens RBH (1985). Deficiency of acyl-CoA: Dihydroxyacetone phosphate acyltransferase in thrombocytes of Zellweger patients: A simple postnatal diagnostic test. Clin Chimica Acta 151:217–221.

Watson SP, McConnell RT, Lapetina EG (1984). The rapid formation of inositol phosphates in human platelets by thrombin is inhibited by prostacyclin. J Biol Chem 259:13199–13203.

Watson SP, Lapetina EG (1985): 1,2 diacylglycerol and phorbol ester inhibit agonist-induced formation of inositol phosphates in human platelets: Possible implications for negative feedback regulation of inositol phospholipid hydrolysis. Proc Natl Acad Sci USA 82:2623–2626.

Wilson JE (1978). Ambiquitous enzymes: Variations in intracellular distribution as a regulatory mechanism. TIPS 3:124–125.

Wilson DB, Bross TE, Hofmann SL, Majerus PW (1984). Hydrolysis of polyphosphoinositides by purified sheep seminal vesicle phospholipase C enzymes. J Biol Chem 259:11718–11724.

Wilson DB, Bross TE, Sherman WR, Berger RA, Majerus PW (1985). Inositol cyclic phosphates are produced by cleavage of phosphatidylinositols with purified sheep seminal vesicle phospholipase C enzymes. Proc Natl Acad Sci USA 82:4013–4017.

Wilson D, Neufeld E, Majerus P (1985b). Phosphoinositide interconversion in thrombin-stimulated human platelets. J Biol Chem 260:275–283.

Wilson DB, Prescott SM, Majerus PW (1982). Discovery of an arachidonoyl Coenzyme A synthetase in human platelets. J Biol Chem 257:3510–3515.

Wilson TM, Connolly TE, Bross PW, Majerus PW, Sherman WR, Tyler AN, Rubin LJ, Brown JE (1985). Isolation and characterization of the inositol cyclic phosphate products of polyphosphoinositide cleavage by phospholipase C. J Biol Chem 260:13496–13501.

Wolf RA, Gross RW (1985). Phospholipase in cardiac tissue. J Biol Chem 260:7295–7303.

Wykle RL, Snyder F (1969). The glycerol source for the biosynthesis of alkyl glyceryl ethers. Biochem Biophys Res Commun 37:658–662.

Wykle RL, Snyder F (1970). Biosynthesis of an O-alkyl analogue of phosphatidic acid and O-alkylglycerols via O-alkyl ketone intermediates by microsomal enzymes of Ehrlich ascites tumor. J Biol Chem 245:3047–3058.

Wykle RL, Snyder F (1976). Microsomal enzymes involved in the metabolism of ether-linked glycerolipids and their precursors in mammals. In Martouosi A (ed): "Enzymes of Biological Membranes." New York: Plenum Press, Vol. 2, pp 87–117.

Wykle RL, Malone B, Snyder F (1980). Enzymic synthesis of 1-alkyl-2-acetyl-sn-glycero-3-phosphocholine, a hypotensive and platelet-aggregating lipid. J Biol Chem 255:19256–10260.

Zavoico GB, Halenda SP, Sha'afi RI, Feinstein MB (1985). Phorbol myristate acetate inhibits thrombin-stimulated Ca^{2+} mobilization and phosphatidylinositol 4,5-bisphosphate hydrolysis in human platelets. Proc Natl Acad Sci USA 82:3859–3862.

Modern Methods in Pharmacology, Volume 4
Methods for Studying Platelets and Megakaryocytes, pages 267–286

Methods of Studying Platelet-Secreted Proteins and the Platelet Cytoskeleton

George P. Tuszynski, Hanna I. Switalska, and Karen Knudsen

INTRODUCTION

The purpose of this chapter is to present methods that we have found useful in the study of the platelet cytoskeleton and platelet-secreted proteins. Each method is prefaced with a short introduction stressing the principle of the method and how the procedure has helped us answer questions concerning the platelet cystoskeleton and platelet-secreted proteins. It is our hope that the reader will benefit from our experience and use these techniques toward the resolution of other problems in the platelet field or in other areas of cell biology.

PREPARATIVE METHODS

Platelet Washing

The most important procedure in the study of platelet-secreted proteins and the platelet cytoskeleton is choosing the best platelet washing procedure. Almost everyone who works with platelets has his or her own procedure that has been adapted from published procedures to suit specialized needs. We routinely use two procedures. For analytical work, platelet aggregation studies, and the studies of the platelet cytoskeleton, we employ the method of gel-filtration based on the procedures described by Tangen et al. [1971] and Timmons and Hawiger [1978]. For isolation of platelet glycoproteins and platelet-secreted proteins, which require a large number of platelets, we employ the centrifugal method of Mustard et al. [1972].

During gel-filtration, plasma proteins are removed from platelets by retention in the included volume of Sepharose 2B while platelets elute in the excluded

From the Departments of Platelet Hematology and Cell Biology, Lankenau Medical Research Center, Philadelphia, Pennsylvania 19151.

H.I. Switalska is on sabbatical leave from the Institute of Hypertension and Angiology, Academy of Medicine, Warsaw, Poland.

volume. Large proteins, such as von Willebrand's factor, are incompletey removed [Koutts et al., 1978] during filtration so that a prior centrifugation step is required. Platelet buffers for gel-filtration must contain at least 1 mg/ml bovine serum albumin (BSA); otherwise, unacceptable platelet activation occurs with concomitant platelet aggregation and loss of most of the platelets at the top of the column. The centrifugal procedure of Mustard et al. [1972] relies on low pH and addition of heparin and apyrase to prevent platelet activation during centrifugation. Heparin and apyrase act to reduce the levels of the platelet-activating agents thrombin and ADP, respectively. One important consideration in this procedure is choosing the proper apyrase concentration, since commercial preparations differ in purity and activity.

Platelet Washing by Gel Filtration

Reagents

HEPES buffered Tyrode's solution, pH 7.3[a]

Compound	Molecular weight	Concentration (mM)	Weight (g/L for 10X sol.)
HEPES[b]	238.3	3.1	9.0
$NaH_2PO_4.H_2O$	137.9	4.00	5.52
NaCl	58.4	137.0	80.0
KCl	74.6	2.6	2.0
$MgCl_2.6H_2O$	203.3	1.0	3.7
Dextrose	180.2	5.6	10.0

[a]Bovine serum albumin (1.0 g/L added to a final concentration to the 1X dilution just before use). This buffer is adjusted to the correct pH with concentrated NaCl and NaOH is stored as a 10× stock with no albumin at −70°.
[b]N-2-hydroxyethylpiperazine-N′-2-ethanesulfonic acid.

Column. A 50-ml plastic syringe is fitted with a porous polyethylene plug. Fifty ml of crosslinked Sepharose 2B is washed by gently slurring with 100 ml of acetone in a Buchner funnel and applying a weak vacuum such that a moist cake is obtained. The washing procedure is repeated once with acetone and twice with distilled water. The column is packed and washed with 150 ml of HEPES buffered Tyrode's solution containing albumin. The column may be used repeatedly. When it is not used for extended periods, it should be stored at 4°C in 10% ethanol-water.

Platelet-rich plasma (PRP). Whole blood is collected by venipuncture into citrate (9 parts blood into 1 part 3.8% Na Citrate, pH 7.4). The blood is centrifuged at room temperature at 140 × g for 15 min (900 rpm for a rotor having a radius of 5.5 in). The top platelet-rich layer is carefully removed, counted for platelets, and used immediately.

Gel-filtration. The buffer level on the equilibrated column is permitted to drop until the top of the resin is just moist. Buffer flow is stopped by pinching shut a short section of latex tubing inserted on the bottom of the column. Five ml of PRP is allowed to flow through the column. After all the PRP solution has entered the resin and the top of the column is still moist, the column is stopped and 10 ml of HEPES-buffered Tyrode's solution containing albumin is carefully layered on the column. Column elution is continued at approximately one drop every second. One-ml fractions are collected. Additional buffer is applied to the top of the column until a total of 20 fractions are collected. Platelets will elute in about 7 fractions, which can be identified by their obvious turbidity. The three most concentrated fractions are pooled and usually give a platelet count of 2 × 10^8 platelets/ml. Columns should be washed with at least 7 column volumes before a second sample of PRP is applied.

Platelet Washing by Centrifugation

Reagents

HEPES buffered Tyrode's solution, pH 7.3 (see above)

Acid-citrate-dextrose (ACD)

Compound	Molecular weight	Concentration (mM)	Weight (g/L for 1× sol.)
Dextrose	180.16	180	32.43
Tri-Na-Citrate	294.10	80	23.53
Citric acid	192.13	52	9.99

Apyrase, 500 units/ml, Grade VII, Sigma.
Heparin, 1,000 units/ml.

Equipment

Centrifuge with 500-ml swinging bucket rotor
500-ml Nalgene screw-top bottles
50-ml screw-top Falcon conical tubes

Procedure. Before drawing blood prepare the following solutions:

Solution 1: 40 ml HEPES containing 500 units of heparin (0.5 ml of 1,000 units/ml stock heparin), 50 μl apyrase, 140 mg BSA, pH to 7.3

Solution 2: 40 ml HEPES containing 50 μl apyrase and 140 mg BSA, pH 7.3

Solution 3: 30 ml HEPES, pH 7.3, containing no $MgCl_2$

Draw 450 ml of blood into a 500-ml Nalgene Bottle containing 60 ml ACD for each unit of blood. Use a 16-gauge needle and tubing from a Travenol blood collection set. With the aid of another person gently mix the blood with the ACD during collection.

Perform all centrifugations at room temperature. Centrifuge the blood for 40 min at 1,100 rpm using a rotor with a radius of 5.0 inches (approximately 140 × g). Remove the top platelet-rich plasma (PRP) and place in 50-ml tubes. If PRP contains numerous red cells, centrifuge 50-ml tubes[1] for 20 min at 2,500 rpm (approximately 3,000 × g) to sediment platelets. Remove supernatants, combine pellets by gently resuspending each pellet in a small volume (e.g., 1–2 ml) of solution 1 with a siliconized glass Pasteur pipette. After the pellets are combined and resuspended, the remaining volume (e.g., 38–39 ml) of solution 1 is added and the platelet suspension incubated in a water bath at 37°C for 20 min. The platelets are centrifuged for 15 min at 2,500 rpm, the supernatant discarded, and the pellet resuspended in solution 2 and the suspension incubated for 20 min at 37°C. After the incubation the platelets are centrifuged again. At this point the pellet can be resuspended either in solution 3 for the isolation of TSP or in HEPES buffer containing BSA for preparation of Triton-insoluble cytoskeletons or for use in aggregation studies.

Preparation of Platelet-Released Proteins

Reagents

Ice water 1 M DFP (diisopropyl fluorophosphate) dissolved in anhydrous dimethylformamide (DMF). Note DFP is highly toxic and should be aliquoted into 0.5-ml samples dissolved in a nonvolatile solvent such as DMF treated with molecular sieves to remove water. Aliquots should be sealed in glass vials and stored in a desiccated container until needed. All operations must be performed in a fume hood and antidotes must be readily available in case of accidental poisoning.

1 M epsilon amino caproic acid (EACA)

Leupeptin (10 mg/ml)

19 mM Ca ionophore A23187 in dimethylsulfoxide (DMSO) (10 mg/ml)

Solution 1, 30 ml HEPES buffer, pH 7.3, containing no albumin and no Mg^{+2} (see above)

Procedure. Suspend the platelet pellet obtained from washing three units of blood obtained in the final step of the centrifugal method (see above) in solution 1. Before aggregating the platelets, check the pH of the suspension and if necessary adjust the pH to 7.3 by addition of a microdrop of 1 M NaOH to the cap of the 50-ml centrifuge tube containing the platelets. Place the cap on the tube and quickly invert several times. In this manner the platelets are not lysed by the NaOH.

Before addition of ionophore solution to the platelets, fill a beaker with ice water and a syringe with a protease inhibitor cocktail containing 150 μl EACA, 20 μl DFP, and 70 μl leupeptin.

[1]At 1,100 rpm for 10 min and remove PRP. Centrifuge PRP in 50 ml tubes.

Add 1.0 μl of ionophore solution to the cap of the tube containing the platelet suspension, secure the cap, and invert the tube gently several times. The platelets should aggregate within 2 min. After maximum aggregation is achieved (i.e., the platelets form large visible clumps), add the inhibitor cocktail and immerse the tube in ice water for 5 min to cool the suspension. Centrifuge the suspension for 20 min at 10,000 $\times$ g at 4°C. Remove the supernatant carefully from the pellet, making sure the supernatant is platelet free. Freeze the supernatant and pellet at −70°C until needed.

Comments. It is essential to prevent platelet lysis during the release reaction induced by ionophore. For example, levels of ionophore above 1–5 μM can induce significant platelet lysis, which results in proteolysis of thrombospondin. Also, if the platelet-released protein solution contains uncentrifuged platelets, platelet lysis can be induced during freezing and thawing of the solution. This proteolysis is presumably due to release of the calcium-activated protease.

Triton-Insoluble Platelet Cytoskeleton (CK)

We have observed the association of numerous platelet alpha granule proteins and cell surface glycoproteins important in platelet aggregation with the Triton-insoluble cytoskeleton of thrombin activated platelets [Tuszynski et al., 1985a]. We postulate that the CK functions to anchor platelet surface receptor systems essential in maintaining the structure of the platelet-fibrin clot. The following procedure has been developed to rapidly isolate the CK from thrombin-activated platelets [Tuszynski et al., 1982].

Reagents

100 ml HEPES buffered Tyrode's solution, pH 7.3, containing 1 mg/ml BSA
100 ml HEPES buffered Tyrode's solution, pH 7.3, containing 0.5% Triton X-100
1 M DFP
Leupeptin (10 mg/ml)
Human thrombin (100 units/ml)
Hirudin (1,000 units/ml)
20% Triton X-100

Equipment

Microcentrifuge
Sonicator with microtip
Column for gel-filtration

Procedure. Gel-filter 5 ml of PRP and combine the peak tubes. Stimulate unstirred platelets for 3 min by adding 10 μl thrombin solution (1 unit/ml) to 1 ml of suspension. Stop the activation and prevent proteolysis by addition of 1 μl of DFP, 10 μl of hirudin, and 2 μl of leupeptin for every ml of suspension. Lyse the platelets by adding 25 μl of the Triton solution per ml of suspension. Vortex the suspension and immediately spin in a microcentrifuge for 2 min at 10,000 × g. Wash the residue from 10^8 platelets two times with 1 ml each of 0.5% Triton in HEPES and one time in HEPES buffer containing albumin. The final pellet is suspended in the buffer of choice by brief sonication. One ml of 10^8 platelets yields 14 μg of washed cytoskeletons.

Comments. The cytoskeletal preparation obtained by this procedure contains actin, myosin, and associated proteins. Microtubules are not preserved. Glycolipid [Schick et al., 1983] and lipids essential for the functional activity of the prothrombinase complex are nearly quantitatively retained [Tuszynski et al., 1984a]. Fibrin and GPIIb-GPIIIa essential for platelet aggregation and clot retraction are also retained [Tuszynski et al., 1984b], as is platelet fibronectin [Niewiarowska et al., 1984].

Protein Purification

Fast protein liquid chromatography (FPLC). We have recently been purifying plasma proteins and platelet-secreted proteins using the Pharmacia system of rapid protein purification. The system offers new high-flow matrix materials that can rapidly perform traditional protein separation by ion exchange, gel-filtration, isoelectric focusing, and hydrophobic affinity chromatography with high resolution. The following procedure is a modification of that described by Clezardin et al. [1984] for the purification of thrombospondin (TSP).

Reagents. 200 ml of 20 mM HEPES, pH 7.3 (buffer A); 200 ml of 20 mM HEPES, pH 7.3, containing 1 M NaCl (buffer B).

Equipment. Mono Q anion exchange column (Pharmacia) and Pharmacia FPLC system.

Procedure. Program the gradient marker for a 20-ml linear gradient starting with buffer A and terminating with buffer B: flow rate 1 ml per min, full scale 0–1 absorbance units. Equilibrate the column with 10 ml of buffer A. Load 30 ml of platelet-released proteins prepared from three units of blood as described above at a flow rate of 1 ml/min. Wash the column in manual mode with buffer A until no absorbance is detected in the wash (about 10 ml). Start the gradient. At the beginning of each peak, manually hold the gradient until the peak has eluted, and then restart the program. After all peaks have eluted, wash the column with 5 M NaOH and 70% acetic acid. Equilibrate system in 10% ethanol-water for prolonged periods or buffer B for overnight.

comments. A typical column elution profile is shown in Figure 1. Approximately 1 mg of highly purified TSP was obtained.

Affinity chromatography. We have developed a rapid procedure for the purification of TSP, utilizing fibrinogen affinity chromatography [Tuszynski et

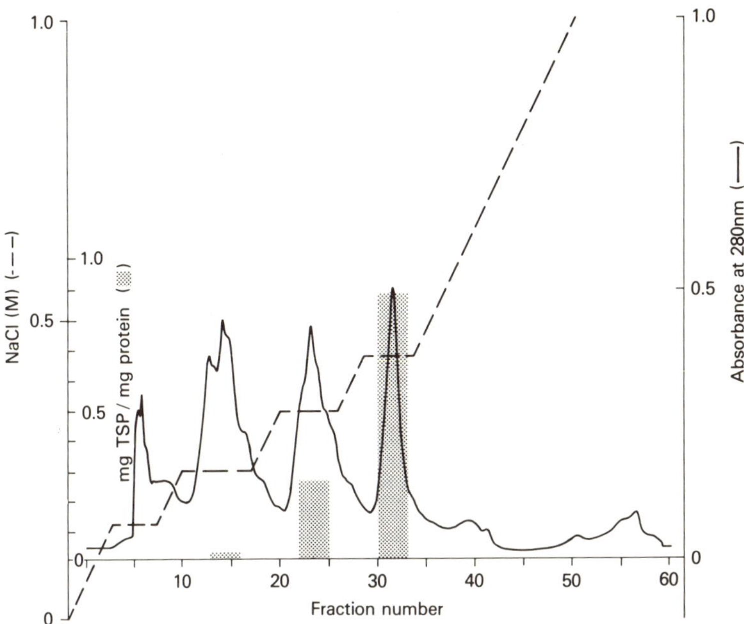

Fig. 1. Elution profile of TSP purification on fast protein liquid chromatography. TSP levels were determined by ELISA.

al., 1985b]. The procedure yields approximately 1.5 mg of highly pure TSP from three units of blood. The technique can also be used to study the interaction of TSP with fibrinogen.

Reagents

Cyanogen bromide-activated Sepharose 4B (Pharmacia)
Fibrinogen (Kabi)
200 ml of 1 mM HCl
500 ml of 0.1 M $NaHCO_3$, pH 8.3, containing 0.5 M NaCl (coupling buffer)
500 ml of 0.1 M Na acetate, pH 4.0, containing 0.5 M NaCl
10 ml of 10 M ethanolamine HCl, pH 8.3 (buffered ethanolamine solution)
100 ml HEPES buffered Tyrode's solution, pH 7.3 (buffer 1)
100 ml buffer 1, containing 0.5% Triton, 1 mM DFP, 50 μM leupeptin, 5.0 mM EACA (buffer 2)
100 ml buffer 1, containing 0.40 M NaCl (buffer 3)

Preparation of column. Weigh 1 g of cyanogen bromide-activated Sepharose and place in sintered glass filter. Wash with 200 ml l-mM HCl using a gentle suction that never permits the swollen gel to go dry. Transfer moist gel to a 5-ml solution of 10 mg/ml fibrinogen dissolved in coupling buffer. Rock the suspension gently overnight at 4°C. At the end of the coupling period, 0.5 ml of ethanolamine solution is added and the suspension rocked for an additional 2 hours. The gel is then filtered and washed successively with 30-ml portions of coupling buffer, acetate buffer, coupling buffer, and HEPES-buffered Tyrode's solution. The gel is stored in HEPES buffer at 4°C and used the following day.

TSP chromatography on fibrinogen-Sepharose. An LKB column (diameter, 1.2 cm, overall length, 13 cm, fitted with flow adaptors) is packed with 5 ml of washed fibrinogen-Sepharose. Apply 30 ml of platelet-released protein solution (see above) at a flow rate of 30 ml/h after addition of 1 mM $CaCl_2$. Calcium ion protects TSP from proteolysis and stabilizes its conformation. After all the extract has passed through the column, reapply it a second and third time to ensure maximum adsorption of TSP. Wash the column with 50 ml of buffer 1. Invert column and elute with buffer 3 at 7.5 ml/h. Peak fractions of TSP are rapidly frozen in liquid nitrogen until further needed. Although the column can be regenerated by washing successively with coupling buffer and acetate buffer as described above, best results are obtained with freshly prepared matrix.

Comments. The SDS-gel of fractions eluted from a fibrinogen-Sepharose column are shown in Figure 2. Peak fractions contained from 200–300 μg/ml TSP.

Gel electrophoresis and protein elution. Gel electrophoresis is a powerful method for the separation of proteins. To complement this technique, we have developed a rapid method for the recovery of proteins from gel slices. The method involves electroelution protein from unfixed, unstained gel slices [Tuszynski et al., 1977]. The procedure was originally designed for SDS-gels but can be adapted for any gel system. A special elution apparatus is required, which can easily be constructed in any machine shop. Plans are available upon request.

Reagents. 5 liters of 0.012 M Tris (Tris(hydroxymethyl)aminomethane)—0.045 M glycine, pH 8.3, containing 0.05% SDS.

Equipment. Elution apparatus.

Procedure. Fill gel chambers with minced gel particles. Fill remainder of apparatus with elution buffer, avoiding the trapping of air bubbles in any chamber of the apparatus. Electroelute gels for 3 hours at 50-mA constant current, 300 volts.

Comments. A diagram of the elution apparatus is shown in Figure 3. We can typically recover 70–80% of protein having less than 50,000 MW. For non-SDS gels that were run under alkaline conditions, use the elution buffer without SDS.

Antibody Production

Production of monospecific antibodies is of paramount importance when these reagents are used in the identification and quantitation of platelet antigens.

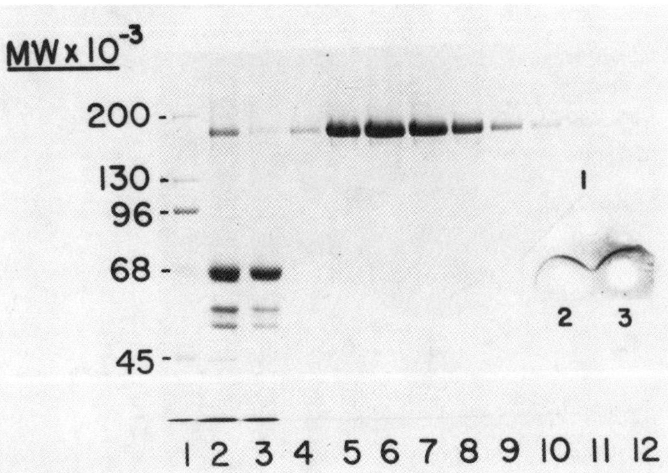

Fig. 2. SDS gel of TSP eluted from fibrinogen-Sepharose and analyzed by double immunodiffusion against anti-TSP antibody. Twenty-μl aliquots of platelet-released proteins before and after passage through fibrinogen-Sepharose and 20μl aliquots of 0.40 M NaCl column eluants were analyzed on an 8% polyacrylamide slab gel. Lane 1, molecular weight standards; lane 2, platelet-released proteins before passage over column; lane 3, platelet-released proteins after passage over column; lanes 4–12, successive fractions eluted with 0.40 M NaCl. Inset, double immunodiffusion against anti-TSP antibody. Well 1, 8 μl of anti-TSP antiserum produced from TSP purified by this procedure; wells 2 and 3, 8 μl of 0.2 μg/ml TSP purified as described by Lawler et al. [1978] and by this procedure, respectively. Reproduced from Tuszynski et al. [1985].

Antigens purified by SDS-gels usually produce high titer and specific antibodies. SDS-gel purified antigens may be eluted from gels as described above and injected to rabbits for antibody production. However, in cases where antigen is scarce and difficult to purify owing to contaminating protein bands of similar molecular weight, a procedure has been developed by Knudsen [1985] that utilizes the transfer of proteins to nitrocellulose paper and injection of the solubilized paper into rabbits. After transfer, the paper is stained to accurately identify the protein bands, which are then excised with a razor blade.

Reagents. Reagents for SDS-gels, see below.

5 liters of transfer buffer—0.027 M NaH_2PO_4, 0.126 M Na_2HPO_4, containing 10% methanol

Staining solution—0.05% amido black in 10% acetic acid and 45% methanol

Nitrocellulose paper

Dimethyl sulfoxide (DMSO)

Freund's complete and incomplete adjuvant

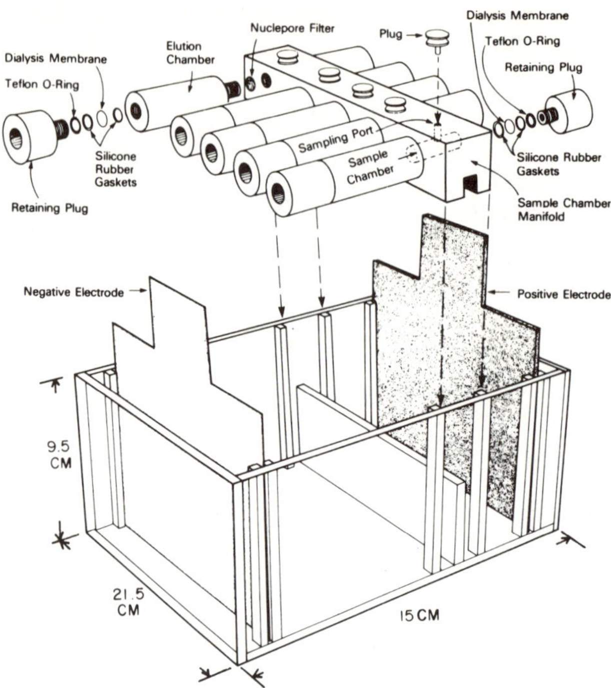

Fig. 3. Apparatus for electrophoretic elution of polyacrylamide gels. Reproduced from Tuszynski et al. [1977].

Equipment. Electrophoretic transblot apparatus and slab gel electrophoresis apparatus.

Procedure. Separate approximately 10–20 μg of antigen on an SDS slab gel using the gel buffer system described by Laemmli [1970]. Transfer the separated protein bands to nitrocellulose paper overnight at 10–15°C at a constant current of 400 mA. After transfer, stain paper for 10 min with staining solution and destain in water, or if proteins are radioactive prepare an autoradiogram. Localize bands of interest, excise, and thoroughly dry under a stream of nitrogen. Dissolve nitrocellulose paper containing the protein of interest in a minimum volume of DMSO. Note the paper must be thoroughly dry in order to completely dissolve in DMSO. Mix dissolved antigen with an equal volume of complete Freund's adjuvant and inject the mixture subcutaneously into a rabbit at four sites. Use incomplete Freund's adjuvant for subsequent injections.

ANALYTICAL METHODS

Gel Electrophoresis

Polyacrylamide gel electrophoresis (PAGE) has greatly advanced the field of protein chemistry by providing protein separation techniques unsurpassed in resolution and speed. The theory of discontinuous gels was first advanced by Ornstein [1964]. Ornstein showed that proteins could be concentrated into thin zones or stacks in the stacking gel region of a discontinuous gel system. In his best known alkaline system, proteins would stack between Cl^-, the ion of highest mobility, and glycinate, the ion of lowest mobility. Once the stack of proteins reaches the running or resolving gel they unstack and separate. Final resolution depends on the intrinsic mobility of the proteins as well as the size of the protein. The highly quoted system of Laemmli [1970] utilizes Ornstein's alkaline system with the addition of SDS, sodium dodecyl sulfate, a denaturing detergent that binds to proteins, equalizing their charge to net negative. Protein-SDS complexes separate in the resolving gel primarily according to size. Most of the gel systems, such as the Laemli system, were originally described for tube gels but have been modified for slab gels essentially according to Studier [1973].

Reagents

100 ml of 40% acrylamide containing 1.05% bisacrylamide

100 ml of 0.5 M Tris-HCl, pH 6.8, containing 0.4% SDS (4× stock stacking buffer)

100 ml of 1.5 M Tris-HCl, pH 8.8, containing 0.4% SDS (4× stock separating buffer)

1,000 ml of 0.25 M Tris, 1.92 M glycine, pH 8.3, containing 1.0% SDS (10× stock electrode buffer)

2% ammonium persulphate prepared fresh weekly

Tetramethylethylenediamine (TEMED)

50 ml of 0.25 M Tris-HCl, pH 6.8, containing 8% SDS, 40% glycerol, 0.004% bromophenol blue (4× sample buffer)

5 liters of 0.025% Coomassie blue R-250 in 25% isopropyl alcohol, 15%acetic acid (staining solution)

5 liters 7% acetic acid (destaining solution)

Equipment. Studier type slab gel electrophoresis chamber.

Procedure. For a typical 8% 1.5-mm-thick polyacrylamide Studier slab gel, prepare a final volume of 25 ml of separating gel solution containing 6.25 ml of 4× separating buffer, 5 ml of the acrylamide stock, 1.25 ml of 2% ammonium persulfate (0.1% final concentration) and 12.5 μl of 100% TEMED added with mixing to the side of the graduated cylinder after the final volume was adjusted with water. The glass plates are filled a distance of 12 cm from the bottom and then carefully overlayered from the sides with water. After the gel has polymerized, the water is poured off, the sample well former (comb) inserted, and 10 ml of 5% acrylamide stacking gel solution poured (prepared by the addition of 1.25 ml acrylamide stock, 2.5 ml of 4× stock stacking buffer, 0.5 ml persulfate, 5 μl TEMED). After polymerization, the well former is removed. Samples are made once in sample buffer containing either no reducing agent or 3 mM dithiothreitol.

Samples are heated in boiling water for 5 min before application to the gel. Slabs are run for 2.5–3.0 hours at 30 mA constant current, stained overnight on an orbital shaker, and destained with 7% acetic acid the following day.

Comments. Do not attempt to adjust the pH of the electrode buffer with HCl if it is not exactly 8.3. The recipe should give a pH within 0.1 pH units of 8.3. Addition of Cl^- to the electrode buffer adversely affects protein stacking and hence resolution of the gel system.

Immunoblotting

The following procedure is a modification of the original procedure described by Towbin et al. [1979]. Proteins are transferred electrophoretically from polyacrylamide gels to nitrocellulose sheets and detected immunologically using peroxidase-conjugated antibodies.

Reagents

5 liters of transfer buffer—0.027 M NaH_2PO_4, 0.126 M Na_2HPO_4, containing 10% methanol

100 ml of TBS (20 mM Tris-HCl, pH 7.5, containing 0.15 M NaCl)

100 ml of TTBS (TBS containing 0.05% Tween 20)

20 ml of 3% BSA in TBS

100 ml of 20 mM Tris-HCl, pH 8.2, containing 0.15 M NaCl (buffer A)

50 ml of developing solution (10 mg 4-chloro naphthol dissolved in 3 ml ethanol added to 47 ml of buffer A containing 50 μl 30% H_2O_2

Equipment. Slab gel apparatus and electrophoretic transfer apparatus.

Procedure. Transfer the separated protein bands from the polyacrylamide slab to nitrocellulose paper overnight at 10–15°C at a constant current of 400 mA. Block unoccupied sites on nitrocellulose paper by incubating paper with 20 ml of BSA in TBS for 20 min. Wash paper three times by soaking for 5 min in TTBS.

Incubate the paper for 2 hours with the first rabbit antibody diluted (usually 1:100) in TTBS containing 1% BSA. Give the paper three 5-min washes in TTBS, and while shaking incubate for 2 hours with peroxidase conjugated goat antirabbit diluted (usually 1:500) in TTBS containing 1% BSA. Give the paper three 5-min washes in TTBS followed by one wash in TBS. Develop paper for 1 hour in developing solution. Rinse paper with TBS and store in dry, dark place.

Comments. This is a very powerful technique that can be used for determination of structure-function relationships. For example, using immunoblotting we demonstrated the specificity of antibodies to various domains of fibrinogen in an effort to characterize the thrombospondin binding domain in fibrinogen [Tuszynski, 1985b]. This experiment is illustrated in Figure 4.

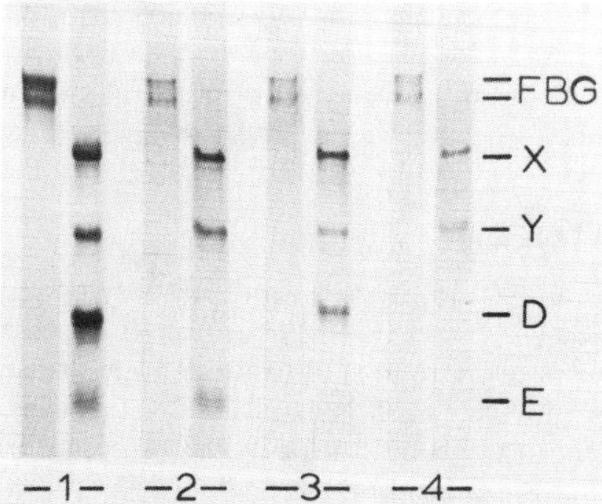

Fig. 4. Characterization of fibrinogen antisera by immunoblotting. Nonreduced fibrinogen (FBG) and its plasmin digestion products, fragments X, Y, D, and E, were separated on a 5% polyacrylamide-SDS slab gel, and the resolved protein bands were transferred to nitrocellulose paper. Within each pair of samples shown, whole fibrinogen is on the left and a mixture of plasmin fragments on the right. The paired samples were treated as follows: lane 1, gel stained with Coomassie Brilliant Blue; lane 2, transfer-stained with anti-E; lane 3, transfer-stained with anti-D; lane 4, transfer stained with anti-A alpha. Reproduced from Tuszynski et al. [1985].

Immunoprecipitation

Immunoprecipitation is a method of isolating proteins based on the ability of a specific antibody to bind a particular antigen even in the presence of numerous unrelated antigens. The method works best when a small subset of radioactive cellular proteins is probed with a highly monospecific antibody. We have used this technique to show that platelet surface proteins labeled with ^{125}I are associated with the platelet cytoskeleton [Tuszynski et al., 1984a]. The following procedure is based on the method described by Kessler [1975], using a fixed suspension of staphylococcal as the source of the protein A immunoadsorbent.

Reagents

100 ml of a 10% formalin fixed suspension of *Staphylococcus aureus,* Cowan I (Staph) in phosphate buffered saline containing 0.2% azide

100 ml of 20 mM Tris-HCl, pH 7.4, containing 0.15 M NaCl 0.5% Nonidet P-40 (buffer 1)

Monospecific rabbit antisera

Radiolabeled antigen solution

Equipment. Microcentrifuge.

Procedure. Wash 5 ml of Staph suspension twice in buffer 1 by centrifugation in a microcentrifuge and keep on ice. Incubate 10 μl of antisera and 10 μl of

^{125}I labeled platelet extract (approximately 200,000 cpm) for 1 hour at 37°C. Add 100 μl of the washed Staph suspension to the incubation mixture to adsorb the antigen-antibody complex. Incubate on ice for 10 min. Wash Staph pellet three times in buffer 1. Elute pellet with SDS sample and analyze proteins by SDS gels.

Platelet Protein Labeling

Platelet surface. We developed a rapid and easy procedure for the ^{125}I-labeling of platelets [Tuszynski et al., 1983]. Platelet suspensions are placed in vials coated with Iodogen, a solid-phase oxidizing agent similar to chloramine-T, and treated with ^{125}I. Analysis of the labeled platelet proteins revealed that the same major protein species were labeled by this procedure as were labeled by procedures utilizing lactoperoxidase.

Reagents

Two-ml septum-capped vials
Iodogen (Pierce Chem. Co.)
Chloroform
Carrier free $Na^{125}I$
Washed platelet suspension containing no more than 1 mg/ml BSA and less than 2×10^8 platelets/ml

Preparation of Iodogen-coated vials. Two-milliliter septum-capped glass vials are coated with 100 μg of Iodogen in the following manner: inject each vial with 100 μl of chloroform containing 100 μg Iodogen. Evaporate the chloroform by means of a syringe needle fitted to a vacuum source. Insert the syringe needle into the septum and with the vacuum on slowly rotate the vial on its side until all the chloroform is evaporated, leaving a thin coat of Iodogen deposited on the sides of the glass. Vials can be stored in a desiccated container at 4°C until needed.

Procedure. Add 1 ml of platelet suspension to glass vial coated with Iodogen. Inject tracer (1 μCi) and wait 15 min. Remove platelets with a syringe and pellet them in a microcentrifuge. Wash the pellet once in HEPES-buffered Tyrode's solution, pH 7.3. The pellet can be dissolved in detergent solution for use in immunoprecipitation or SDS-gels.

Comments. Optimum platelet labeling is achieved if the platelets are suspended in albumin free solution or buffers containing less than 1 mg/ml BSA. Dilute platelet suspensions on the order of 10^8 platelets/ml show the highest incorporation of label.

Purified proteins. Iodogen-coated vials can be also used to label isolated proteins. Usually glass vials give excellent recovery of protein; however, if problems are encountered with glass, Iodogen-coated plastic vials can be substituted. Labeling will take place over a wide range of neutral and alkaline pH. Most buffers will not interfere. Reducing agents such as dithiothreitol will interfere, however. Labeling best occurs at protein concentrations in excess of 1 mg/ml. Unreacted tracer can be removed by centrifugation through small columns of G-25 [Tuszynski et al., 1980].

Reagents

Iodogen-coated vials

Sephadex G-25 medium grade equilibrated in buffer in which protein is dissolved

Carrier free ^{125}I-Iodide

Procedure. The protein solution is placed in an Iodogen-coated vial, the ^{125}I added with a syringe, and the reaction allowed to continue for 15 min. The labeled protein is removed from the vial with a syringe and added to a small volume of carrier protein such as albumin, which brings the protein concentration of the sample to 5 mg/ml. This allows for efficient recovery of tracer during the removal of unbound iodine.

Unbound iodine is removed by centrifuging the protein solution a small column of G-25. To do this a small microcentrifuge tube is pierced at the bottom and plugged with a small ball of siliconized glass wool. The tube is then filled with 1.3 ml of G-25 slurry and placed piggyback into a 12 $\times$ 75mm plastic culture tube (Falcon 2058), which serves as holder and collection tube during centrifugation. The combination is spun at 200 $\times$ g in either a fixed-angle rotor or swing-out rotor for 2 min. After centrifugation the tube should have at least 1 ml of packed resin. If necessary additional slurry is added and the column is centrifuged and the collection tube emptied. The column is now ready for removal of unbound iodine. No more than 200 μl of reaction mixture is added to the column and spun. Free iodine is retained in the column and the protein travels with the void volume into the collection tube.

QUANTITATIVE METHODS

Enzyme Linked Immunosorbent Assay (ELISA)

The ELISA utilizes the sensitivity of an enzyme reaction to measure antibody-antigen complex formation [Engval, 1980]. In the ELISA, antibody in solution binds to an antigen immobilized in the well of a microtiter plate. The antigen-antibody complex on the plate is recognized by an enzyme-conjugated second antibody specific against the first antibody. After addition of the appropriate substrate solution, the second antibody generates a colored product (by means of its bound enzyme) in proportion to the amount of the first antibody.

In a competitive ELISA, antigen in solution competes for binding of the first antibody to the antigen immobilized on the plate. Therefore, an increase in free antigen (standard or unknown solution) results in a decrease binding of first antibody and, thus, decrease binding of second antibody and decrease generation of the colored product.

The following competitive ELISA has been developed for the quantitation of thrombospondin in plasma and other solutions.

Reagents

200 ml of Voller's buffer, 15 mM Na_2CO_3, 34.8 mM $NaHCO_3$, 0.02% NaN_3, pH 9.6, stored at 4°C up to 2 weeks

1.0 liter PBS-T, 0.02 M Na_2HPO_3, pH 7.2, containing 0.15 M NaCl, 0.05% Tween-20, stored at room temperature up to 4 weeks

100 ml of 1% BSA in Voller's buffer

Thrombospondin (TSP) solutions: 20 ml of 0.375 μg TSP/ml in Voller's buffer (TSP plate coating solution), 0.5-40 ng TSP/110 μl in PBS-T (TSP standard solution)

5 ml of 1:1,000 dilution of rabbit antihuman TSP in PBS-T

1 liter Zn-Mg buffer: 0.1 M glycine, pH 10.4, containing 1 mM $ZnCl_2$

1 mM $MgCl_2$, stored for 4 weeks at room temperature or freeze in aliquots

5 ml of a 1:800 dilution of alkaline phosphatase-conjugated goat antirabbit IgG in PBS-T

40 ml of 1 mg/ml p-nitrophenylphosphate in Zn-Mg buffer

40 ml of 2 M NaOH

96-well microtiter plates (Costar #3590)

Equipment. ELISA microplate reader and ELISA washer (optional).

Procedure. Prepare several 96-well plates coated with albumin or TSP by incubating each well with either 200 μl of TSP in coating solution (75 ng TSP/well) or 250 μl of 1% BSA in Voller's buffer overnight at 4°C. After removal of solutions and three 300-μl/well washes with PBS-T, coated plates can be stored at 4°C for up to 1 month.

One hundred ten μl of TSP standard solution containing TSP amounts of 0.5 to 40 ng or 110 μl of various dilutions of the unknown solution in PBS-T are added to wells of BSA-coated plates followed by 110 μl of anti-TSP solution (1:1,000). The plate is covered with parafilm and incubated overnight at 4°C. The next morning, the solutions are transferred to TSP-coated wells and incubated at room temperature for 30 min. Wells are then emptied, washed three times with 300 μl of PBS-T, and incubated for 90 min at room temperature with 200 μl of a 1:800 dilution of alkaline phosphatase conjugated goat antirabbit IgG solution. Wells are again emptied, washed three times with 300 μl of PBS-T, and incubated for 30 min at room temperature with 200 μl of substrate solution. The reaction is stopped by the addition of 50 μl of 2 M NaOH and the resulting color read at 405 nm in a microplate ELISA reader. Appropriate controls for each assay should include samples containing antibody and no TSP, TSP alone, TSP and second antibody, substrate alone, and second antibody alone. Concentrations of unknown samples are calculated from comparison to the standard curve.

Comments. The optimum dilution of first and second antibody and optimum amount of TSP covering the plates should be determined empirically by each new investigator. This is accomplished by preparing standard curves using cells coated with varying amounts of TSP and TSP incubated with various amounts of first antibody. The concentration of the second antibody is usually not limiting but must be low enough not to give high background absorbance readings. An example of a standard curve obtained with TSP is shown in Figure 5. The assay can detect levels of TSP in plasma on the order of 50 ng/ml.

Radioimmunoassay (RIA)

The technique of RIA [Yalow and Berson, 1960] is a highly sensitive method for measuring the concentration of antigen in solution. The procedure is based on the ability of cold antigen to compete with radiolabeled antigen (tracer) for antibody binding. Typically, radioactive antigen is incubated with limiting amounts of antibody such that 30–50% of the tracer is bound in an antibody-antigen complex in the absence of cold competing antigen. With the addition of increasing cold antigen, less radioactive antigen is bound in the antibody-antigen complex. The antibody-antigen complex is isolated by immunoprecipitation, and the decrease in immunoprecipitated radioactivity is proportional to the cold antigen added. RIA procedures have been developed to measure the concentration of platelet-secreted proteins such TSP [Dawes et al., 1983] and platelet factor 4-related antigens [Rucinski et al., 1979]. The following is a procedure developed in our laboratory for the measurement of TSP by RIA [Switalska et al., 1985].

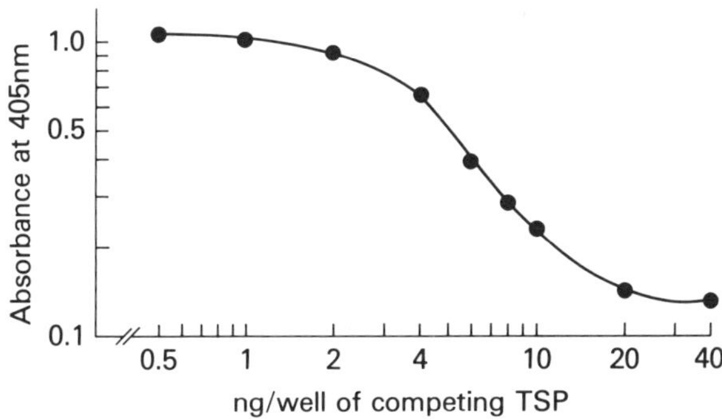

Fig. 5. Standard TSP competition curve for TSP ELISA assay.

Reagents

Borate buffer: 100 ml of 0.10 M borate buffer, pH 8.3, containing 2% normal rabbit serum (NRS) and 1% Triton X-100 (borate buffer)

Purified TSP dissolved in borate buffer, final concentrations of 0.75–50 ng/ml

^{125}I labeled TSP (see below)

Rabbit antihuman-thrombospondin antiserum (1 ml)

100 ml of goat antirabbit IgG diluted 1:5 with saline and used as the second antibody

Equipment. Gamma counter and general-purpose centrifuge.

Preparation of radiolabeled TSP. Although any method for the iodination of TSP can be used, we routinely employ the modified chloramine-T method [Greenwood et al., 1963]. In a septum-capped vial, 20 μg of TSP in 20–50 μl of TSP elution buffer (see above) is mixed with 10 μl of 0.20 M phosphate buffer, pH 7.3, 0.5 mCi ^{125}I, and 10 μl chloramine-T (1 mg/ml in 0.20 M phosphate buffer). The reaction is allowed to proceed for 30 sec at room temperature and then stopped by the addition of 10 μl sodium metabisulfite (1 mg/ml in 0.20 M phosphate buffer) and 20 μl 1% KI in phosphate buffer. Fifty μl of 1% BSA in 0.20 M phosphate buffer containing 0.5 M NaCl (gel-filtration buffer) is added to the sample and the sample gel-filtered on G-25 equilibrated with the gel-filtration buffer. The ^{125}I-labeled TSP is stable for up to 10 days at −70°C. After 10 days, the labeled TSP can be repurified on a small column of heparin-agarose equilibrated in 0.20 M phosphate buffer and eluted with gel-filtration buffer.

Procedure. All reagents and samples are prepared in borate buffer. Each sample tube contains 100 μl ^{125}I-TSP (10,000 cpm), 100 μl of sample (either a standard TSP solution or an unknown), and 100 μl of a 1:30,000 dilution of rabbit anti-TSP antiserum. The samples are incubated overnight at 4°C. The following day 100 μl of goat antirabbit IgG is added to each sample and incubation continued for 2 hours at room temperature. The samples are centrifuged for 20 min at 3,000 × g and the supernatants counted to determine the amount of radioactivity precipitated. Results are expressed as percent tracer bound versus concentration of unlabeled TSP in the incubation mixture. Unknown TSP concentrations may be determined from comparisons of standard curves plotted by the log-logit transformation as described by Rodbard [1974]. Using this method [Switalska et al., 1985], normal levels of TSP in platelet-poor plasma and serum in healthy donors were found to be 60.6 ± 10.7 ng/ml (n = 6) and 10.1 ± 6.8 μg/ml (n = 8), respectively.

ACKNOWLEDGMENTS

This work was supported by the Department of Health Services Grant CA33209, National Science Foundation grant DCB-8409571, grants RD-218 and

PDT-287 from the American Cancer Society, and grants from the Muscular Dystrophy Association and W.W. Smith Charitable Trust.

REFERENCES

Clezardin P, McGregor JL, Manach M, Robert F, Dechavanne M, Clemetson KJ (1984). Isolation of thrombospondin released from thrombin-stimulated human platelets by fast protein liquid chromatography on an anion-exchange mono-Q column. J Chromatogr 296:249–246.

Dawes J, Clemetson KJ, Gogstad GO, McGregor JL, Clezardin P, Provse CV, Pepper DS (1983). A radioimmunoassay for thrombospondin used in a comparative study of thrombospondin, beta-thromboglobulin, and platelet factor 4 in healthy volunteers. Thromb Res 29:569–582.

Engval E (1980). Enzyme immunoassay ELISA and EMIT. Meth Enzymol Immunochemical techniques part A 70:419–439.

Greenwood FC, Hunter WM, Glover JS (1963). The preparation of ^{131}I-labeled human growth hormone of high specific activity. Bioch J 89:114–123.

Kessler S (1975). Protein A-antibody adsorbent for isolation of cellular antigens. J Immunol 115:1617–1622.

Knudsen KA (1985). Proteins transferred to nitrocellulose for use as immunogens. Anal Bioch 147:285–188.

Koutts J, Walsh PN, Plow EF, Fenton J, Bouma BN, Zimmerman TS (1978). Active release of human platelet factor VIII-related antigen by adenosine diphosphate, collagen and thrombin. J Clin Invest 62:1255–1263.

Laemmli UK (1970). Cleavage of structural proteins during the assembly of the head of bacteriophage T4. Nature 227:680–685.

Lawler JW, Slayte HS, Coligan JE (1978). Isolation and characterization of a high molecular glycoprotein from human blood platelets. J Biol Chem 253:8609–8616.

Mustard JF, Perry DW, Ardlie NG, Packman MA (1972). Preparation of suspensions of washed platelets from humans. Br J Haematol 22:193–204.

Ornstein L (1964). Disc electrophoresis—I. Background and theory. Ann NY Acad Sci 121:321–349.

Niewiarowska J, Cierniewski CS, Tuszynski GP (1984). Association of fibronectin with the platelet cytoskeleton. J Biol Chem 259:6181–6186.

Rodbard D (1974). Statistical quality control and routine data processing for radioimmunoassays and immunoradiometric assays. Clin Chem 20:1255–1270.

Rucinski B, Niewiarowski S, James P, Walz DA, Budzynski AZ (1979). Antiheparin proteins secreted by human platelets. Purification and characterization and radioimmunoassay. Blood 53:47–62.

Schick PK, Tuszynski GP, VanderVort PW (1983). Human platelet cytoskeletons: Specific content of glycolipids and phospholipids. Blood 61:163–166.

Studier FW (1973). Analysis of bacteriophage T7 early RNAs and proteins on slab gels. J Mol Biol 79:237–248.

Switalska HI, Niewiarowski S, Tuszynski GP, Rucinski B, Schmaier AH, Morinelli TH, Cierniewski CS (1985). Radioimmunoassay of human platelet thrombospondin: Different patterns of thrombospondin and beta-thromboglobulin antigen secretion and clearance from the circulation. J Lab Clin Med 106:690–700.

Tangen O, Berman HR, Marfey P (1971). Gel filtration: A new technique for separation of blood platelets from plasma. Thromb Diathesis Haemorrhagica 25:268–278.

Timmons S, Hawiger J (1978). Separation of human platelets from plasma proteins including factor VIII by a combined albumin gradient-gel filtration method using Hepes buffer. Thromb Res 12:297–301.

Towbin H, Staehelin T, Gordon J (1979). Electrophoretic transfer of proteins from polyacrylamide gels to nitrocellulose sheets: Procedure and some applications. Proc Natl Acad Sci USA 76:4350–4354.

Tuszynski GP, Damsky CH, Fuhrer JP, Warren L (1977). Recovery of concentrated protein samples from sodium dodecyl sulfate-polyacrylamide gels. Anal Bioch 83:119–129.

Tuszynski GP, Knight L, Kornecki E, Srivastava S (1983). Labeling of platelet surface proteins with ^{125}I-Iodine by the Iodogen method. Anal Bioch 130:166–170.

Tuszynski GP, Knight L, Piperno JR, Walsh PN (1980): A rapid method for removal of ^{125}I Iodide following iodination of protein solutions. Anal Bioch 106:118–122.

Tuszynski GP, Kornecki E, Cierniewski CS, Knight L, Koshy A, Niewiarowski S, Walsh PN (1984a). Association of fibrin with the platelet cytoskeleton. J Biol Chem 259:5247–5254.

Tuszynski GP, Mauco GP, Koshy A, Schick PK, Walsh PN (1984b). The platelet cytoskeleton contains elements of the prothrombinase complex. J Biol Chem 259:6947–6951.

Tuszynski GP, Srivastava S, Switalska HI, Holt JC, Cierniewski CS, Niewiarowski S (1985a). The interaction of human platelet thrombospondin with fibrinogen. Thrombospondin purification and specificity of interaction. J Biol Chem 22:12240–12245.

Tuszynski GP, Daniel JL, Stewart G (1985b). Association of proteins with the platelet cytoskeleton. Semin Hematol 22:303–312.

Tuszynski GP, Walsh PN, Piperno JR, Koshy A (1982). Association of coagulation factor V with the platelet cytoskeleton. J Biol Chem 257:4557–4563.

Yalow RS, Berson SA (1960). Immunoassay of endogenous plasma insulin in man. J Clin Inv 39:1157–1162.

Modern Methods in Pharmacology, Volume 4
Methods for Studying Platelets and Megakaryocytes, pages 287–304

Methods of Studying Contractile Behavior of Platelets: The Platelet Strip

LEON SALGANICOFF

INTRODUCTION

The platelet strip is a biological preparation made with platelets activated by thrombin. This preparation may be used for the in vitro study of stimulus-contraction coupling and its biochemical correlates subsequent to the stages of irreversible aggregation and release. The predecessor of the platelet strip model is the platelet-rich plasma clot, which has permitted the study of certain relaxation responses [Bottecchia and Fantin, 1973; Cohen and DeVries, 1973; DeGaetano et al., 1974; Majno et al., 1972]. However, a detailed analysis of stimulus-contraction coupling is difficult in a preparation where the active responses of the platelets are dissipated in a large mass of a passive plastic component like fibrin [Niewarowsky et al., 1972]. The platelet strip is characterized by a high ratio of platelets to fibrin and can be conditioned not only to relax after the irreversible contraction but also to maintain this relaxed state in the presence of external Ca^{++}.

This preparation thus allows the analysis of the final stages of the platelet function under conditions that were not testable before and describes a new state of the activated platelet. Thrombin treated platelets retain an intact stimulus-contraction coupling mechanism even after secretion of granule contents and contraction, and respond with characteristic kinetics and force changes to known platelet agonists and inhibitors. When in a conditioned state the preparation relaxes on washout of the contracting agonists, allowing the study of stimulus-contraction under reversible conditions. Further, a state similar to the original irreversible contraction can be reproduced in the conditioned preparation using the adequate combination of agonists. The platelet strip is useful for understanding the physiology and pharmacology of activated platelets in a stage that is characteristic of the white thrombus [Salganicoff et al., 1977, 1985a].

From the Department of Pharmacology and the Thrombosis Research Center, Temple University School of Medicine, Philadelphia, Pennsylvania 19140.

METHODOLOGY

Preparation of Strips

Summary of operations. Immediately after neutralization and recalcification, cold platelet-rich plasma (see below for preparation) is centrifuged in a specially made flat bottom tube in which a highly elastic nylon mesh has been previously mounted on a plastic hoop. The platelets are deposited in the crevices of the mesh. After decantation of the residual platelet-poor plasma, thrombin formation in the interstitial plasma of the pellet is accelerated by warming the tube to 37°C. Activation of the tightly packed mass of platelets results in the formation of a large flat aggregate. This is followed by the release of platelet granule contents and by peripheral fibrin formation (fibrin strands are not visible among the platelets). The mesh remains embedded in the platelet aggregate but does not adhere to it and therefore does not interfere markedly with the contractile response. The formed platelet disk can now be unmounted and cut into strips, which are hung in an organ bath. The platelet strips are relaxed with a saline solution containing EGTA as a chelating agent. When the strips are totally relaxed, external Ca^{2+} is added to preparation in a stepwise manner to produce a relaxed preparation suspended in a calcium-containing milieu. The preparation is functional for up to 18 hours at 37°C and may be stored in the cold for 24 hours with little loss of responsiveness. As the methodology is new and some aspects are quite critical, the technical considerations for successful preparation and handling of the strips are described here in detail [Salganicoff and Sevy, 1985b].

Special centrifuge and plastic hoops. The centrifuge tube (Fig. 1) consists of a top and bottom section that, when fitted together, form a tube with the same shape and external dimensions as the 50 ml centrifuge tube used in the rotor HB4 of the Sorvall centrifuge or equivalent (Dupont, Newton, CT). The top section is an open cylinder cut from a 50 ml polycarbonate or polysulfone tube (28 mm external diameter, 87 mm long). The bottom part is a modified plug of aluminum that has been passivated by anodization. In section, the plug has an upper pedestal to fit a hoop and mesh assembly and a neck grooved to contain two rubber O ring seals, which fit tightly into the upper section. The upper pedestal ends in a flat, high polished surface section. The stem of the pedestal is 19.8 mm diameter × 4.0 mm long and accepts a pair of close-fitting concentric polycarbonate rings (hoop). The outer ring has an external diameter of 25.0 mm and an internal diameter of 22.7 mm. The inside ring has an external diameter of 22.55 mm and an internal diameter of 20 mm. Both rings are 3.7 mm long.

Nylon mesh. Plain single-knit jersey stocking fabric made of 15/3 denier nylon yarn texturized by the Agilon™ process (Round-the-Clock Stocking, Milliken Marietta, SC). The nylon mesh selected is very critical owing to the

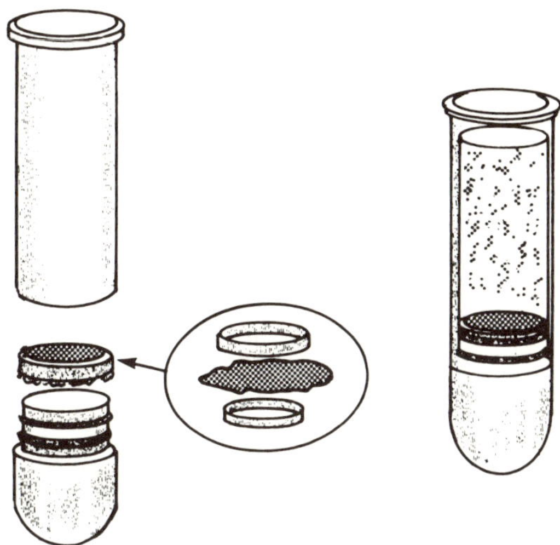

Fig. 1. Special centrifuge tube for preparing platelet disks. Components are shown in the sequence of assembly. A nylon mesh, previously marked with stiffened stripes is fitted on a hoop and the assembly is mounted on the pedestal of the upper section of the aluminum plug bottom section. The assembly is fitted in the upper polycarbonate cylinder. After filling the tube with a measured volume of cold recalcified platelet-rich plasma, centrifugation, decantation, and activation are performed. The tube is disassembled, the hoop dismounted, and the nylon mesh containing the giant platelet aggregate is cut into strips.

texturization process. Agilon™ processing stretches the nylon yarn over a sharp hot edge, producing a nick deformation in the cylindrical fiber that forces the yarn filaments to acquire a spiral springlike form, giving a high compliance to the woven tissue. The mesh is washed with detergent in an ultrasonic cleaner, rinsed multiple times, soaked in distilled water for 24 hours, and dried for storage.

Strengthening of strip ends. A quick-drying, dark, pigment-loaded, cellulose acetate or nylon paint is used to create nonstretching stiffened ends that help the mounting of the strips to the transducer clamps. A square piece of mesh (5 cm × 5 cm) is laid flat on a filter paper without stretching. Two parallel stripes, each 20 mm long × 1 mm wide, 10 mm apart, are impregnated with the paint, using a homemade rubber stamp. The paint has to glue and stiffen the nylon filaments but not cover the mesh spaces. To attain good reproducibility from day to day the stripes should be printed along the same general axis in the mesh.

Assembly of the hoops. The hoops are used to support the mesh just as embroidery hoops hold cloth. The mesh is placed over the inner hoop so that the stripes are centered and parallel, then the external hoop is slid on. The friction between the hoops and the mesh has to stretch the stripes 1 mm apart, assuring, therefore, the complete flatness of the mesh. The excess material is trimmed, using a razor blade or sharp scissors. It is necessary to make sure that when the trimmed hoops are mounted on the platform a free space remains between the bottom of the hoops and the periphery of the platform. This precaution assures that the mesh will lie flat against the platform during centrifugation. Failure to insure this will cause the pellet to form below the mesh instead of filling it.

The assembly is now fitted on the pedestal of the aluminum plug, and the base is fitted into the top cylindrical section. The tube is filled with ice-cold saline and centrifuged at 10,000g for 5 min to eliminate trapped air bubbles and make sure that the mesh lies flat on the pedestal base. The tube is kept with the saline in an ice bath until used.

Platelet-rich plasma. Blood is collected from normal human donors by venipuncture using a 16 gauge venotube leading into a 1/10 volume of ACD solution (2.5% sodium tricitrate, 1.5% citric acid, 2% dextrose). The anticoagulated blood is centrifuged at 150 g for 20 min to isolate platelet-rich plasma (PRP). Platelets are counted, and a volume of plasma containing 10^{10} platelets is cooled to 4°C in a plastic tube.

Neutralization and recalcification of the PRP. Making absolutely sure that the PRP is at 4°C or less, neutralization and recalcification is done by adding, while rapidly vortexing, an amount of equal parts of cold 1.5M tris-Cl pH 7.4 and 0.5M $CaCl_2$ equivalent to 0.04 of the measured plasma (final pH 7.4 and pCa 4.8). The special centrifuge tube is emptied of the cold saline, filled with the recalcified neutralized plasma, and centrifuged without delay at 4°C for 10 min at 10,000g in a precooled HB4 rotor. It is of utmost importance that the whole operation: neutralization, recalcification, and centrifugation, be done at low temperatures to avoid platelet aggregation or fibrin formation before the platelets are sedimented. After centrifugation, the platelet-poor plasma is decanted and the tube is kept covered at a slight angle in crushed ice. After 10 min any additional plasma that has collected is siphoned off without disturbing the platelet pellet. The tube is then covered with a saline-dampened cotton plug, covered with parafilm, and immersed in a water bath for 20 min at 37°C (to permit full activation of the recalcified platelet pellet by the thrombin formed in the residual plasma). Aggregation, release, fibrin formation, irreversible polymerization, and contraction occur in this period. After activation, the tube is put back in the ice for about half an hour and then disassembled. The hoop with the aggregated platelets embedded in the nylon mesh is removed from the pedestal with a slow rotation while pulling. Special care has to be taken in this step to avoid the undue stretching caused by the interfacial adhesion of the wet disk to the flat bottom of the pedestal. Overstretching may fissure the preparation. A good sign of a successful operation is: 1) a clean separation of the disk from the pedestal and 2) the presence of a hairline crack that follows the inner perimeter of the hoop (this crack results from the contraction of platelets aggregate). The disk is immediately submerged in saline to avoid desication. The retaining rings are demounted with the help of the column shown schematically in Figure 2. The hoop is inverted (the upper face of the mesh facing the column) and the external ring is slid down. The disk is separated from the internal ring using tweezers and submerged flat in a petri dish containing cold Krebs-Henseleit saline (K-H).

Cutting of strips. To prepare the strips, the platelet disk is floated on a thin plastic sheet. A rectangular section bound by the two external edges of the stiffening stripes is cut first. Then 4-mm-wide strips are cut, using very sharp scissors. (We use fine, iris scissors mounted in tandem to make 4 equal strips in a single operation (Fig. 3). Each strip contains 1.8×10^8 platelets (approximately 1.25 mg of protein). The cut strips are stored in cold K-H until used. For more prolonged storage, it is convenient to cover the tube containing the strips with parafilm to avoid alkalinization of the saline due to the loss of CO_2.

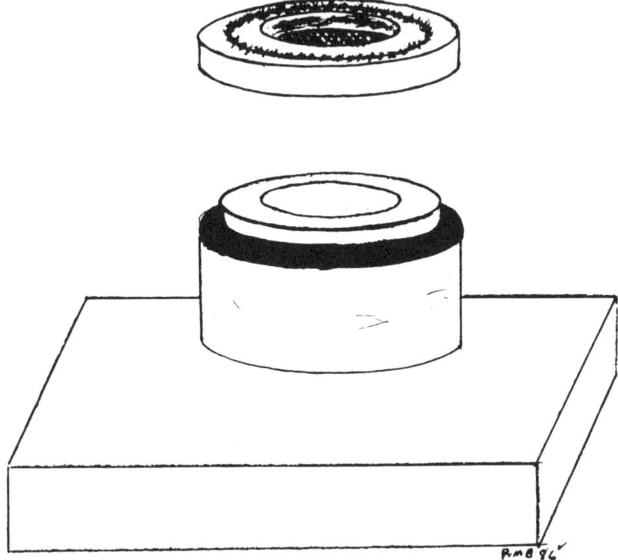

Fig. 2. Column for dismounting the hoop. The hoop is inverted (face down) and centered over the rim of the plastic column. The outer ring is pushed down and the exposed side of the mesh is separated from the inner ring, using tweezers.

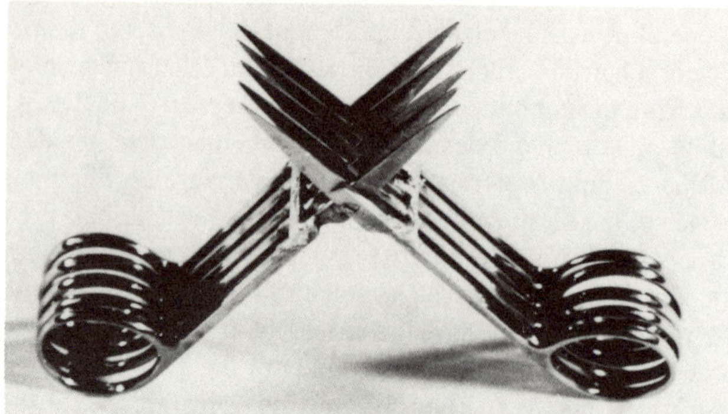

Fig. 3. Tandem assembled scissors used to cut platelet strips. Fine iris scissors are assembled with a distance between blades of 4 mm and the pivot points aligned. They are soldered as a unit, using a bar across the handles. This device is quite useful to obtain equal force generating strips.

Mounting. The strips are mounted vertically in thermostated organ baths, the upper end is attached via a stainless steel (or plastic clamp) and a gold chain to a force transducer, the bottom is pressed on to an anchor made by forming a miniature comb in the edge of a #40, 4-mm-wide stainless steel wire mesh that has been sandwiched in a support or attached to a fixed inverted clamp. The anchors are mounted at the end of a 10-cm-long #17 hypodermic tubing that is attached via an acrylic bar to a micrometer (Mitutoyo MHK-25R 153-201 non rotating shaft or equivalent). The tubing is closed in the bottom but has a small hole opposite the anchor that is used to oxygenate the saline. The 95% O_2 – 5% CO_2 mixture is introduced from the upper part of the tubing (Fig. 4). The strips weigh only 20–25 mg but may be manipulated without undue trauma by floating them onto a small piece of plastic that can be used as a handle. The transducer clip is attached first and then the preparation is left hanging over the comb placed exactly at the height of the lower stripe. The preparation is then pushed against the comb, using the edge of the the plastic sheet as a tool, until the wire teeth protrude across the stripe. The organ bath filled with KH at 4°C is now elevated to cover the strip.

Recording of contractile activity. Contractile activity is recorded either isometrically or isotonically. We prefer isometric measurements because the passive elasticity of the nylon mesh is kept constant under these conditions. We have used either Statham UC2 transducers (Gould, Cleveland, OH) or Bioscience 52–9545 (Harvard Instruments, MA) or equivalent. The apparatus consists of four or eight transducers, which after electronic amplification are fed into a Multiplex Recorder (Gould 816, Cleveland, OH) or 2 four-channel potentiometric

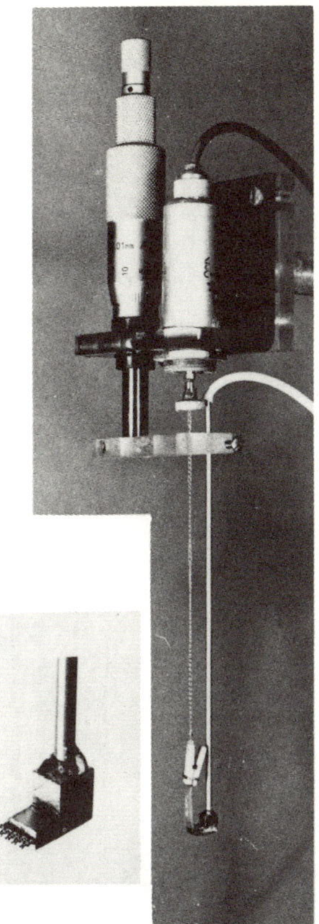

Fig. 4. Components for mounting the platelet strips. Assembly of micrometer, hypodermic tube for gassing, comb and transducer for holding and stretching the preparation. The insert shows a detailed view of the comb.

recorders. Each strip generates forces of up to 1.0 g.

Adjustment of strips for force measurement. The transducers are balanced with strips immersed in the bath at a slack length of 0 mg and then the strips are stretched to an initial nonslack force of 25 mg with the help of the micrometer. The length of the strips at this force is measured with a caliper (to the nearest 1/10 of a mm) or with the micrometer. The strips are left in the organ bath at 0°C for 30 min and then stretched again to a force of 70 mg. The force is readjusted after 1 hour. The ratio of actual length to the slack length is from 1.05–1.1. Then the temperature of the organ bath is changed to 37°C to start the contraction. We use two water baths with circulating pumps that are at 0°C and 37°C respectively. They are switched by a three-way stopcock assembly.

The organ bath saline solutions are changed by an overflow method, admitting the saline through a port in the bottom of the organ bath. Because of the low forces generated, strong bubbling with CO_2-O_2 for mixing purposes generates noise in the recording traces. We prefer to use a flat base organ bath coupled to a magnetic stirrer (Fig. 5) to avoid noise.

Heating the strips to 37°C generates forces of up to 500–600 mg. We have found that the best behavior is attained when forces not larger than 500–600 mg are demanded from the preparation. If the force generated is larger, a small decrease in the L/LS is performed.

Expression of data. To express the data in a unified manner muscle physiology conventions are used (mg/cm^2) (newton/m^2). The apparent sectional

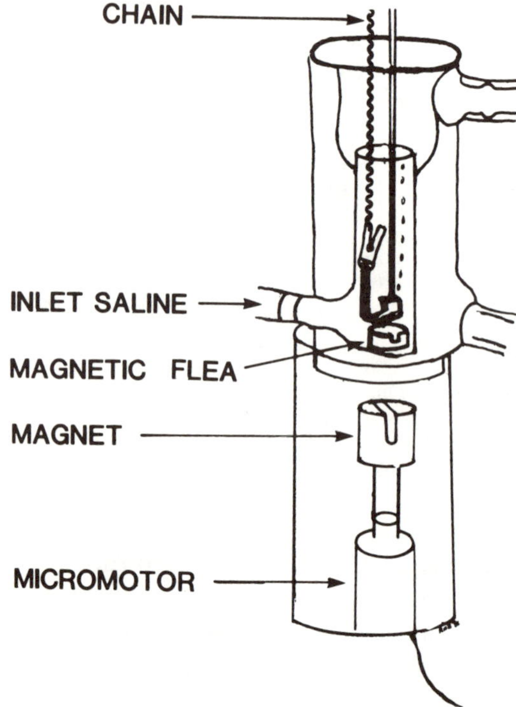

Fig. 5. Organ bath for the platelet strip. The internal cup (12.5 × 60 mm) is filled from the bottom. Suction at the angle between the protuding lip of the cup and the thermostated mantle allows rapid wash by overflow and reproducible filling volume. The magnetic stirrer is adjusted to allow the fastest mixing compatible with low noise in the recorder trace.

area (A) of the strip is calculated from the equation $A=(W_s - W_m)$ L where W_s is the wet weight of the strip, W_m is the weight of the mesh, δ is the average density of platelets (1.049), and L is the length of the strips as obtained from the caliper measurement. Extracellular space is assumed to be 30% (Salganicoff, unpublished) and should be subtracted from the calculated data.

Salines. Modified K-H solution (in mM):N_aCl:119.0; KCl 4.7; $MgCl_2$: 2.0; KH_2PO_4 1.2; $NaCO_3H$: 25.O; EGTA: 0.05; glucose: 5.0; Ca^{2+} or chelants are omitted and added afterward for the particular protocols. The EGTA is added to remove residual free Ca^{2+} and traces of heavy metals. The saline is gassed with 95% O_2-5% CO_2 to adjust the pH to 7.4.

Modified K-H. EGTA solution (pCa 9.6). The EGTA concentration of the previous saline is increased to 2 mM.

Modified K-H. Ca^{2+} solution: The Ca^{2+} concentration of the K-H is increased to 1.0mM.

KCl depolarizing solution (in mM): KCl 60.0; NaCl 70.0; $NaCO_3H$ 25.0; $MgCl_2$ 2.0; K_2 PO_4H 1.2; EGTA 0.05; glucose: 5.0.

K_2SO_4-depolarizing solution (in mM): K_2SO_4 113.0; KCO_3H 25.0; $MgSO_4$ 2.0; EGTA 2.0; glucose 5.0.

PHYSIOLOGY AND PHARMACOLOGY

Behavior of the Non-Conditioned Strips

The platelet strips, like platelet-rich plasma clots, remain contracted after activation. If not perturbed by pharmacological or other treatments, they will retain contracted for their useful lifetime as indicated by the length-tension relationship. Platelet strips can be mounted at 37°C immediately after activation. When this approach is used, platelet strips suspended in a Ca^{2+}-containing saline generate a force of 400–500 mg (approximately 100g/cm^2) when stretched to an L/L_s of 1.05–1.1. Instead, if the preparation is kept for 1 hour at 0°, the same amount of stretching will only generate a force of 100 mg. Warming the preparation to 37°C generates a rapid contraction and a generation of forces of 400–500 mg. After this force is attained it will be maintained steadily for approximately 1 hr before starting to decrease. The decrease is slow and biphasic ($t_{1/2}$) of the first phase 120–150 min; $t_{1/2}$ of the second phase 500 min). Small contractile response may be observed on addition of agonists. As soon as the preparation enters the first phase of relaxation, responses can be elicited by agents like ADP or epinephrine. When added to the incubation medium these agents will restore part of the lost tension, acting therefore like contracting agonists. The size of the response to the agonist increases in proportion to the total force generated until the preparation enters the second phase of relaxation. In the second phase, the size of the response to the agonist remains proportional to the total force generated by the preparation but is never higher than 20–30% of the total force generated (Fig. 6). Therefore, the nonconditioned platelet strip can be compared to smooth muscle with a high degree of tonus. Washout of the agonist relaxes the preparation to its previous force [Salganicoff et al., 1985].

Conditioning of the Platelet Strip

Rational. Techniques have been devised to induce full relaxation of the preparation. Two basic approaches are described: the first is based on the decrease of cytoplasmic Ca^{2+} to basal levels using chelants; the second is based on the increase, by pharmacologic means, of the cAMP levels of the preparation. We will consider first the Ca^{2+} chelation methods: The use of chelating agents establishes an outward gradient for Ca^{2+} ions. The decrease of cytoplasmic Ca^{2+} has a dual effect: 1) inactivation of the set of enzymes linked to contraction and 2) return of the phospholipase A_2 to basal levels to avoid the release of arachidonate for synthesis of TXA_2. It is important to remember that prolonged washout with chelants will complete emptying the receptor operated pools [Bolton, 1979] and therefore uncouple stimulus from contraction.

Treatment with K-H EGTA. When the contracted platelet strip is treated with K-H containing 2 mM EGTA the preparation starts to relax immediately. The relaxation is monophasic (t½: 60–90 min), although oscillations of force are sometimes seen. In approximately 2–4 hours a stable relation is attained. When a stable relaxation is achieved a decrease in force larger than 80% of the initial value is measured (Fig. 6) [Salganicoff and Sevy, 1985b].

Treatment with K_2SO_4-EGTA. The combination of depolarization by increase in external K^+ coupled to the substitution of the Cl^- for the impermeable anion $SO_4^=$ in the K-H, rapidly relaxes the preparation (t ½ = 20 min). After maintaining the preparation in a fully relaxed state for 30 min, the depolarizing saline is changed to K-H and left for another 30 min (Fig. 7).

Rapid relaxation is related only to the impermeable anion, since substitution of the Cl^- with other impermeable anion also leads to relaxation. Extraction of Ca^{2+} from the cytoplasm is however related to the cation. When the preparation is treated with Na_2 SO_4-EGTA rapid relaxation is seen, but return to K-H contracts the preparation again. The strong depolarization by potassium thus appears to maintain high levels of cytoplasmic Ca^{2+} independently of receptor deactivation allowing Ca^{2+} extraction [Salganicoff and Sevy, 1980].

Impermeabilization of the Membrane

Rationale. After treatment with chelants, the cell membrane is in what has been defined as a "hyperpermeable state." Large additions of Ca^{2+} to the

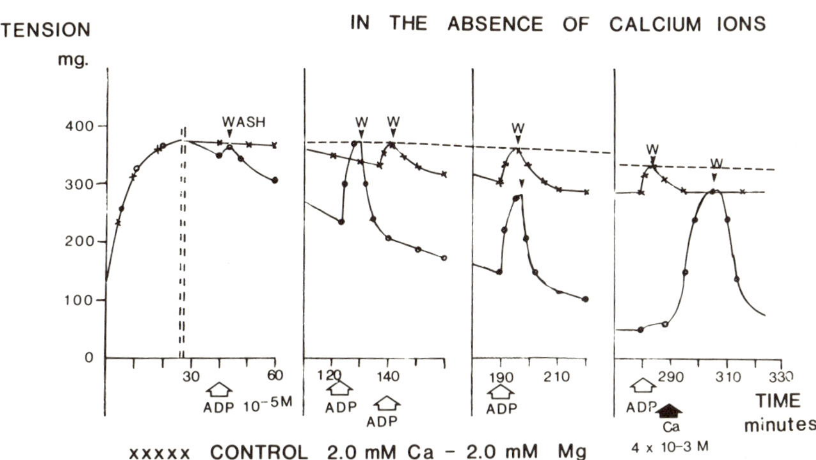

Fig. 6. General contractile behavior of the platelet strip. Two platelet strips have been mounted in parallel and allowed to contract until maximal force generation. The control preparation continues to be maintained in the presence of external Ca^{2+} while in the experimental strip, the saline is changed to a Krebs-Henseleit containing 2 mM EGTA. ADP is used as agonist, W: washing out of the drug. Notice the rapid relaxation, increase in the size, and the reversibility of the response on washout. After 5 hours of incubation the response to the agonist decreases in size owing to the exhaustion of the Ca^{2+} pools (4th frame).

medium allow the influx to increase intracellular Ca^{2+} to levels which induce contraction in the preparation before the membrane regains its impermeability. If the cellular buffering mechanisms allow the return of the increased internal Ca^{2+} to basal levels, the preparation will relax. However, it is possible to impermeabilize the membrane without contraction by making small Ca^{2+} additions in a stepwise fashion, therefore avoiding the creation of large gradients before the membrane regains its impermeability. This approach also helps in maintaining the phospholipase A_2 in an unactivated state, avoiding further liberation of arachidonate from phospholipids and generation of TXA_2.

Preparations relaxed in K-H EGTA. Once the preparation has reached a stable relaxation state the medium is changed to K-H for 15 min. If no contraction occurs, extracellular Ca^{2+} is increased in a geometric progression starting at $10\mu M$ allowing an adaption period of 3–5 min between additions. When the concentration of free extracellular Ca^{2+} is near 200 μM, doubling the concentration may initiate a slow but steadily increasing contraction. If this occurs it is necessary to rapidly wash out the Ca^{2+} and continue with a lower Ca^{2+} concen-

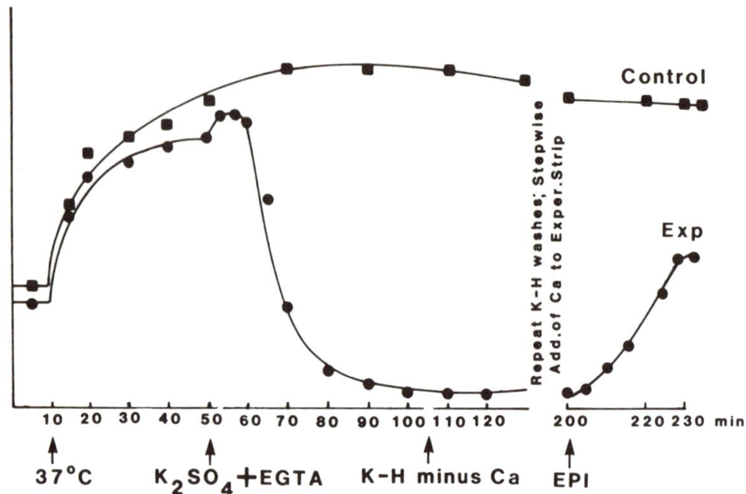

Fig. 7. Relaxation kinetics of the platelet strip in a K_2SO_4 depolarizing saline. The preparation has been contracted in a K-H containing 1 mM Ca^{2+}. When the force has stabilized the saline has been changed to a K_2SO_4 depolarizing saline (see text). The preparation contracts further for a brief period and starts to relax rapidly. When the relaxation is stable the preparation is changed back to a K-H without Ca^{2+}. Relaxation is maintained and the preparation is capable of responding to agonists. (Epinephrine 10^{-6}M.)

tration. Also, when the concentration of Ca^{2+} is low the preparation may start to contract but will then relax spontaneously to the baseline. If such a contraction is observed, it is necessary to stop the addition of Ca^{2+} and wait for the stabilization of force before the next Ca^{2+} addition (Fig. 8).

Preparations Relaxed With K_2SO_4-EGTA

The problems of contraction during membrane impermeabilization appear more frequently with the use of K_2SO_4-EGTA.

The approach used is identical to that for the preparations relaxed in K-H-EGTA. However, the preparation may recontract when changed to the K-H. When this occurs the treatment with depolarizing saline has to be reinitiated. Similar events may occur when small amounts of Ca^{2+} are added in the initial stages of impermeabilization. As a rule, preparations relaxed in K_2SO_4 are more unstable than the ones relaxed with K-H EGTA. It is therefore recommended for the beginner to start with the K-H EGTA approach.

Relaxation Induced by Agents That Increase cAMP

Rationale. Relaxation of the platelet strip is also induced by agents activating adenylcyclase (PGE_1, PGI_2, PGD_2) or by inhibition of phosphodiesterase (papav-

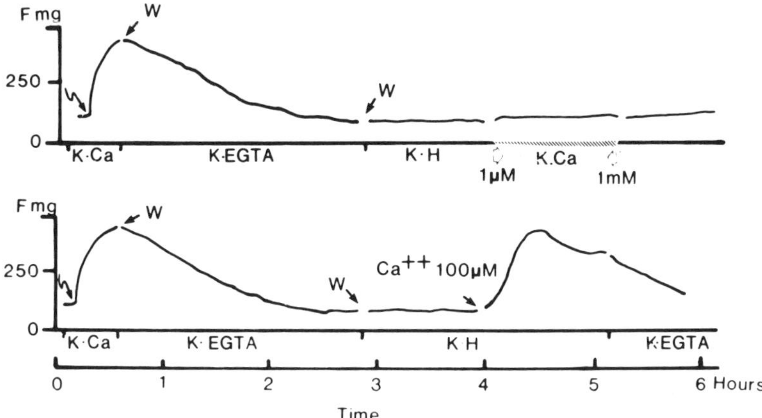

Fig. 8. Impermeabilization of the membrane. Conditions are similar to Figure 1 (experimental strip). After the preparation has fully relaxed the saline is changed to a Krebs-Henseleit (see text) and Ca^{2+} is added in an incremental manner (dashed region). Relaxation is maintained. *Lower trace*. For demonstration we include the behavior of a strip responding with an active contraction or addition of a bolus of 100 μM Ca^{2+}.

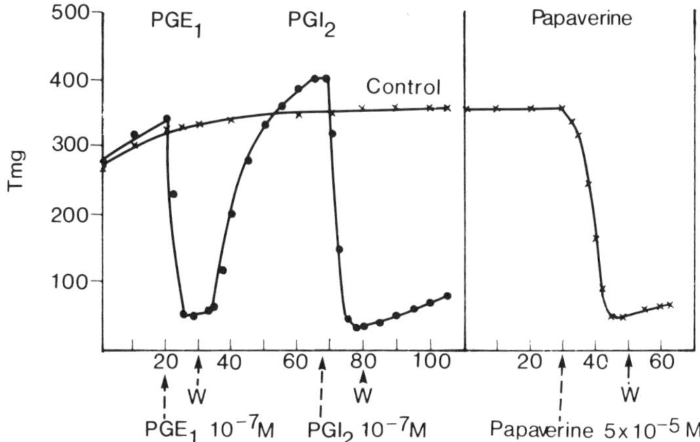

Fig. 9. Relaxation induced by agents increasing platelet cAMP. Conditions are as in Figure 1 (control). When contraction is maximal addition PGE_1 (1μM) induces a fast relaxation. Washout of the drug allows for a spontaneous contraction. Similar results are obtained with PGI_2 or with papaverine.

erine, dipyridamole). Studies with agents acting on cycling AMP metabolism can be carried out with the contracted, nonconditioned platelet strip (Fig. 9). The suggestion that increases in cyclic AMP, acting through a cyclic AMP-dependent protein kinase, lead to the phosphorylation of myosin kinase, and, through this event, to a decrease in the sensitivity of the enzyme to Ca^{2+}, appears to be valid for the platelet strip [Bromberg, 1984]. However, other parameter changes add complexity to this picture: 1) cyclic AMP levels depend very tightly on the ratio of the activities of adenylcyclase and phosphodiesterase. Full activation of adenylcyclase can easily overpower phosphodiesterase catabolism leading rapidly to a 200-fold increase in intracellular cyclic AMP levels [Bromberg, 1984]. Under these conditions the preparation shuts off and maintains its relaxation for as long as the cyclic AMP is above the control region. It may take hours to regain its reactivity. 2) In addition, the increase in cyclic AMP appears to alter the state of the interplatelet material, leading to a reversible disorganization of its anatomical components. This event is highly sensitive to the force generated by the preparation before the increase in cyclic AMP. If the force is too high (over 500 mg), a permanent damage to cell-to-cell associations will occur, and a loss of reversibility will be the result [Salganicoff, 1985c]. 3) A decrease in the outward flux of Ca^{2+} occurs with cyclic AMP increase. This appears to be due to either the closing of channels or the creation of new binding sites. The mechanism of these events is not yet understood.

These complexities suggest that cyclic AMP-induced relaxation ought to be considered as a special problem whose interpretation must be made quite cautiously.

The technique recommended for cyclic AMP-induced relaxation is by titration with PGE_1 or papaverine until an 80% reduction of the initial force occurs and a steady state is maintained (Fig. 9). It must be remembered that PGE_1 or papaverine has to always be present to avoid spontaneous contraction of the preparation on washout. An L/L_S not larger than 1.05 or forces not higher than 400 mg during the initial contraction are recommended to maintain a reversible behavior (Fig. 9) [Salganicoff et al., 1985; Bromberg, 1984].

The Model

Description of the anatomy of the platelet strip and the overall biochemical events that lead to its contractile behavior allows the development of a mechanistic model that, although provisional, has been shown useful in the formulation of working hypotheses. We can thus begin to predict behavior and to understand the molecular events leading to contraction, relaxation, and impermeabilization of the membrane and the pharmacologic responses of the conditioned platelet strip.

From an architectural point of view, the platelet strip can be thought of as being formed by a honeycombed assembly of columns of aggregated platelets surrounded by aqueous channels. The geometry of this system is organized by the nylon mesh contained within the platelet mass. The relationship of the platelets and the nylon filaments, while intimate in the packed pellet, is quite limited after thrombin activation. Electron microscopy studies show that the aggregated platelets are separate from the nylon filaments. The reason for this is a combination of poor adherence of the platelets to the nylon filaments and contraction of the platelet mass. As a result, the mesh, while partially filling the aqueous channels, is mechanically uncoupled from the platelets' mass. The number of platelets used in the preparation of the strip has been calculated to allow an aggregate thickness that allows the protrusion of curved segment of the nylon filaments above the surface of the aggregate. Stretching the preparation allows the formation of small fissures at the interphase between the filament and the aggregate that act as channels to the external medium. These channels are useful in accelerating the diffusion of drugs or metabolites to and from the platelet aggregate columns [Salganicoff et al., 1985].

From an electronmicroscopic point of view, the platelet columns are homogeneous aggregates. The platelets maintain their structural integrity. As expected, they also show a decreased number of granules and a conversion of the cytoplasm from the largely granular structure typical of nonactivated state to an organization of microfilament bundles. The filament reorganization is especially visible when the preparation is fixed under stretching. The external membranes appear intact and show close apposition with the microfilaments. There is a pattern of continuity from platelet to platelet through areas of electron dense material which fills all interplatelet spaces. This organization appears to be responsible for the transmission of force.

From a physiological point of view, the platelet strip can be thought of as a smooth muscle in a highly tonic state. Several pieces of evidence suggest that the energy source utilized for the contraction is mainly ATP derived from anaerobic glycolysis. The preparation relaxes rapidly with glucose deprivation and recontracts when glucose is added to the saline. Inhibition of mitochondrial function decreases the force generated only by 25%, suggesting that while oxidative phosphorylation is functional, glycolytic ATP generation plays an important role in the energetics of contraction [Salganicoff et al., 1985a].

The biochemical mechanisms directly involved in force generation appear to fit the model described for smooth muscle, i.e., after an increase in cytoplasmic Ca^{2+}, the Ca^{2+} calmodulin myosin kinase-dependent phosphorylation of the light chain of myosin activates actomyosin ATPase and the sliding of filaments occurs. Control of myosin kinase by the cyclic AMP-dependent protein kinase is apparently operational in the platelet strip [Adelstein et al., 1981; Bromberg et al., 1984; Bromberg et al., 1985]. The receptor-linked functions either for the cyclic AMP or Ca^{2+}-linked responses are also operational, such as those produced by PGE_1 (receptor activation) or forskolin (catalytic unit). Other modes of regulation, such as phosphodiesterase inhibition, that lead to increases in cell cyclic AMP and to relaxation are also operative. ADP, epinephrine, TXA_2, and angiotensin induce contraction. The deactivation mechanisms also are intact, as shown by the reversal of the events on washout of the agonists. With reference to the specific amplification pathways related to cyclooxygenase, both TXA_2 and prostaglandin synthesis appear to be intact. The platelet strip utilizes arachidonic acid for the synthesis of TXA_2 and prostaglandins: Inhibition of TXA_2 synthetase leads to relaxation and an increase in the cytoplasmic cyclic AMP levels. Therefore the channeling of PGG_2 either into TXA_2 (contraction) or PGD_2 (activation of adenylcyclase) is operational [Wang et al., 1983].

Furthermore, we have demonstrated that the increased permeability to external Ca^{2+}, thought to be an irreversible effect of the proteolytic effects of thrombin on the platelet membrane, can be reversed when cytoplasmic Ca^{2+} is decreased to basal levels.

From the limited exploration completed to date, it seems that most of the pathways related to energy metabolism, activation, and deactivation of contractile processes and the specific amplification pathways remain functional after strong thrombin activation. To complete the picture of the biochemical organization of the preparation, the only irreversible change appears to be the crosslinking of the platelet membrane with fibrin monomers or with other proteins either secreted from the platelets or originating from plasma. This crosslinking is maintained during the life of the preparation and is modulated by increases in cyclic AMP. The crosslinking probably occurs at specialized places in the membrane that do not affect the overall behavior, permeability, or receptor-linked functions.

The conditioned platelet strip shows great pharmacologic similarities to contractile tissues that operate through pharmacomechanical coupling [Bolton, 1979; Somlyo and Somlyo, 1968]. However, it still maintains some unique characteristics of the platelet such as: 1) the specialized kinetics of response to agonists, 2) the specialized amplification pathways, and 3) the handling of cytoplasmic Ca^{2+}. The slow exhaustion of the amplification pathways allows also the observation of the dynamics of the interaction between the activation of the different receptors and the amplification pathways. The platelet strip contracts with ADP, epinephrine, TXA_2, and angiotensin, but the contraction with supramaximal amounts of each dose of agonist is incomplete and full force is attained when two or three receptors of different class are stimulated. Differences in the kinetics of relaxation are found on washout of the agonists. Relaxation is fast and reversible for ADP and epinephrine, slow and incomplete for TXA_2 and its analogs, and incomplete with a tendency to become irreversible as a function of time for thrombin and angiotensin [Salganicoff and Sevy, 1985b]. As a result of these differences it is found that when ADP, TXA_2, and thrombin are used simultaneously the preparation does not relax on washout of the agonists and behaves in a similar manner to nonactivated platelets stimulated with thrombin, where of course ADP and TXA_2 are made available during activation by secretion and cyclooxygenase metabolism. Therefore, the special kinetics of the receptors, the amplification pathway and the control of cytoplasmic Ca^{2+} appears to determine the reversibility or irreversibility of the platelet response to agonists. Reversibility is observed when the receptor stimulus (intensity time) is below a certain level. In this case, the increase in cytoplasmic Ca^{2+} can be compensated for by the cellular buffering of the ion (membrane pumps, uptake by mitochondria, and dense tubular system) on disappearance of the stimulus. Irreversibility (defined as the maintenance of the response after the disappearance of the stimulus) is associated with the increase of Ca^{2+} to levels that fully activate phospholipase A_2 and therefore the continuous controlled liberation of arachidonate. Its metabolism to TXA_2 leads to Ca^{2+} liberation from the TXA_2 receptor-dependent pools and to the maintenance of cytoplasmic Ca^{2+} at high levels while Ca^{2+} synthesis lasts.

Platelet secretion may occur by any of the proposed mechanisms. However, for the prolonged maintenance of platelet contraction, as it probably occurs under in vivo conditions, the irreversibility is needed. It appears also that external Ca^{2+} influx taxes the kinetics of the extrusion of the increased cytoplasmic Ca^{2+}. It is clear that the influx is slow and that the mechanisms controlling the levels of the cytoplasmic Ca^{2+} appear still functional although incompetent even under rigorous activation conditions [Russo and Salganicoff, 1985; Salganicoff, 1979].

ACKNOWLEDGMENTS

To Remus Berretta for graphic work and to Carol Francis for excellent typography and infinite patience. To Drs. R. Colman and J.B. Smith for careful editing.

REFERENCES

Adelstein RS, Pato MD, Conti MA (1981). The role of phosphorylation in regulation contracticle proteins. Adv Cyclic Nucleotides Res 14:362–373.

Bolton, TB (1979). Mechanisms of action of transmitters and other substances on smooth muscle. Physiol Rev 5:606–718.

Bottecchia D, Fantin G (1973). Platelets and clot retraction. Effects of divalent cations and several drugs. Thromb Diath Haemorrh 30:567–576.

Bromberg ME, (1984). Studies on the regulation of contractility in thrombin activated platelet. Doctoral Thesis 8419745. Temple University School of Medicine. University microfilms, Ann Arbor, Michigan.

Bromberg ME, Sevy RW, Daniel JW, Salganicoff L (1985). Role of myosin phosphorylation in contractility of a platelet aggregate. Am J Phys Cell Physiol 249: C297–303.

Cohen I, DeVries A (1973). Platelet contractile regulation in an isometric system. Nature 246:36–37.

deGaetano G, Franco R, Donati M, Bonaccorsi A, Garattini S (1974). Mechanical recording or reptilase-clot retraction: Effect of adenosine-5′ -diphosphate and prostaglandin E_1. Thromb Res 4:189:192.

Majno G, Bouvier CA, Gabbiani G, Ryan GB, Statkov P (1972). Kymographic recording of clot retraction: Effects of papaverine, theophylline and cytochalasin B. Thromb Diat Haemorr 28:49–53.

Niewarowsky S, Regoeczi E, Stewart G, Mustard JF (1972). Platelet interaction with polymerizing fibrin. J Clin Inv 51:685–700.

Russo MA, Salganicoff L (1985). Calcium dependent disorganization of thrombin aggregated platelets (platelet strip). In Alia E, Arena N, Russo M (eds): "Contractile Proteins in Muscle and Non-muscle Systems." New York: Praeger Scientific.

Salganicoff L (1979). A deficient platelet Ca^{++} pump as the cause of the irreversibility of clot retraction. Thromb Haemost 42:215:1979.

Salganicoff L, Sevy R (1980). Reversible relaxation of a contracted platelet aggregate with sulfate. Fed Proc 39:582.

Salganicoff L, Loughnane M, Sevy R, Russo M (1985a). The platelet strip: low fibrin contractile model of thrombin-activated platelets. Am J Physiol (Cell Physiology) 249: C279–285.

Salganicoff L, Russo M, Loughnane M (1977). The platelet strip: A new model for the study of the mechanochemical properties of a platelet aggregate (Abstract). Thromb Haemost 38:155.

Salganicoff L, Sevy R (1985b). II. The platelet strip: stimulus-contraction coupling in thrombin-activated human platelets. Am J Physiol (Cell Physiology) 249: C288–296.

Salganicoff L, Sevy RW, Russo M (1985c). New aspects of the behavior of irreversibly aggregated platelets. Semin Haem 22:135–150.

Somlyo A, Somlyo AP (1968). Electromechanical and pharmacomechanical coupling in vascular smooth. J Pharmacol Exp Ther 159–145.

Wang T, Sevy R, Salganicoff L (1983). Arachidonic acid metabolism in thrombin activated platelets. Pharmacologist 25:144.

Index